Esophageal Diseases: Diagnosis and Treatment

Esophageal Diseases: Diagnosis and Treatment

Edited by Alexander Hopper

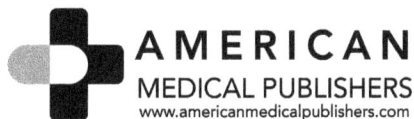

AMERICAN
MEDICAL PUBLISHERS
www.americanmedicalpublishers.com

American Medical Publishers,
41 Flatbush Avenue,
1st Floor, New York,
NY 11217, USA

Visit us on the World Wide Web at:
www.americanmedicalpublishers.com

ISBN: 978-1-63927-137-5

Cataloging-in-Publication Data

Esophageal diseases : diagnosis and treatment / edited by Alexander Hopper.
    p. cm.
Includes bibliographical references and index.
ISBN 978-1-63927-137-5
1. Esophagus--Diseases. 2. Esophagus--Diseases--Diagnosis.
3. Esophagus--Diseases--Treatment. I. Hopper, Alexander.
RC815.7 .E76 2022
616.32--dc23

Table of Contents

Preface

Every book is initially just a concept; it takes months of research and hard work to give it the final shape in which the readers receive it. In its early stages, this book also went through rigorous reviewing. The notable contributions made by experts from across the globe were first molded into patterned chapters and then arranged in a sensibly sequential manner to bring out the best results.

The esophagus can be affected by many diseases, whether congenital or acquired. The burning sensation caused in the chest due to acid reflux is a very common esophageal disease. Prolonged exposure to the gastric acids may erode the lining of the esophagus, leading to Barrett's esophagus. It is a clinical condition which is considered a high risk factor for adenocarcinoma. Some of the other conditions of esophagus are Chagas disease, esophageal cancer, esohageal dysphagia, esophagitis, Killian–Jamieson diverticulum, neurogenic dysphagia, Zenker's diverticulum, etc. An X-ray of swallowed barium is generally used to assess the shape and size of the esophagus and any underlying mass. Through a procedure called endoscopy, it is possible to visualize the interior of the esophagus. It also allows a biopsy to be taken that is useful for the diagnosis of cancer. Esophageal cancer is usually managed with chemotherapy, radiotherapy or the partial surgical removal of the esophagus. The topics included in this book on esophageal disease are of utmost significance and bound to provide incredible insights to readers. This book presents researches and studies performed by experts across the globe on the diagnosis and treatment of esophageal diseases. It will prove to be immensely beneficial to students and researchers involved in gastroenterology.

It has been my immense pleasure to be a part of this project and to contribute my years of learning in such a meaningful form. I would like to take this opportunity to thank all the people who have been associated with the completion of this book at any step.

Editor

Discussing the influence of electrode location in the result of esophageal prolonged pH monitoring

Valter Nilton Felix[1,3]*, Ioshiaki Yogi[2], Daniel Senday[2], Fernando Tadeu Vannucci Coimbra[2], David Pares[2], Vinicius Garcia[2] and Carlos Eduardo Garcia[2]

Abstract

Background: There is a large consensus to preserve the distance of 5 cm above the proximal border of the lower esophageal sphincter (PBLES) as appropriate to the location of the electrode of the pH-metry. The main objective of this study is to determine whether placement of the electrode below the recommended location achieves a significant difference in the calculation of the DeMeester score.

Methods: The study was made up of 60 GERD patients and 20 control subjects. They were submitted to esophageal manometry and to pH-metric examination with two pH-metric catheters contained antimony electrodes - the distal was positioned 3 cm above the PBLES, leaving the other 5 cm away from it.

Results: LES pressure (LESP) in the GERD group was significantly lower than in the control group (P = 0.005). Normal mean DeMeester score was observed simultaneously in the control group, by both the electrodes, but abnormal DeMeester score was much more expressive when observed by the distal electrode in the GERD group. There were significant differences as for DeMeester score, of patients with GERD from that of the control group and of distal from the proximal electrode in the GERD group.

Conclusions: Acid reflux is directly related to lower levels of LESP. Lower location of the catheter may strongly affect the results of prolonged esophageal pH monitoring in GERD patients.

Keywords: Gerd, Esophageal ph monitoring, Ph-metric electrode location

Background

Gastroesophageal reflux disease (GERD) is a multifaceted disease, defined as chronic symptoms or mucosal damage produced by the abnormal reflux of gastric contents into the esophagus and close to 50% of the population will have some type of GERD symptom during a calendar year. In the patient presenting with heartburn and/or regurgitation, the diagnosis of GERD is highly likely and a reference standard of pH monitoring and/or endoscopy has been used to establish a diagnosis of GERD [1].

Endoscopy is the single best test to answer the question of whether mucosal injury or BE (Barrett esophagus) is present [2], but the overall sensitivity of endoscopy for the diagnosis of GERD is less than 50%; that is, less than half of GERD patients will have esophagitis at the time of endoscopy.

Ambulatory esophageal pH monitoring documents the pattern, frequency, and duration of esophageal acid exposure and allows correlation between reflux events and symptoms; thus it is the best test to answer the question: are these symptoms due to reflux of acid? [3]. Early studies found sensitivity and specificity of this test to be extremely high (over 90% sensitive and specific) [4], although other studies, particularly in endoscopy-negative patients, report lower accuracy of the pH-metry [5].

In 1969 the idea of a prolonged intra-esophageal pH measurement (18 hours) [6] was introduced. It was later standardized to a 24 h test [7], with the intention of obtaining data that quantitatively expresses the gastro

* Correspondence: v.felix@terra.com.br
[1]Digestive Surgery Division, São Paulo University, and Head of the Nucleus of General and Specialized Surgery, São Paulo, Brazil
[3]School of Medicine, São Paulo University, R. Frei Caneca, 1407 – cj 221, São Paulo, SP, Brazil

esophageal reflux (GER), the ability to identify esophageal clearance, observing the duration of each reflux episode, and mimic the acid perfusion test of the esophagus, since the reflux episodes could be correlated with the patient's symptoms, indicated on the graphic by the touch of a specific button in the registration equipment and reported in the journal of the examination.

The possible interference of the presence of the electrode in the esophageal lumen, increasing saliva production and frequency of contractions of the organ was discarded by a classic project [8], while another [9] removed any doubt as to the possibility of electromagnetic interference altering the final result of the exam.

Then the hypothesis of possible food flows, outside of the main meals, clearly marked on the charts, being able to alter significantly the total time of pH less than 4 was rejected [10]. The use of pH 4 as the threshold of normality was established in 1987 [8] and DeMeester score began to be used widely.

As for the positioning of the electrode 5 cm above the proximal border of lower esophageal sphincter (PBLES), as made by Johnson & DeMeester [7] to define the normal exam, with scores less than 14.72, there were always disputes. Some authors prefer to measure it at a distance of 3 cm [11], while others put the lower limit of LES as a starting point for the measurement of 5 cm [12].

These changes were not well received, although some occasional question as for the classic positioning of the electrode remains, for example arguing that if the reflux did not reach that level it could go unnoticed, even when causing GERD complicated by the emergence of Barrett's epithelium in the more distal esophagus [13].

However, there is a large consensus both in Brazil [14] and in the exterior [15] to continue preserving the distance of 5 cm above the upper border of the LES, preferably located by prior esophageal manometry, as appropriate to the location of the electrode of the pH-metry.

The main objective of this study is to determine whether placement of the electrode, below the recommended location, achieves a significant difference in the calculation of the DeMeester score. The secondary objective includes verifying correlations of pH monitoring and LES pressure in GERD.

Methods

The study was made up of 60 patients (28 men and 32 women, average age: 39.29 ± 10.04 years), with BMI never exceeding 25 Kg/m^2, who were all suffering from a heartburn complaint, presenting episodical extra-esophageal symptoms, in which digestive endoscopy previously identified erosive esophagitis Los Angeles B without hiatal hernia. Clinical and endoscopic criteria, after a minimum period of one year under unsuccessful heartburn clinical control tentative including PPI,

procinetics, postural and habits orientation, established indication for surgery. Incomplete control of symptoms or almost immediate recurrence after suspension of treatment occurred even using PPI at a dose of 80 mg/day. Twenty control subjects (8 men and 12 women, mean age: 43.3 ± 11.50 years), volunteers, without esophageal complaints, with normal esophagoscopy, were submitted to the same study protocol.

All subjects signed a consent form following the standards of the Helsinki Convention. This study was approved by the ethics committee of São Paulo – Rio Preto Faculty of Medicine.

The first procedure was esophageal manometry. With the patients in semi-recumbent position, the catheter was pulled out by 1 cm steps, crossing the high pressure zone of the gastro-esophageal junction. This procedure was preceded by suspension of all medicines prescribed for palliation of peptic symptoms for 72 hours and fasting for 8 hours, and followed by the installation of two pH-metric catheters through one nostril with the patient in a sitting position.

The catheters contained antimony electrodes and, after appropriate calibration, the distal was positioned 3 cm above PBLES, leaving the other 5 cm away from that anatomical and functional reference.

From then on the procedure followed the usual pattern of the pH-metric examination. The patients were instructed to keep their habitual daily activities and to record food and fluid consumption, and posture changes, on a diary card. Two Digitrapper Mark III pH recorder Synectics, Medtronics® were employed and after about 24 hours the data collected in the register were translated and processed in the Synectics® program, each electrode providing an independent database. Acid reflux was defined as a sudden drop in esophageal pH below 4.

With the processed data, a search was made to determine:

- The length and resting pressure of LES (LESP) obtained from the average of the records of the four distal circumferential manometric sensors, and the location of PBLES, in patients and control subjects;
- If there were significant differences between the mean length and resting pressure of the LES in both groups;
- The DeMeester scores corresponding to the data collected by the electrodes positioned 3 cm and 5 cm from PBLES and if there was a significant difference between their averages, enabling an intra and intergroup analysis.

The data were subjected to statistical analyzes, using the Student t test to compare quantitative data, accepting $P \leq 0.05$, with a confidence limit of 95%.

Results

No patient or control had an extension of LES less than 3 cm, always with at least 1 cm located below the diaphragm, while the average LESP in the group of patients with GERD (12.24 ± 7.02 mmHg) was significantly lower ($P = 0.005$) than that noted in the control group (18.4 ± 7.76 mmHg) (Table 1).

No discrepancy with respect to DeMeester score was observed, when considering the results obtained simultaneously in the control group, by the electrodes situated 3 cm and 5 cm from PBLES, normal in both and without statistical difference between averages (11.27 ± 1.69 and 10.10 ± 2.33) ($P = 0,37$). The mean scores corresponding to the data captured by electrodes placed 3 cm and 5 cm from PBLES in patients with GERD (respectively, 25.67 ± 12.23 and $15,87 \pm 11.71$) were significant different from one to other ($P = 0.008$) (Table 2).

Both for the electrode positioned 3 cm, and for the one located 5 cm from PBLES, there were significant differences as to the DeMeester score, of patients with GERD from that of the control subjects (respectively $P = 0.001$ and $P = 0.022$) (Table 2).

The catheter located 5 cm above the PBLES registered a normal DeMeester score in 26/60 patients (43.33%) and in 20/20 control subjects, implying sensitivity of 56.66% and specificity of 100% of conventional prolonged esophageal pH monitoring. The catheter located 3 cm above PBLES increased sensibility to 80%, upholding specificity of 100% (from normal DeMeester score in 12/60 (20%) patients and in 20/20 control subjects).

Discussion

Ambulatory esophageal pH monitoring is classically performed by placing a pH electrode 5 cm above the proximal border of the lower esophageal sphincter [3]. The most useful parameter for documentation of pathologic reflux is the DeMeester score, but the test has its limitations, with reported sensitivities ranging from 60% to 100% [16] through to indexes as low as 28% [17].

Ferdinandis et al. [18] found pathological acid reflux in 43 patients (31%) at the esophageal pH monitoring, helping to establish a cause for the morbidity in a significant number of patients with GERD symptoms, but not in the majority of patients referred for the test.

Table 1 Averages of extension (EXT) and resting pressure of the lower esophageal sphincter (LESP)

Group	EXT (cm)	LESP (mmHg)
GERD	3.61 ± 0.38	12.24 ± 7.02
Control	3.97 ± 0.49	18.4 ± 7.76
P	0.622	0.005

Table 2 DeMeester score for different levels of the pH-metry probe above the proximal border of the lower esophageal sphincter (PBLES)

GROUP	3 cm above PBLES	5 cm above PBLES	P
GERD	25.67 ± 12.23	15.87 ± 11.71	0.008
CONTROL	11.27 ± 1.69	10.10 ± 2.33	0.37
P	0.001	0.022	

The inconstant sensibility of the exam can make its methodology doubtful and then some points need to be considered if it´s normal:

- A non-reflux diagnosis, such as achalasia, gastroparesis or functional heartburn, or non-acid reflux. Currently available technology, such as impedance monitoring, bilimetry, esophageal manometry and/or gastric scintigraphy, might help us to identify many patients who have non-reflux disease or non-acid reflux [19,20];
- The patients could have missed acid reflux that was not picked up on a single day study: 25% of cases monitored by capsule pH testing could have normal findings one day and abnormal findings the next day in a 48 h study [21]. However, Hakanson et al. [22] report that no studies were cited in the published guidelines that indicate superior outcomes for patients for treatment guided by wireless pH testing versus traditional pH testing. The major advantage for the wireless system cited was patient tolerability;
- The pH probe might have missed distal acid reflux [13];
- Alternatively, noxious effect of the nasal catheter could have limited both eating and activity and resulted in a false-negative test.

The latter possibility could perhaps be overcome with better explanation of the background of the examination to the patients, giving them greater involvement and ensuring their cooperation, thus resulting in more effective testing.

Traditionally, the pH probe is placed 5 cm above the proximal border of the lower esophageal sphincter. One study found that over a period of 24 h, the amount of acid exposure in 11 endoscopy-negative dyspeptic patients was greater if measured 5 mm above the squamo-columnar junction than when measured at the conventional 5 cm above the squamo-columnar junction (11.7% vs 1.8%; P <0.001) [23]. These authors suggested a lower placement of the electrode to better detect the gastro-esophageal reflux.

The problem, however, is how much this reflux can be aggressive to the region most distal of the esophagus, which may have increased resistance and much faster clearance. This without mentioning the fact that drastic change in catheter placement requires new standards of quantitative interpretation of the examination.

This was the starting point of this study, considering that the validity of pH monitoring scores is currently linked to the positioning of the electrode 5 cm from PBLES. Therefore, it is necessary to discuss whether a slight change that would alter this methodological aspect interferes with the result of the examination, taking care to use manometric equipment and esophageal pH monitoring, as well as catheters with a recognized technical reliability.

We excluded patients with hiatal hernia to avoid distortion of the results due to the mobility of esophago-gastric junction, inherent to that anatomical condition.

The results showed that electrodes located either 3 or 5 cm from PBLES show similar normal DeMeester scores, in the control group, reflecting that, in fact, as previously reported [24], placing the electrode slightly below the conventional 5 cm from PBLES tends not to alter the pH-metric final result in normal subjects. However, in patients with GERD, there is a significant difference between the averages obtained by the electrodes placed 3 cm or 5 cm above PBLES, much more reflux being registered by the distal electrode, although abnormal averages have been observed in both.

LESP may not be the only determinant factor in LES competency, but it could be of great importance. DeMeester, using three criteria (LES hypotony, intra-abdominal sphincter length < 1 cm or total sphincter length < 2 cm), found that there was a 70% chance of abnormal reflux if one of the three above factors was present. If all three criteria were met, reflux was seen in 92% of patients [25].

In this series a reduction in length of the LES in patients or control subjects was not observed, but resting sphincter pressure, in fact, proved be directly related to reflux, so that the average LESP in the group of patients with GERD (12.24 ± 7.02) was significantly lower (P = 0.005) than that noted in the control group (18.4 ± 7.76 mmHg).

Particularly among normal individuals, LESP seems to provide a so good anti-reflux protection that normal DeMeester score can be observed even with the electrode positioned 3 cm above the PBLES. On the other hand, in GERD patients, its lower value can determine significant difference between distal and proximal electrodes measurements. Therefore it can be observed that acid reflux is directly related to lower levels of resting sphincter pressure, and that sensibility of the conventional prolonged esophageal pH monitoring could be increased with lower location of the pH-metric electrode. Charbel et al. [26] must be recollected, because they stated that pH monitoring is most likely to be normal using conventional and the most stringent methodological criteria [26].

Conclusions
Placement of the electrode below the recommended location could be harmful in some GERD patients, simulating a much more severe gastroesophageal reflux, maybe implying unnecessary fundoplicature. However we could eventually underestimate the reflux locating the catheter at 5 cm, too far from the PBLES. New studies could help to clarify this doubtful and important matter.

Helsinki statement
All subjects signed a consent form, after receiving detailed informations about all aspects of the work and about the observation of the standards of the Helsinki Convention.

Abbreviations
GERD: Gastroesophageal reflux disease; GER: Gastroesophageal reflux; PBLES: Proximal border of lower esophageal sphincter; LESP: Resting pressure of lower esophageal sphincter.

Competing interests
The authors declare that they have no competing interests.

Authors' contributions
VNF conceived of the study and drafted the manuscript. VNF, IY, DS, FTVC and DP carried out the exams. DP, VNG and CEG participated in the design of the study and performed the statistical analysis. IY, DS and FTVC participated in its design and coordination. All authors read and approved the final manuscript.

Acknowledgements
None.

Author details
[1]Digestive Surgery Division, São Paulo University, and Head of the Nucleus of General and Specialized Surgery, São Paulo, Brazil. [2]Nucleus of General and Specialized Surgery, São Paulo, Brazil. [3]School of Medicine, São Paulo University, R. Frei Caneca, 1407 – cj 221, São Paulo, SP, Brazil.

References
1. Felix VN, Viebig RG: Simultaneous bilimetry and pHmetry in GERD and Barrett's patients. Hepato-Gastroenterology 2005, 52:1453–1455.
2. Caygill CP, Dvorak K, Triadafilopoulos G, Felix VN, Horwhat JD, Hwang JH, Upton MP, Li X, Nandurkar S, Gerson LB, Falk GW: Barrett's esophagus: surveillance and reversal. Ann N Y Acad Sci 2011, 1232:196–209.
3. Kahrilas PJ, Quigley EM: Clinical esophageal pH recording: a technical review for practice guideline development. Gastroenterology 1996, 110(6):1982–1996.
4. Johnson LF: A 24-hour pH monitoring in the study of gastroesophageal reflux. J Clin Gastroenterol 1980, 2:387–399.
5. Dent J, Brun J, Fendrick A, Fennerty M, Janssens J, Kahrilas P, Lauritsen K, Reynolds J, Shaw M, Talley N: An evidence-based appraisal of reflux disease management: the Genval Workshop report. Gut 1999, 44:1–16.
6. Spencer J: The use of prolonged pH recording in the study of gastroesophageal reflux. Br J Surg 1969, 56:912–914.
7. Johnson LF, DeMeester TR: Twenty-four hour pH monitoring of the distal esophagus. Am J Gastroenterol 1974, 62:325–329.
8. Schindlbeck NE, Heinrich C, Konig A, Dendorfer A, Pace F, Muller-Lissner SA: Optimal thresholds, sensitivity and specificity of long term pH-metry for the detection of gastroesophageal reflux disease. Gastroenterology 1987, 93:85–90.
9. Evans DF: Twenty-four hour ambulatory oesophageal pH monitoring: an update. Br J Surg 1987, 74:157–161.

10. de Caestecker JS, Blackwell JN, Pryde A, Heading RC: **Daytime gastroesophageal reflux is important in esophagitis.** *Gut* 1987, **28:**519–526.
11. Kaye MD: **Postprandial gastroesophageal reflux in healthy people.** *Gut* 1977, **18:**709–712.
12. Vitale GC, Cheadle WG, Sadek S, Michel ME, Cushieri A: **Computerized 24 hour ambulatory pH monitoring and esophagogastroduodenoscopy in the reflux patient.** *Ann Surg* 1984, **200:**724–728.
13. Richter JE: **How to manage refractory GERD.** *Nat Clin Pract Gastroenterol Hepatol* 2007, **4:**658–664.
14. Moraes Filho JPP, Cecconello I, Gama-Rodrigues JJ, Brazilian Consensus Group: **Brazilian Consensus on Gastroesophageal Reflux Disease: proposals for assessment, classification and management.** *Am J Gastroenterol* 2002, **97:**241–248.
15. DeVault KR, Castell DO: **Updated guidelines for the diagnosis and treatment of gastroesophageal reflux disease.** *Am J Gastroenterol* 1999, **94:**1434–1442.
16. Jamieson JR, Stein HJ, DeMeester TR: **Ambulatory 24-h esophageal pH monitoring: normal values, optimal thresholds, specificity, sensitivity, and reproducibility.** *Am J Gastroenterol* 1992, **87:**1102–1111.
17. Shay S, Richter J: **Direct comparison of impedance, manometry, and pH probe in detecting reflux before and after a meal.** *Dig Dis Sci* 2005, **50:**584–590.
18. Ferdinandis TG, Amarasiri L, De Silva HJ: **Use of ambulatory oesophageal pH monitoring to diagnose gastrooesophageal reflux disease.** *Ceylon Med J.* 2007, **52:**130–132.
19. Martinez SD, Malagon IB, Garewall HS, Cui H, Fass R: **Non-erosive reflux disease (NERD) – acid reflux and symptom patterns.** *Aliment Pharmacol Ther* 2003, **17:**537–545.
20. Pohl D, Tutuian R: **Reflux monitoring: pH-metry, Bilitec and esophageal impedance measurements.** *Best Pract Res Clin Gastroenterol* 2009, **23:**299–311.
21. Pandolfino JE, Richter JE, Ours T: **Ambulatory esophageal pH monitoring using a wireless technique.** *Am J Gastroenterol* 2003, **98:**545–550.
22. Hakanson BS, Berggren P, Granqvist S: **Comparison of wireless 48-h (Bravo) versus traditional ambulatory 24-h esophageal pH monitoring.** *Scand J Gastroenterol* 2009, **44:**276–283.
23. Fletcher J, Wirz A, Henry E, McColl KEL: **Studies of acid exposure immediately above the gastro-oesophageal squamocolumnar junction: evidence of stat segment reflux.** *Gut* 2004, **53:**168–173.
24. Hirano I, Richter JE: **Practice Parameters Committee of the American College of Gastroenterology. ACG practice guidelines: esophageal reflux testing.** *Am J Gastroenterol* 2007, **102:**668–685.
25. DeMeester TR: **Gastroesophageal reflux disease.** In *Esophageal Disorders.* Edited by DeMeester TR, Skinner DB. New York: Raven; 1985:132–158.
26. Charbel S, Khandwala F, Vaezi MF: **The Role of Esophageal pH Monitoring in Symptomatic Patients on PPI Therapy.** *Am J Gastroenterol* 2005, **100:**283–289.

The prognostic influence of body mass index, resting energy expenditure and fasting blood glucose on postoperative patients with esophageal cancer

Ning Wu[1†], Yongjun Zhu[1†], Dhruba Kadel[2], Liewen Pang[1], Gang Chen[1] and Zhiming Chen[1*]

Abstract

Background: Body mass index (BMI), resting energy expenditure (REE) and fasting blood glucose (FBG) are major preoperative assessments of patients' nutrition and metabolic state. The relations and effects of these indices on esophageal cancer patients' postoperative short-term and long-term outcomes remain controversial and unclear. We aimed to study the impact of BMI, REE and FBG in esophageal cancer patients undergoing esophagectomy.

Methods: Three hundred and six esophageal cancer patients who underwent esophagectomy were observed retrospectively. Clinical characteristics, postoperative complications and survival analysis were compared among different BMI, REE and FBG groups.

Results: There were significant linear relationships between REE, BMI and FBG indices, patients with low BMI tended to have low REE ($p < 0.001$) and low FBG ($p = 0.003$). No significant difference was found in case of mortality and postoperative complications among different groups. Low BMI ($X^2 = 6.141$, $p = 0.046$), REE ($X^2 = 6.630$, $p = 0.010$) and FBG ($X^2 = 5.379$, $p = 0.020$) were related to poor survival. FBG ≤90 mg/dL was independently associated with poor survival (HR = 0.695; 95 % CI 0.489–0.987, $p = 0.042$). BMI and REE came to be stronger prognostic factors on lymph node-negative patients and proved to be independent prognostic indicators (HR = 0.540; 95 % CI 0.304–0.959, $p = 0.035$ and HR = 0.457; 95 % CI 0.216–0.967, $p = 0.041$, respectively).

Conclusions: BMI, REE and FBG are important prognostic factors in patients with esophageal cancer undergoing esophagectomy and preoperative evaluation of these indices help to determine the prognosis in these patients.

Keywords: Esophageal cancer, Body mass index, Resting energy expenditure, Fasting blood glucose, Prognosis

Background

Esophageal cancer (EC) is the eighth most common cancer and the sixth leading cause of cancer mortality worldwide [1]. Esophageal adencarcinoma (EAC) and esophageal squamous cell carcinoma (ESCC) are the most frequent histological subtypes. ESCC is the dominant histological subtype in china [2]. The potential prognostic indicators of esophageal cancer include histological variants (histological grading, differentiation, invasion

depth and classification of lymph node metastasis) and nutrition or inflammation based prognostic factors (total lymphocyte counts, neutrophil to lymphocyte ratio (NLR), serum albumin and so on). BMI, REE and FBG, which are widely used to assess preoperative nutritional and metabolic status, have also been described to be prognostic predictors in several tumors [3].

Previous studies reported that high BMI was associated with increased risk of EAC while low BMI with ESCC [4]. High BMI in surgical patients is thought to be associated with increased comorbidities and postoperative complications, but the influence of high BMI on survival in patients undergoing esophagectomy is controversial. Hayashi found patients with high BMI showed

* Correspondence: czm_md@163.com
†Equal contributors
[1]Department of Cardio-thoracic Surgery, HuaShan Hospital of Fudan University, Shanghai 200040, People's Republic of China

better overall survival (OS) and disease-free survival (DFS) because of the early clinical diagnosis [5]. In contrast to this, Yoon pointed out that high BMI was independently associated with two-fold worsening of DFS, and OS after surgery for EAC [6]. Blom concluded that BMI had no prognostic value on short-term and long-term outcomes [7]. Compared with the previous studies, the mean BMI in Western populations was higher and had a greater incidence rate of EAC whereas the mean BMI in Chinese population was found to be lower with predominant ESCC. The effect of low BMI on postoperative complications and long-term survival remains unclear. So our study assessed the relationship between BMI and postoperative complications and long-term survival in Chinese population.

Disorder of energy metabolism is a common phenomenon in cancer patients. The energy metabolic status among different cancers may not be the same. Many researchers assessed the resting energy expenditure on cancer patients and no unanimous conclusions have been drawn. In this study, patients' preoperative REE was an estimated variable, and calculated by the Mifflin-St. Jeor equation [8]. REE is the sum of the metabolic activities of internal body and can reflect patient's physiques and muscle volumes, and REE per kg total body weight (REE/kg) may reflect the diffusion and metabolic rate of muscle more accurately. So both REE and REE/kg were used to explore its effects on short-term and long-term outcomes on esophageal cancer patients.

Epidemiologic evidence suggests that elevated blood glucose is associated with many forms of cancer [9]. However, opinions toward the association between elevated blood glucose and outcomes are mixed. Elevated blood glucose may promote cancer progression and lead to poor outcomes via pathways mediated high levels of insulin and insulin-like growth factor [10]. On the other hand, some studies proposed that diabetes-related microvessel changes might play a protective role against "neoplastic" cell metastasis in cancer patients and enhance cancer prognosis [11]. For EC, the relationship between the circulating glucose levels and prognosis has never been reported. To examine effects of fasting glucose levels at time of cancer diagnosis on postoperative outcomes is another aim of this study.

So the purpose of the study is to investigate the prognostic value using combined assessment of BMI, REE and FBG in esophageal cancer patients.

Methods

Patients

Patients who underwent esophagectomy and lymph node dissections during Sep 1, 2003 to Dec 31, 2008 were observed. Twenty-three patients who had palliative or R1/R2 resections were excluded. Patients who had histology other than SCC or AC (one lymphoma, one melanoma, one neuroendocrine carcinoma, one stromal tumor and two small cell carcinoma) were excluded. Patients who received neoadjuvant therapy were also excluded. Three hundred and six patients with histologic documentation of AC or SCC were included. All patients provided written consent and this retrospective study was approved by the Institutional Review Board of Huashan Hospital, Fudan University.

Clinical data

Preoperative staging was performed in all patients by means of barium meal test, fibro-gastroscopy, computed tomography of the chest and abdomen and ultrasound of the neck and retroperitoneal lymph nodes. Some patients also received whole body positron emission tomography (PET)-CT scanning. All patients were assessed for physiological ability to undergo esophagectomy. These evaluations included pulmonary function test, cardiac function test and nutritional assessment.

One hundred and eighty-six patients with tumors in middle or lower thoracic esophagus and no evidence of lymph node involvement in the superior mediastinum or neck region received transthoracic esophagectomy via left thoracotomy which also included a two-field lymphadenectomy; 53 patients with tumors in the middle or upper thoracic esophagus and possible lymph node metastasis in the superior mediastinum or neck region received McKeown 3-hole esophagectomy with three-field lymphadenectomy; 67 patients with tumors in the esophagogastric junction received esophagogastrectomy through median laparotomy.

TNM staging was performed according to the AJCC 7th edition guidelines. Patients were followed up every 6 months for the first 3 years and then annually. Survival time was measured as the time from the date of surgery to the date of death or the latest follow-up time. Endoscopy, CT, PET-CT and Radionuclide bone scan were performed if recurrent or metastatic disease was suspected.

Patients' weight and height were measured at their first hospitalization. BMI was calculated as weight in kilograms divided by height in meters squared.

REE was calculated by Mifflin-St. Jeor equation. The applied technique to calculate BMI is as follows: for males = 10 * weight (kg) + 6.25 * height (cm) - 5 * age (y) + 5; for females = 10 * weight (kg) + 6.25 * height (cm) - 5 * age (y) - 161. Both REE and REE/kg were calculated.

The serum FBG concentration of patients was measured in the morning during the first hospitalization by hexokinase method after fasting for 10 h. Serum albumin was measured by means of the bromocresol purple method using automated equipments, and all patients were screened and excluded from acute and chronic liver disease. The complete blood count test (leukocyte, neutrophil, lymphocyte, monocyte, eosinophil, basophil, platelet counts, and hemoglobin) was carried out by an automated haematology analyser within one week prior to surgery. NLR was calculated as the ratio of neutrophils to lymphocytes in peripheral blood. These reagents and equipments were convenience-validated and standardized in our central clinical laboratory.

The 6-month preoperative weight loss was also measured and patients were divided into three categories: No/Little (loss of 0 to 5 % body weight), Middle (loss of 5 to 10 % body weight) and Large (loss more than 10 % body weight).

During the first few days after surgery, patients were treated with total parenteral nutrition. An initial dose of 5–10 $kcal.day^{-1}.kg^{-1}$ of enteral nutrition was supplied via a duodenum or jejunum feeding tube from the 2nd or 3rd postoperative day and gradually increased to the full dose of 25–30 $kcal.day^{-1}.kg^{-1}$. Some patients with low BMI or low serum albumin levels were treated with full dose of enteral nutrition from one week before surgery to the tenth day after surgery.

Statistical analysis

All statistical analysis was performed with SPSS 16.0. Spearman rank order correlation coefficient (Spearman's rho) for nonparametric data was used. Univariate analysis of survival was performed using Kaplan-Meier method and log-rank test to estimate the prognostic value. Multivariate analysis of survival was performed using Cox-regression model to estimate hazard ratios (HRs) with 95 % confidence intervals (CI) and identify independent prognostic factors. The level of significance was set to $p < 0.05$.

Results

Patient characteristics

The clinical characteristics and 5-years survival rate are summarized in Table 1. The median follow-up time was 37 months. The overall 1-, 3- and 5-year survival rate was 86.6, 60.8 and 47.1 % respectively.

The BMI distribution was as follows: low (<20 kg/m^2), $n = 81$ (26.5 %); normal (20–25 kg/m^2), $n = 186$ (60.8 %) and high (>25 kg/m^2), $n = 39$ (12.7 %). The median REE was 1387.5 $kcal\ day^{-1}$ for male and 1064.0 $kcal\ day^{-1}$ for female where we defined the median REE as the cutoff point and stratified patients into low REE group (male < 1387.5 and female <1064.0), $n = 154$ (50.3 %) and high REE group (male ≥1387.5 and female ≥1064.0), $n = 152$ (49.7 %). The median REE/kg was 21.49 $kcal.day^{-1}.kg^{-1}$. Compared with 245 (80.1 %) patients with REE/kg < 23.2, 61 (19.9 %) patients with REE/kg ≥23.2 had

significant worse survival, so 23.2 $kcal.day^{-1}.kg^{-1}$ was set as the cutoff point. We divided the patients into two groups according to serum FBG concentration where 108 patients (35.3 %) with low FBG (≤90 mg/dL) and 198 patients (64.7 %) with high FBG (>90 mg/dL).

Patient characteristics by BMI, REE, REE/kg and FBG

As shown in Table 2. Spearman's rho indicated that patients with age > 65 years ($p < 0.001$) and advanced T-stage ($p = 0.040$) were more likely to fall in the low REE class. Smoking patients were more likely to be associated with low BMI class ($p = 0.013$), low FBG class ($p = 0.039$) but high REE/kg class ($p = 0.001$).

It was interesting to explore the relationship between REE and REE/kg. Both high REE and low REE/kg patients were found to have better survival, which was consistent with the spearman correlation analysis that found patients with high REE tended to have lower REE/kg ($p < 0.001$).

There were significant linear relations between BMI, REE, and FBG, patients with low BMI tended to have low REE ($p < 0.001$) and low FBG ($p = 0.003$). The trend of a linear association between REE and FBG could also be seen ($p = 0.011$).

There were close relations between REE/kg and weight lost or BMI, patients with high REE/kg have been found to lose more weight ($p = 0.006$) and have lower BMI ($p < 0.001$).

Low FBG was more likely to be seen in patients with high REE/kg ($p = 0.025$) and low albumin ($p < 0.001$).

Comorbidities, postoperative mortality and postoperative complications

Preoperative comorbidities, mortality and postoperative complications among different groups of BMI, REE, REE/kg and FBG were presented in Table 2. COPD appeared to be more frequent in low REE patients ($p = 0.022$), and diabetes was more common in high BMI patients ($p = 0.006$). All the seven patients with cardiovascular disease belonged to low FBG class ($p < 0.001$). Observing the short-term outcomes, no significant difference was found in postoperative mortality and major postoperative complications among different BMI, REE, REE/kg and FBG groups.

Nutrition or inflammation-based prognostic factors

Univariate analysis of nutrition or inflammation-based prognostic factors found to be serum albumin ($p < 0.001$), but not Total lymphocyte counts ($p = 0.780$) or NLR ($p = 0.787$), which was positively related to survival. The spearman correlation analysis found higher serum albumin levels were observed in high BMI, REE and FBG but in low REE/kg groups.

Table 1 Patient characteristics and univariate analysis

Factors		N	5-year survival (%)	p
Age, year	≤65	210	53.3	**0.003**
	>65	96	34.6	
Sex	Male	235	44.0	**0.039**
	Female	71	57.8	
Histology	AC	98	49.7	0.590
	SCC	208	45.7	
Surgical type	Transthoracic	186	47.0	0.701
	McKeown	53	40.4	
	Transabdominal	67	51.2	
Differentiation	Well	38	61.9	**0.000**
	Moderately	173	55.1	
	Poorly	95	24.9	
T stage	Tis/T1	31	82.2	**0.000**
	T2	65	62.1	
	T3	159	43.3	
	T4a	51	17.1	
N stage	N0	156	67.5	**0.000**
	N1	73	38.6	
	N2	52	14.2	
	N3-4	25	9.5	
TNM stage	0-I	42	80.5	**0.000**
	II	118	66.5	
	III	146	21.3	
Weight lost	No/Little	203	46.5	0.555
	Middle	50	56.8	
	Large	53	41.7	
Adjuvant Chemoradiation	Yes	78	41.7	0.187
	No	228	48.8	
Albumin	<35 g/l	36	26.7	**0.000**
	35–40 g/l	132	41.6	
	>40 g/l	138	57.8	
Lymphocyte	<1.1*10^9	42	48.7	0.780
	1.1–3.2*10^9	228	47.5	
	>3.2*10^9	36	42.6	
NLR	<5	289	47.1	0.787
	≥5	17	47.1	
REE/kg	<23.2	245	50.4	**0.024**
	≥23.2	61	35.2	
REE	Low	154	40.4	**0.010**
	High	152	55.3	
FBG	Low	108	35.0	**0.020**
	High	198	51.7	

Table 1 Patient characteristics and univariate analysis *(Continued)*

BMI	Low	81	36.8	**0.046**
	Normal	186	49.1	
	High	39	62.8	

CI confidence interval, *OR* odds ratio
The results were in bold, if the 95 % CI excluded 1 or p<0.05

Univariate, multivariate and subgroup analysis

To evaluate the prognostic factors potentially related to survival, univariate analysis was applied (Table 1) and found no statistical associations of histologic subtype, surgical type, weight loss and adjuvant chemoradiation with OS. The prognostic factors were age, sex, differentiation, T-stage, N-stage, BMI ($X^2 = 6.141$, $p = 0.046$, Fig. 1), albumin ($X^2 = 19.761$, $p < 0.001$, Fig. 2), REE ($X^2 = 6.630$, $p = 0.010$), REE/kg ($X^2 = 5.063$, $p = 0.024$, Fig. 3) and FBG ($X^2 = 5.379$, $p = 0.020$, Fig. 4). Patients with low BMI, REE, FBG and high REE/kg had significant worse survival.

Variables significant (age, sex, differentiation, T-stage, N-stage, albumin, BMI, REE, REE/kg and FBG) in Univariate analysis were included in a multivariate analysis (Table 3), which did not show a significant association between BMI (HR = 0.945; 95 % CI 0.660–1.351, $p = 0.755$), REE (HR = 1.101; 95 % CI 0.718–1.688, $p = 0.660$) or REE/kg (HR = 1.164; 95 % CI 0.717–1.890, $p = 0.540$) and OS. Age, differentiation, T-stage, N-stage, albumin (HR = 0.757; 95 % CI 0.589–0.973, $p = 0.030$) and FBG (HR = 0.695; 95 % CI 0.489–0.987, $p = 0.042$) were independent prognostic factors.

In order to assess the impact of BMI and REE on different tumor stages, we divided patients into subgroups on the basis of N-stage (N0 vs. N1-4). Patients with higher BMI and REE had significantly better OS in subgroup of N0 ($X^2 = 15.507$ $p < 0.001$ and $X^2 = 14.717$, $p < 0.001$, respectively), but no statistical significance in subgroup of N1-4 ($X^2 = 1.952$, $P = 0.377$ and $X^2 = 0.386$, $p = 0.534$, respectively). Multivariate analysis of subgroups revealed BMI (HR = 0.540; 95 % CI 0.304–0.959, $p = 0.035$) and REE (HR = 0.457; 95 % CI 0.216–0.967, $p = 0.041$) were independent prognostic factors for N0 patients but not for N1-4 patients.

Discussion

Our study identified that FBG level ≤90 mg/dL was independently associated with poor survival and also confirmed that advanced cancer stages remain the most powerful prognostic factors. In addition, we observed that BMI, REE and FBG were significant prognostic factors, but the prognostic value of BMI and REE is not the same between different lymph node metastasis statuses. For metastatic esophageal cancers, the most important prognostic factors were FBG, albumin and cancer staging including differentiation and invasion depth

Table 2 Associations among characteristics, BMI, REE, REE/kg and FBG

Factors	BMI, kg/m^2				REE, kcal day^{-1}			REE/kg, kcal day^{-1}			FBG, mg/dL		
	<20	20–25	>25	p	Low	High	p	Low	High	p	≤90	>90	p
	81	186	39		154	152		245	61		108	198	
Age													
≤ 65	50	134	26	0.332	87	123	**0.000**	157	53	**0.001**	73	137	0.774
> 65	31	52	13		67	29		88	8		35	61	
Sex													
Male	65	141	29	0.408	118	117	0.942	174	61	**0.000**	88	147	0.153
Female	16	45	10		36	35		71	0		20	51	
Histology													
SCC	54	132	22	0.561	103	105	0.682	165	43	0.639	81	127	0.052
AC	27	54	17		51	47		80	18		27	71	
Differentiation													
Well	7	28	3	0.869	19	19	0.507	31	7	0.552	14	24	0.557
Moderately	50	98	25		91	82		140	33		63	110	
Poorly	24	60	11		44	51		74	21		31	64	
T stage													
Tis/T1	8	19	4	0.172	12	19	**0.040**	27	4	0.124	12	19	0.499
T2	14	42	9		30	35		54	11		22	43	
T3	42	93	24		81	78		126	33		50	109	
T4a	17	32	2		31	20		38	13		24	27	
N stage													
N0	36	98	22	0.241	73	83	0.476	131	25	0.262	54	102	0.551
N1	20	44	9		42	31		55	18		28	45	
N2	20	27	5		26	26		38	14		22	30	
N3-4	5	17	3		13	12		21	4		4	21	
Bad habits													
Smoking	51	86	17		77	77	0.909	112	42	**0.001**	63	91	**0.039**
Drinking	26	60	11		46	51	0.490	74	23	0.261	38	59	0.355
Comorbidities													
Highblood	12	35	12	0.063	27	32	0.437	50	9	0.318	16	43	0.145
Copd	12	18	5	0.478	24	11	**0.022**	29	6	0.662	13	22	0.809
Cardiovascular disease	2	5	0	0.551	6	1	0.058	5	2	0.564	7	0	**0.000**
Arrhythmia	7	16	8	0.129	14	17	0.546	27	4	0.303	14	17	0.227
Diabetes	15	41	18	**0.006**	35	39	0.551	66	8	0.024	0	74	**0.000**
Mortality	1	5	1	0.970	6	1	0.058	6	1	0.706	3	4	0.673
Postoperative complications													
Fistula	6	6	3	0.083	12	3	0.182	9	6	0.259	6	9	0.825
Sepsis	9	6	6	0.208	15	6	0.260	12	9	0.125	9	12	0.673
Pneumonia	7	11	8	0.615	16	10	0.892	20	6	0.676	8	18	0.233
Respiratory insufficiency	6	9	6	0.846	14	7	0.692	18	3	0.504	7	14	0.122
Arrhythmia	14	33	8	0.661	30	25	0.419	45	10	0.720	18	37	0.491
Cardiac insufficiency	8	38	4	0.068	30	20	0.950	42	8	0.125	12	38	0.136
Albumin													
< 35 g/l	16	19	1	**0.001**	29	7	**0.000**	26	10	**0.009**	20	16	**0.000**

Table 2 Associations among characteristics, BMI, REE, REE/kg and FBG *(Continued)*

35–40 g/	38	78	16		68	64		99	33		55	77	
> 40 g/l	27	89	22		57	81		120	18		33	105	
Lymphocyte													
< 1.1*109	13	26	3	0.092	23	19	0.031	34	8	0.305	15	27	0.401
1.1–3.2	64	133	32		121	108		179	50		84	145	
> 3.2	4	27	4		10	25		32	3		9	26	
NLR													
< 5	73	179	37	0.135	144	145	0.473	233	56	0.316	101	188	0.603
≥ 5	8	7	2		10	7		12	5		7	10	
Weight lost													
No/Little	45	125	33	**0.001**	103	100	0.731	171	32	**0.006**	66	137	0.543
Middle	14	33	3		21	29		38	12		25	25	
Large	22	28	3		30	23		36	17		17	36	
FBG													
Low	37	64	7	**0.003**	65	43	**0.011**	79	29	**0.025**			
High	44	122	32		89	109		166	32				
REE													
Low	71	82	1	**0.000**				107	47	**0.000**			
High	10	104	38					138	14				
REE/kg													
Low	32	174	39	**0.000**									
High	49	12	0										

CI confidence interval, *OR* odds ratio
The results were in bold, if the 95 % CI excluded 1 or *p*<0.05

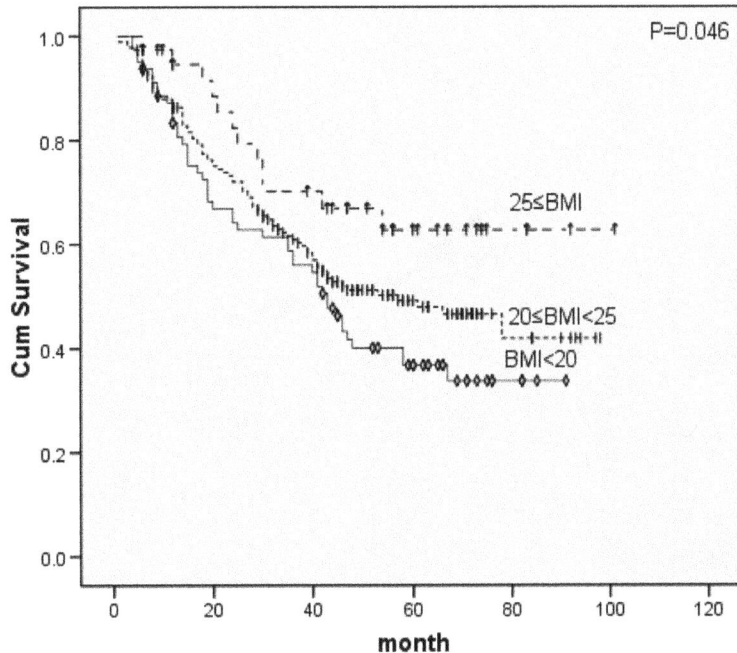

Fig. 1 Survival curves of BMI classes

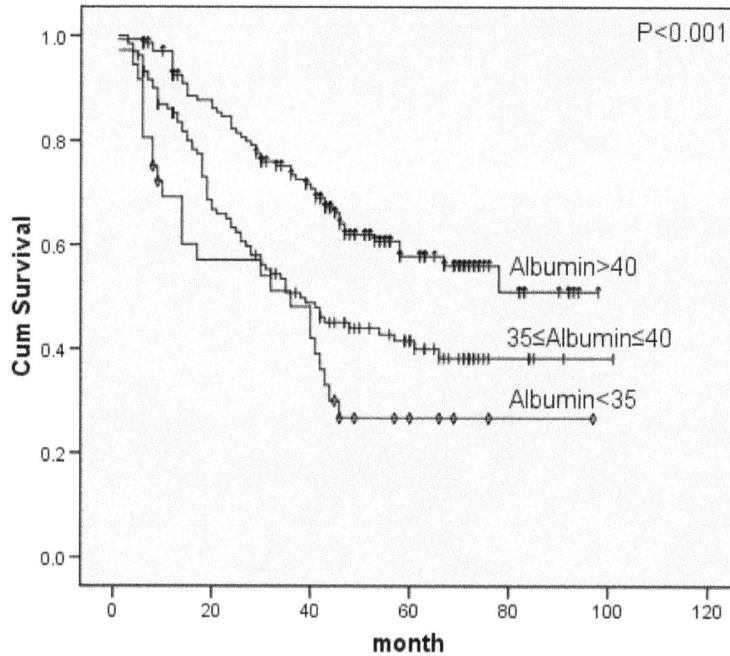

Fig. 2 Survival curves of albumin classes

whereas BMI and REE did not significantly affect the OS. However, for non-metastatic esophageal cancers, BMI and REE were important risk factors and proved to be independent prognostic indicators.

Total lymphocyte counts, NLR and serum albumin were recognized as nutrition based or inflammation-based prognostic factors. Among the cancer patients, those with digestive tract malignancies were more likely to suffer from hypoalbuminaemia, which has been attributed to increased catabolism, obstruction of the digestive tract and the systemic inflammatory response [12]. The combined use of albumin and serum C-reactive protein

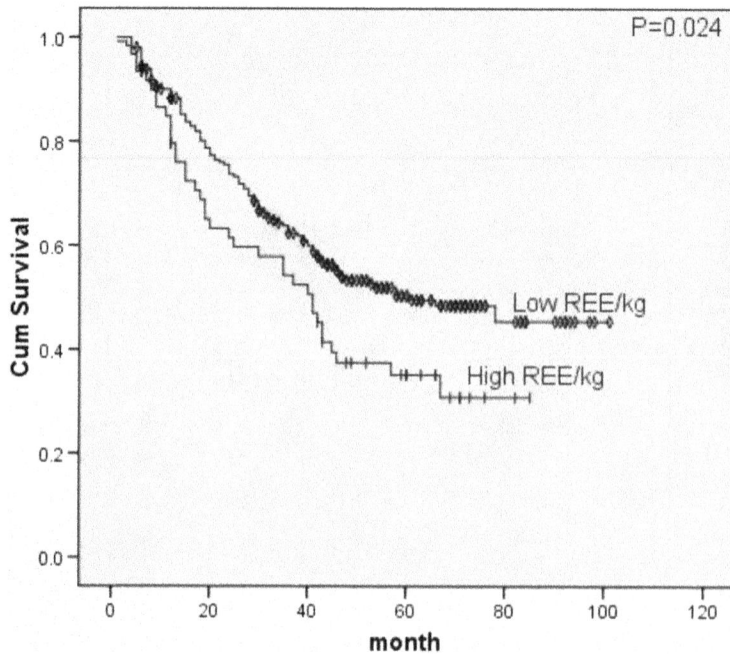

Fig. 3 Survival curves of REE/kg classes

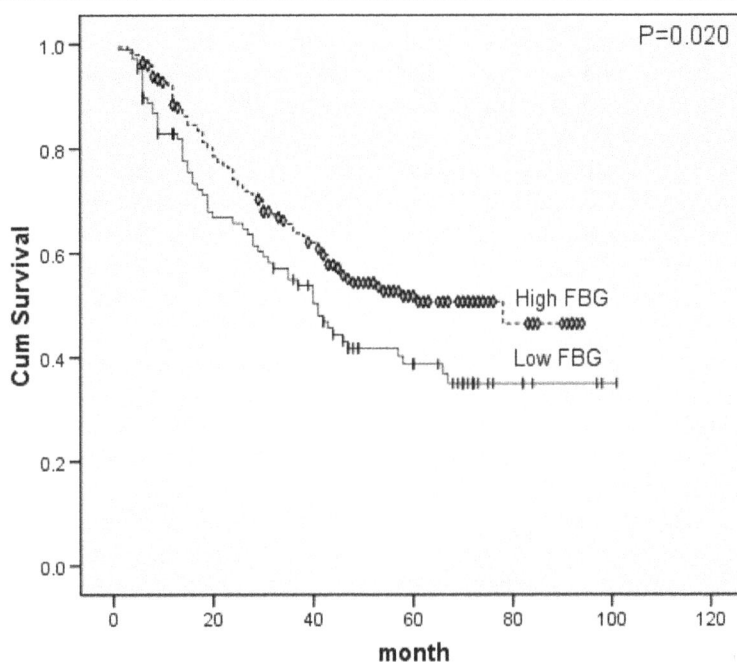

Fig. 4 Survival curves of FBG classes

were introduced by the Glasgow prognostic score [13, 14] and the combined use of albumin and lymphocyte counts have been mentioned by the Onodera's prognostic nutritional index [15]. Hypoalbuminaemia has been shown to correlate with ideal body weight, weight loss, body cell mass and poor prognostic in cancer patients [16]. In our cohort, hypoalbuminaemia associated with weight loss, low REE and low FBG. Patients with serum albumin levels <35 g/l had the 5-year survival rate of 26.7 %, compared to 57.8 % in patients with serum albumin > 40 g/l. Serum albumin was proved to be an independent significant prognostic factor by multivariate analysis even after adjusting for potential confounding factors. To assess the impact of albumin on different tumor stages, we divided patients into subgroups by N-stage (N0 vs. N1-4), and found hypoalbuminaemia as a worse survival factor in both N0 group ($X^2 = 11.078$, $p = 0.004$) and N1-4 group ($X^2 = 7.236$, $p = 0.027$). But the multivariate prognostic analysis for subgroups of N0 and N1-4 exhibited that serum albumin as a weaker prognostic value than other potential prognostic factors. It may be explained by the different clinical characteristics of each subgroup which may impact on the prognostic value.

Table 3 Multivariate prognostic analysis

Factors	All patients			N0 patients			N1-4 patients		
	P	OR	95 % CI	P	OR	95 % CI	P	OR	95 % CI
Age	**0.001**	1.844	1.279–2.661	0.286	1.417	0.747–2.689	**0.005**	1.982	1.228–3.200
Sex	0.229	0.757	0.481–1.191	**0.016**	0.309	0.119–0.803	0.465	0.818	0.478–1.401
Differentiation	**0.004**	1.560	1.154–2.107	0.761	0.921	0.542–1.564	**0.002**	1.885	1.267–2.805
T stage	**0.005**	1.463	1.125–1.903	**0.024**	1.611	1.065–2.436	**0.018**	1.528	1.076–2.168
N stage	**0.000**	1.610	1.366–1.898	-	-	-	0.056	1.317	0.992–1.749
BMI	0.755	0.945	0.660–1.351	**0.035**	0.540	0.304–0.959	0.789	0.939	0.594–1.485
REE	0.660	1.101	0.718–1.688	**0.041**	0.457	0.216–0.967	0.163	1.493	0.851–2.619
REE/kg	0.540	1.164	0.717–1.890	0.060	2.054	0.971–4.343	0.739	0.905	0.503–1.628
FBG	**0.042**	0.695	0.489–0.987	0.632	0.863	0.474–1.574	**0.043**	0.627	0.399–0.985
Albumin	**0.030**	0.757	0.589–0.973	0.863	0.960	0.605–1.524	0.198	0.819	0.604–1.110

CI confidence interval, OR odds ratio
The results were in bold, if the 95 % CI excluded 1 or p<0.05

As a particular nonspecific marker of systemic inflammation, an elevated NLR is hypothesized to be associated with poor survival in various solid tumors [17]. But for esophageal cancer, its effect on long-term outcome is still controversial [18, 19]. Most of previous studies did not find the positive predictive values of NLR in patients with esophageal cancer [20, 21]. In this study, there was no significant difference in survival as the NLR cutoff value taken as five because many previous literatures reported optimal cutoff value as five [22]. We also did not find the prognostic value of total lymphocyte counts in patients with esophageal cancer.

A few studies focused on the influence of BMI on postoperative outcomes in patients with EC and had shown contradictory results, varying from no differences in postoperative complications and mortality to a higher incidence of individual complications (such as respiratory complications and anastomotic leak) in high BMI patients [5–7]. In our study, we found no difference of the frequency of postoperative complications and mortality among different BMI patients. In addition, patients with a high BMI had a higher frequency of diabetes. Smoking patients appeared to have a lower BMI. Although smoking is the preventable cause for esophageal cancer, but it was not observed to be a poor prognostic factor in our finding.

Previous studies had revealed contradictory results regarding the association between BMI and long-term outcome in esophageal cancer patients [4–7, 23–25]. Most of these studies were conducted in western populations that have a high incidence rate of EAC, which occurs more frequently in patients with a high BMI. But the main type in Chinese populations is ESCC (67.9 % in our data). The population is prone to be lean (26.5 % with BMI < 20 and only 12.7 % with BMI > 25 in our data) compared to Western populations. Based on our data, compared with normal patients, we found a significantly worse OS in low BMI patients and a significantly better OS in high BMI patients on a univariate analysis. The prognostic effect of BMI seems to be more valuable on lymph node-negative patients than lymph node-positive patients and proved to be independent prognostic indicators.

High blood glucose level makes patients more susceptible to certain postoperative complications such as surgical site infections, sepsis, myocardial ischemia and so on [26]. But no similar studies were reported concerning esophageal cancer. Based on our date, FBG did not affect the risk of all-cause mortality and postoperative complications. Our study found low FBG level and hypoalbuminaemia are inter-related. In the class of albumin <35 g/l, only 44.4 % (16/36) patients had the FBG > 90 mg/dL, but in the class of albumin >40 g/l, almost 76.1 % (105/138) patients had the FBG > 90 mg/dL,

and both hypoalbuminaemia and low FBG level were proved to be worse survival factors. It is easy to measure and monitor FBG or serum albumin in clinical research, so both FBG and serum albumin can easily be used for survival prognosis, and researchers can choose the appropriate method according to their laboratory conditions. To assess the impact of FBG on prognosis in patients with esophageal cancer, both the univariate and multivariate analysis proved that low FBG level (≤90 mg/dL) was independently associated with poor OS. These finding is consistent with previous studies which suggested that hyperglycemia related microvessel changes may have a protective effect against neoplastic cell spread and metastasis in patients with malignant tumors such as non-small cell lung cancer and so on [27, 28].

REE is believed to be elevated in several types of tumors, It has been hypothesized that increased energy expenditure may contribute to the development of malnutrition and weight loss [29]. Our study found patients with a low REE had significantly worse survival compared with high REE (5-year survival rate: 40.4 % vs 55.3 %, $p = 0.010$). In addition, there was no significant association of REE with postoperative complications and mortality. To our knowledge, it is the first demonstration of the prognostic value of estimated REE in postoperative patients with EC. Our study also observed a significant linear correlation between BMI and REE ($p < 0.001$), showing that patients with low BMI tended to have low REE. As the estimated REE largely depends on patients' weight and height, the worse prognosis for low REE patients may reflect that these patients are under-nourished and are likely to have poor prognosis as a result. In addition, patients with low REE tended to be associated with advanced T-stages, so we concluded that the advanced tumor stages may be another reason to explain the low REE patients' worse survival.

We also explore the relationship between REE and REE/kg. We found the effect of REE on patient survival was opposite to that of REE/kg. Low REE as well as high REE/kg was found to be a potential worse prognostic indicator. The existing hypothesis of REE is, the sum of the metabolic activities of internal organs, muscle, bone, and adipose tissue and can reflect patient's physiques and muscle volumes, but REE/kg may reflect the diffusion, consumption and metabolic rate of muscle. So patients with high REE/kg have been found to lose more weight, have lower BMI and have a worse survival, this finding is consistent with the hypothesis.

In this research, low FBG was significantly associated with low BMI, albumin and REE, a potential explanation might be proposed. Individuals with esophageal cancer commonly experience metabolic abnormalities. The abnormal state of insulin (hyperinsulinemia or insulin resistance) is one cause, and it promotes cancer growth and progression through its effects on the insulin and insulin-like growth factor pathways [30]. Meanwhile, diabetic microangiopathy render the vascular basal membrane less digestible by tumor cells, which may play a role in impeding neoplastic cell spread and metastasis.

Following are the main limitations in our study. First, this is a retrospective study and the sample size is not large. Second, all-cause mortality is used instead of disease-specific deaths, the latter is difficult to confirm. Third, we only chose R0 patients, so our results may not be suitable for all patients.

Conclusion

In conclusion, it is the first article to explore the prognostic significance of BMI, REE and FBG among patients with EC. FBG level ≤90 mg/dL was independently associated with poor survival for all patients. BMI and REE were important prognostic factors and the value was significant on lymph node negative patients. Therefore it is advisable that the combined assessment of BMI, REE and FBG can be used for a better preoperative assessment and prognostic evaluation in esophageal cancer patients.

Abbreviations
AC: Adencarcinoma; BMI: Body mass index; CI: Confidence interval; CT: Computer tomography; DFS: Disease-free survival; EAC: Esophageal adencarcinoma; EC: Esophageal cancer; ESCC: Esophageal squamous cell carcinoma; FBG: Fasting blood glucose; HR: Hazard ratio; NLR: Neutrophil to lymphocyte ratio; OS: Overall survival; PET: Positron emission tomography; REE: Resting energy expenditure; SCC: Squamous cell carcinoma

Acknowledgements
Not applicable.

Funding
None.

Authors' contributions
NW, YJZ and ZMC: study design; NW, DK, LWP, GC and ZMC: data acquisition, data analysis, drafting of manuscript; All authors read and approved the final manuscript.

Competing interests
The authors declare that they have neither financial competing interests nor non-financial (political, personal, religious, ideological, academic, intellectual, commercial or any other) competing interests. The authors declare that they have no competing interests.

Author details
[1]Department of Cardio-thoracic Surgery, HuaShan Hospital of Fudan University, Shanghai 200040, People's Republic of China. [2]Department of General Surgery, HuaShan Hospital of Fudan University, Shanghai 200040, China.

References

1. Kamangar F, Dores GM, Anderson WF. Patterns of cancer incidence, mortality, and prevalence across five continents: defining priorities to reduce cancer disparities in different geographic regions of the world. J Clin Oncol. 2006;24:2137–50.
2. Jemal A, Bray F, Center MM, Ferlay J, Ward E, Forman D. Global cancer statistics. CA Cancer J Clin. 2011;61:69–90.
3. Harvie MN, Howell A, Thatcher N, Baildam A, Campbell I. Energy balance in patients with advanced NSCLC, metastatic melanoma and metastatic breast cancer receiving chemotherapy-a longitudinal study. Br J Cancer. 2005;92:673–80.
4. Smith M, Zhou M, Whitlock G, Yang G, Offer A, Hui G, et al. Esophageal cancer and body mass index: results from a prospective study of 220,000 men in China and a meta-analysis of published studies. Int J Cancer. 2008; 122:1604–10.
5. Hayashi Y, Correa AM, Hofstetter WL, Vaporciyan AA, Rice DC, Walsh GL, et al. The influence of high body mass index on the prognosis of patients with esophageal cancer after surgery as primary therapy. Cancer. 2010;116:5619–27.
6. Yoon HH, Lewis MA, Shi Q, Khan M, Cassivi SD, Diasio RB, et al. Prognostic impact of body mass index stratified by smoking status in patients with esophageal adenocarcinoma. J Clin Oncol. 2011;29:4561–7.
7. Blom RL, Lagarde SM, Klinkenbijl JH, Busch OR, van Berge Henegouwen MI. A high body mass index in esophageal cancer patients does not influence postoperative outcome or long-term survival. Ann Surg Oncol. 2012;19:766–71.
8. Mifflin MD, St Jeor ST, Hill LA, Scott BJ, Daugherty SA, Koh YO. A new predictive equation for resting energy expenditure in healthy individuals. Am J Clin Nutr. 1990;51:241–7.
9. Rapp K, Schroeder J, Klenk J, Ulmer H, Concin H, Diem G, et al. Fasting blood glucose and cancer risk in a cohort of more than 140,000 adults in Austria. Diabetologia. 2006;49:945–52.
10. LeRoith D, Novosyadlyy R, Gallagher EJ, Lann D, Vijayakumar A, Yakar S. Obesity and type 2 diabetes are associated with an increased risk of developing cancer and a worse prognosis; epidemiological and mechanistic evidence. Exp Clin Endocrinol Diabetes. 2008;116:S4–6.
11. Nerlich AG, Hagedorn HG, Boheim M, Schleicher ED. Patients with diabetes-induced microangiopathy show a reduced frequency of carcinomas. In Vivo. 1998;12:667–70.
12. Diakos CI, Charles KA, McMillan DC, Clarke SJ. Cancer-related inflammation and treatment effectiveness. Lancet Oncol. 2014;15:493–503.
13. Proctor MJ, Morrison DS, Talwar D, Balmer SM, O'Reilly DS, Foulis AK, et al. An inflammation-based prognostic score (mGPS) predicts cancer survival independent of tumour site: a Glasgow Inflammation Outcome Study. Br J Cancer. 2011;104:726–34.
14. McMillan DC. The systemic inflammation-based Glasgow Prognostic Score: a decade of experience in patients with cancer. Cancer Treat Rev. 2013;39:534–40.
15. Onodera T, Goseki N, Kosaki G. Prognostic nutritional index in gastrointestinal surgery of malnourished cancer patients. Nihon Geka Gakkai Zasshi. 1984;85:1001–5.
16. McMillan DC, Watson WS, O'Gorman P, Preston T, Scott HR, McArdle CS. Albumin concentrations are primarily determined by the body cell mass and the systemic inflammatory response in cancer patients with weight loss. Nutr Cancer. 2001;39:210–3.
17. Templeton AJ, McNamara MG, Šeruga B, Vera-Badillo FE, Aneja P, Ocaña A, et al. Prognostic role of neutrophil-to-lymphocyte ratio in solid tumors: a systematic review and meta-analysis. J Natl Cancer Inst. 2014;106:dju124.
18. Han LH, Jia YB, Song QX, Wang JB, Wang NN, Cheng YF. The prognostic significance of preoperative lymphocyte-monocyte ratio in patients with resectable esophageal squamous cell carcinoma. Asian Pac J Cancer Prev. 2015;16:2245–50.
19. Xie X, Luo KJ, Hu Y, Wang JY, Chen J. Prognostic value of preoperative platelet-lymphocyte and neutrophil-lymphocyte ratio in patients undergoing surgery for esophageal squamous cell cancer. Dis Esophagus. 2014;19. doi: 10.1111/dote.12296
20. Rashid F, Waraich N, Bhatti I, Saha S, Khan RN, Ahmed J, et al. A pre-operative elevated neutrophil: lymphocyte ratio does not predict survival from oesophageal cancer resection. World J Surg Oncol. 2010;8:1.

21. Dutta S, Crumley AB, Fullarton GM, Horgan PG, McMillan DC. Comparison of the prognostic value of tumour- and patient-related factors in patients undergoing potentially curative resection of oesophageal cancer. World J Surg. 2011;35:1861–6.
22. Guthrie GJ, Charles KA, Roxburgh CS, Horgan PG, McMillan DC, Clarke SJ. The systemic inflammation-based neutrophil-lymphocyte ratio: experience in patients with cancer. Crit Rev Oncol Hematol. 2013;88:218–30.
23. Grotenhuis BA, Wijnhoven BP, Hotte GJ, van der Stok EP, Tilanus HW, van Lanschot JJ. Prognostic value of body mass index on short-term and long-term outcome after resection of esophageal cancer. World J Surg. 2010;34:2621–7.
24. Melis M, Weber JM, McLoughlin JM, Siegel EM, Hoffe S, Shridhar R, et al. An elevated body mass index does not reduce survival after esophagectomy for cancer. Ann Surg Oncol. 2011;18:824–31.
25. Morgan MA, Lewis WG, Hopper AN, Escofet X, Harvard TJ, Brewster AE, et al. Prognostic significance of body mass indices for patients undergoing esophagectomy for cancer. Dis Esophagus. 2007;20:29–35.
26. Rehman HU, Mohammed K. Preoperative management of diabetic patients. Curr Surg. 2003;60:607–11.
27. De Giorgio R, Barbara G, Cecconi A, Corinaldesi R, Mancini AM. Diabetes is associated with longer survival rates in patients with malignant tumors. Arch Intern Med. 2000;160:2217.
28. Bartling B, Simm A, Sohst A, Silber RE, Hofmann HS. Effect of diabetes mellitus on the outcome of patients with resected non-small cell lung carcinoma. Gerontology. 2011;57:497–501.
29. Johnson G, Salle A, Lorimier G, Laccourreye L, Enon B, Blin V, et al. Cancer cachexia: measured and predicted resting energy expenditures for nutritional needs evaluation. Nutrition. 2008;24:443–50.
30. Cannata D, Fierz Y, Vijayakumar A, LeRoith D. Type 2 diabetes and cancer: what is the connection? Mt Sinai J Med. 2010;77:197–213.

A randomized controlled trial of endoscopic steroid injection for prophylaxis of esophageal stenoses after extensive endoscopic submucosal dissection

Hiroaki Takahashi[1], Yoshiaki Arimura[2]*, Satoshi Okahara[1], Junichi Kodaira[1], Kaku Hokari[3], Hiroyuki Tsukagoshi[3], Yasuhisa Shinomura[2] and Masao Hosokawa[4]

Abstract

Background: Esophageal stenosis following endoscopic submucosal dissection (ESD) is a serious adverse event that makes subsequent management more difficult.

Methods: This parallel, randomized, controlled, open-label study was designed to examine whether local steroid injection is an effective prophylactic treatment for esophageal stenoses following extensive ESD. This single center trial was conducted at the Keiyukai Hospital, a tertiary care center for gastrointestinal disease in Japan [University Hospital Medical Network Clinical Trial Registry (UMIN-CTR) on 15 September 2011 (UMIN000006327)]. Thirty-two patients with mucosal defects involving ≥75% of the esophageal circumference were randomized to receive a single dose of triamcinolone acetonide injections (n = 16) or be treated conventionally (n = 16). The primary outcome was the frequency of stricture requiring endoscopic dilatation; the surrogate primary endpoint was the number of dilatation sessions needed. Secondary outcomes included adverse event rates, the minimum diameter of the stenotic area and the duration of the course of dilatation treatments.

Results: The frequency of stricture was not significantly different between the groups because of insufficient statistical power, but the number of dilatation sessions required was significantly less in the steroid group (6.1 sessions [95% confidence interval, CI 2.8–9.4] *versus* 12.5 [95% CI 7.1–17.9] sessions in the control group; $P = 0.04$). The perforation rate was similar in both groups. The minimum diameter of stenotic lumens was significantly greater in the treatment group than controls (11.0 mm *versus* 7.1 mm, respectively; $P = 0.01$). The perforation rate was not significantly different between the groups (1.0% *versus* 0.5% in the treatment and control group, respectively). Steroid injection was effective in cases of mucosal defects encompassing the entire esophageal circumference.

Conclusions: Prophylactic endoscopic steroid injection appears to be a safe means of relieving the severity of esophageal stenoses following extensive ESD.

Keywords: Esophageal stenosis, Steroid, Local injection, Endoscopic submucosal dissection (ESD), Early squamous cell carcinoma of esophagus

* Correspondence: arimura@sapmed.ac.jp
[2]Department of Gastroenterology, Rheumatology, and Clinical Immunology, Sapporo Medical University, S-1, W-16, Chuo-ku, Sapporo 060-8543, Japan
Full list of author information is available at the end of the article

Background

In Japan, endoscopic submucosal dissection (ESD) is widely accepted as a standard treatment for early esophageal squamous cell carcinomas without documented metastasis. The ESD technique has been shown to reduce the risk of local recurrence, and perforations arising as a consequence of treatment are generally well tolerated [1]. As ESD can excise larger lesions than endoscopic mucosal resection, it is becoming increasingly popular, but esophageal stenosis after removal of large lesions by ESD is a major concern. Mucosal defects extending over three-quarters of the circumference of the esophagus after endoscopic resection are closely associated with the subsequent development of esophageal stenosis [2], which can cause dysphagia and impair quality of life.

Patients with esophageal stenosis are frequently treated by endoscopic dilatation therapy. The risk of perforation complicating the procedure increases with the number of therapeutic sessions [3]. It is important to identify ways of preventing esophageal stenosis after ESD, and minimizing the complications associated with treatment when it does arise. Treatment options for esophageal stenosis include mechanical dilatation with a bougie or balloon, stent placement and autologous keratinocyte implantation [4]. Dilatation therapies may, however, have a higher incidence of adverse events and recurrence rates than previously thought [5-7]. Therefore, simple, safe, reliable and inexpensive approaches are needed to cope with iatrogenic esophageal stenoses.

Systemic [8] or local [9,10] administration of steroids is reported to be an effective means of addressing esophageal stenosis after ESD, as well as for peptic stenosis [11-13]. Although systemic steroids should be avoided in patients with diabetes mellitus or hypertension, locally administered steroids appear to be safe in the vast majority of patients [10]. Locally administered steroids have minimal systemic effects owing to the small dose administered and short duration of exposure [10]. Previous retrospective and controlled prospective studies of endoscopic steroid injection therapy have found that the incidence of esophageal stenosis following ESD in patients treated with steroid was 10–19%, compared with 66–75% in untreated control groups. In addition, steroid injection therapy significantly reduced the number of required dilatation sessions.

To our knowledge, no randomized studies to date have analyzed the potential preventative benefits of endoscopic steroid injection therapy, or whether it is safe and effective, for stenosis caused by a mucosal defect involving the entire circumference of the esophagus after ESD. We undertook a prospective, randomized controlled trial to analyze the prophylactic effects of endoscopic steroid injection therapy for esophageal stenoses complicating extensive ESD.

Methods

This randomized, controlled, open-label study was performed at Keiyukai Sapporo Hospital, Japan. All participants gave their written informed consent, based on the Helsinki Declaration (1964, 1975, amended in 1983, 2003 and 2008) of the World Medical Association, and the Ethics Committee of Keiyukai Sapporo Hospital approved the study protocol. The study was designed according to the CONSORT guidelines and was registered with the University Hospital Medical Network Clinical Trial Registry (UMIN-CTR) on 15 September 2011 (UMIN000006327).

Study groups

Patients who had undergone ESD to treat histologically confirmed early squamous cell carcinoma of the esophagus from February 2010 to October 2011 and who were expected to have a mucosal defect encompassing ≥75% of the circumference of the esophageal mucosa after ESD were eligible for the study. Patients who received additional adjuvant treatments, such as surgery or chemoradiation therapy, and patients who were not regularly or adequately followed-up were excluded. Depth of tumor invasion was determined based on the findings of endoscopy and/or endoscopic ultrasonography. Mucosal to slightly invasive submucosal cancers (of invasion less than 200 μm in depth) were regarded as indications for ESD. Removal of a carcinoma involving two-thirds of the circumference of the esophagus by ESD was expected to result in a mucosal defect spanning more than three-quarters of the circumference. Patients enrolled in the study were randomized to receive steroid injection therapy or to be treated conventionally. Randomization was computer-generated with concealed allocation using sequentially numbered containers. Data were collated at Sapporo Medical University and independently analyzed by one author (Y.A.). The baseline demographic and clinical characteristics of the study population were compared on the basis of age, sex, tumor location, proportion of the esophageal circumference involved, number of multiple Lugol voiding lesions [14], clinical T factor [15] and follow-up period (Table 1). All ESD procedures (Figure 1A–C) were performed as described in our previous report [1]. The characteristics of the ESD procedures undertaken in the treatment and control groups were compared on the basis of the size of the tumor and resected specimen, depth of invasion, operation time, pathological margin, mucosal circumferential defect and peri-procedural perforation (Table 2).

Protocol for endoscopic steroid injection and dilatation therapy

As previously described [9,10], patients who did not develop immediate complications, such as perforation or bleeding, during the ESD procedure and who had been

Table 1 Baseline characteristics of the study population

	Treatment group	Control group	p-value
	n = 16	n = 16	
Age, years mean ± SD (range)	70.0 ± 9.7 (48–89)	71.0 ± 7.1 (58–83)	0.74
Sex, male/female	13/3	12/4	0.99
Tumor location, n (upper/middle/lower)	1/10/5	2/9/5	0.72
Proportion of esophageal circumference involved, n (≥2/3 to <3/4/≥3/4 to <1/1)	4/7/5	6/5/5	0.57
Multiple Lugol voiding lesions, n (%)	8 (50.0)	7 (43.8)	0.99
Clinical T factor, n (m1/m2/m3/sm1)	1/12/3/0	3/8/4/1	0.40
Follow-up period, month mean ± SD (range)	16.1 ± 5.6 (10–27)	16.9 ± 5.4 (9–27)	0.66

Abbreviation: SD, standard deviation.

allocated to the steroid injection group were endoscopically injected with triamcinolone acetonide (Kenacort-A®, 40 mg/ml, Bristol-Myers Squibb, Anagni, Italy) immediately after the procedure. Triamcinolone was diluted with 0.9% NaCl to a final concentration of 10 mg/ml, then 0.5 ml aliquots were injected at the base of the artificial ulcer using a 25-gauge, 3 mm needle (TOP Corporation, Tokyo, Japan; Figure 1D). Injection commenced at the distal edge of the ulcer base and was repeated evenly at points 10 mm apart towards the proximal edge, taking care to avoid injuring the muscularis propria.

Esophagogastroduodenoscopy (EGD) was performed to assess for stenosis, bleeding or perforation at the injected sites 6 days after treatment (Figure 2). Barium contrast esophagography was performed in patients who complained of dysphagia, or 4 weeks after the last EGD if patients were asymptomatic, to quantitatively assess stenosis (Figure 3). Esophageal stenosis was defined as an esophageal diameter <11 mm, rather than the inability to pass the gastroscope (which had a diameter of 9.8–11.0 mm) or inability to achieve or maintain a diameter of 14 mm despite dilatation every 2–4 weeks [5,16]. The luminal diameter was estimated by measurement of the minimum diameter of the stricture on esophagography (for examples, see Figures 3 and 4). Dilatation therapy was performed every 1–4 weeks as previously described [3]. Briefly, dilatation was performed in the outpatient department under fluoroscopic guidance using a Maloney (Medovations, Milwaukee, WI) or Savary (Wilson Cook Medical, Winston-Salem, NC) wire-guided dilator [17]. Dilatation therapy was considered successful when patients did not report any symptoms of dysphagia

without having needed dilatation in the previous 4 weeks (Figure 5).

Statistical analysis

The incidence of esophageal stenoses and the frequency of dilatation sessions required were compared in the treatment and control groups. Independent t tests were used to compare age, resection size and procedure time. The primary study endpoint was the frequency of stricture requiring endoscopic dilatation for esophageal stenosis after ESD. A surrogate primary endpoint, the number of dilatation sessions required, was subsequently included in the analysis because the primary endpoint did not reach statistical significance. Secondary endpoints included the frequency of complications that occurred as a consequence of either local steroid injection or endoscopic dilatation, the minimum diameter of the stenotic area and the duration of the course of dilatation treatments (Tables 3 and 4). The number of patients to be enrolled was determined in advance using a power calculation for two-sample proportions test based on expected bougienage rates of 13% with and 60% without steroid injection, informed by previous reports of esophageal peptic stricture rates [13], with an α error of 0.05 (two-tailed) and a β error of 0.2. Consequently, the number of patients required in each group was calculated as 16 using R statistical software [18]. *Post hoc* analysis was also undertaken to compare the group of patients with whole circumferential mucosal defects (WCMD) with the group of those with lesions that involved less than the whole circumference (non-WCMD, NWCMD; Table 4), and a further analysis of the characteristics of patients with WCMDs was made (Table 5). All other statistical analyses were performed using IBM SPSS Statistics version 21 (IBM Japan, Tokyo, Japan). Chi-square tests were used to compare nominal and ordinal variables, with the exact P value based on Pearson's statistics or the Monte Carlo method applied as appropriate. We used t tests or Mann–Whitney tests for ratio scale variables, and for all tests a two-tailed P value of <0.05 was considered statistically significant.

Results

Recruitment began in February 2010 and the last follow-up was in October 2011. The trial ended because data were considered complete. During the study period, 209 patients with 256 lesions underwent ESD in our hospital, 42 of whom (20.1%) were enrolled in the study because they were expected to have mucosal defects extending over three-quarters of the esophageal circumference due to the ESD. Since one of these 42 patients declined to participate, in total 41 were enrolled and randomized. 21 were allocated to the injection (treatment) group whereas 20 were allocated to the non-injection (control) group. However, after ESD, nine patients were excluded from the

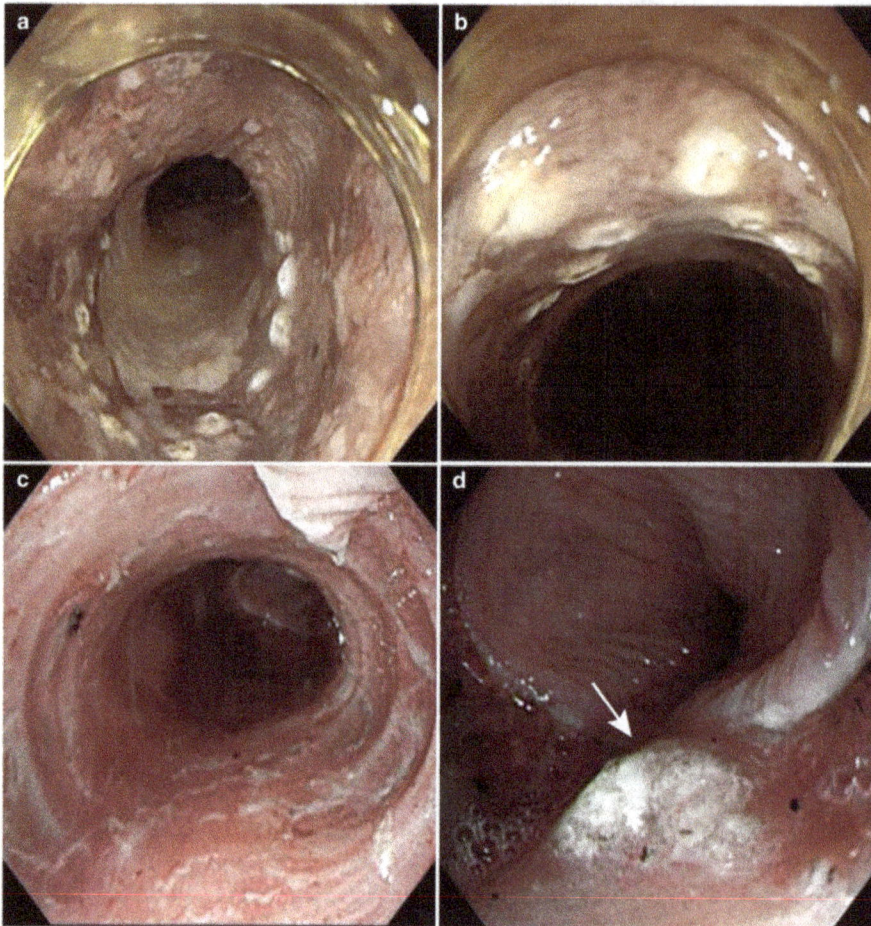

Figure 1 Typical endoscopic views of the esophagus in a patient in the injection group. a. A superficial esophageal carcinoma in the middle esophagus. The entire circumference of the lesion was marked out by electrocautery using a needle-knife at least 1 mm from the tumor border, confirmed by a Lugol-unstained region. **b**. This tumor encompasses half the circumference of the esophagus, as seen in the center of the lesion. **c**. The artificial ulcer encompassed the entire circumference after ESD. **d**. Injection of triamcinolone into the ulcer (white arrow).

study: one whose follow-up was inadequate and eight who received additional therapy. Of the latter eight patients, seven had submucosal invasion that exceeded 200 μm and one had lymphatic invasion despite a depth of invasion of only 180 μm. Ultimately, 16 patients were allocated to each group (Figure 6).

Comparison of treatment and control groups

Patients' baseline demographic and clinical characteristics (Table 1) and those of the ESD procedures (Table 2) were not significantly different between the groups. No patient experienced perforation caused by steroid injection or any other side effects of steroids. The frequency of stricture was not significantly different between the treatment (n = 10, 62.5%) and control (n = 14, 87.5%) groups ($P = 0.22$, Table 3). The mean number of sessions of dilatation therapy was significantly lower in the treatment than in the control group (6.1 sessions [95% confidence interval, CI 2.8–9.4 sessions] *versus* 12.5 sessions [95% CI 7.1–17.9

sessions]; $P = 0.04$). The perforation rate caused by dilatation procedures was 1.0% (one out of 97 sessions) in the steroid injection group and 0.5% (one out of 200 sessions) in the control group. The mean minimum diameter of stenotic lumens just before dilatation therapy was greater in the treatment group than controls (11.0 mm [95% CI 8.5–13.4 mm] *versus* 7.1 mm [95% CI 5.5–8.6], $P = 0.01$; Figure 4). The duration of dilatation therapy was 3.5 months in the treatment group and 6.1 months in the control group, but the difference was not statistically significant ($P = 0.11$, Table 3).

Post hoc comparison between patients with whole and non-whole circumferential mucosal defects

There were no significant differences in the baseline demographic, clinical or ESD characteristics of the 10 patients with WCMDs compared with the remaining 22 with NWCMDs (data not shown). The incidence of stricture was significantly more frequent (100% *versus* 63.6%,

Table 2 Characteristics of endoscopic submucosal dissection procedures

	Treatment group n = 16	Control group n = 16	p-value
Size of carcinoma, mm mean ± SD (range)	58 ± 16 (28–92)	53 ± 19 (30–90)	0.40
Size of resected specimen, mm mean ± SD (range)	68 ± 14 (43–97)	62 ± 17 (39–101)	0.29
Depth of invasion, n (m1/m2/m3/sm1/sm2*)	2/11/2/0/1	2/6/6/0/2	0.35
Operation time, min mean ± SD (range)	89.6 ± 37.5 (36–176)	88.3 ± 44.5 (44–235)	0.93
Pathological margin free, n (%)	15 (93.8)	15 (93.8)	0.99
Mucosal defect of circumference, n (<75% / ≥75%)	11/5	11/5	0.99
Perforation by ESD, n (%)	0/16 (0)	0/16 (0)	0.55

Abbreviations: m1, carcinoma *in situ*; m2, intramucosal invasive carcinoma limited to the lamina propria mucosa; m3, carcinoma limited to the muscularis mucosa; sm2, submucosal invasion between sm1 (slight invasion less than 200 μm in depth) and sm3 (massive invasion); SD, standard deviation; ESD, endoscopic submucosal dissection.
*Three patients with sm2 invasion had relative contraindications for surgical intervention for one or more of the following reasons: age considerations (the patients were 76, 79 and 89 years old), serious medical conditions (cerebral vascular disease, multiple primary cancers, low performance status), and/or patients' decisions to decline surgery. A treatment plan for these patients was carefully chosen under full informed consent.

$P = 0.035$) and the mean number of dilatation therapy sessions required was significantly more (16.3 *versus* 6.1 sessions, $P = 0.013$) in those with WCMD lesions. The perforation rate caused by dilatation procedures was similar: 0.6% (one out of 163 sessions) in the WCMD group compared with 0.7% (one out of 134 sessions) in the NWCMD group. The mean minimum diameter of stenotic lumens immediately before dilatation therapy was smaller in the WCMD group (7.2 *versus* 9.9 mm in the NWCMD group) but the difference was not significant ($P = 0.10$). The mean duration of dilatation therapy was significantly longer (8.1 *versus* 3.3 months, $P = 0.047$) in the WCMD group (Table 4).

Subgroup analysis of the whole circumference mucosal defect group

Comparisons of patients in the WCMD subgroup treated with steroid (n = 5) and those treated conventionally (n = 5) revealed no significant differences in baseline demographic, clinical or ESD characteristics (data not shown). The only treatment-related factor that differed significantly between the groups was the mean number of dilatation therapy sessions required, which was lower in those treated with steroids compared with controls (10.4 sessions [95% CI 6.0–14.8 sessions] *versus* 22.2 sessions [95% CI 9.0–35.4 sessions], respectively, $P < 0.05$; Table 3).

Discussion

Strictures have been observed to develop when the mucosal defect extends beyond three-quarters of the esophageal circumference in 68–92% of patients [2,5,9]. Because of the recent trend of treating larger lesions by extensive ESD, the number of patients with post-ESD strictures is increasing. These strictures interfere with subsequent management and impair quality of life. We therefore designed a randomized, controlled trial to examine the efficacy of endoscopic triamcinolone injection in preventing esophageal stenoses after extensive ESD, including patients with mucosal defects encompassing the entire circumference of the esophagus.

We found that endoscopic triamcinolone injection did not reduce the frequency of stricture formation, but

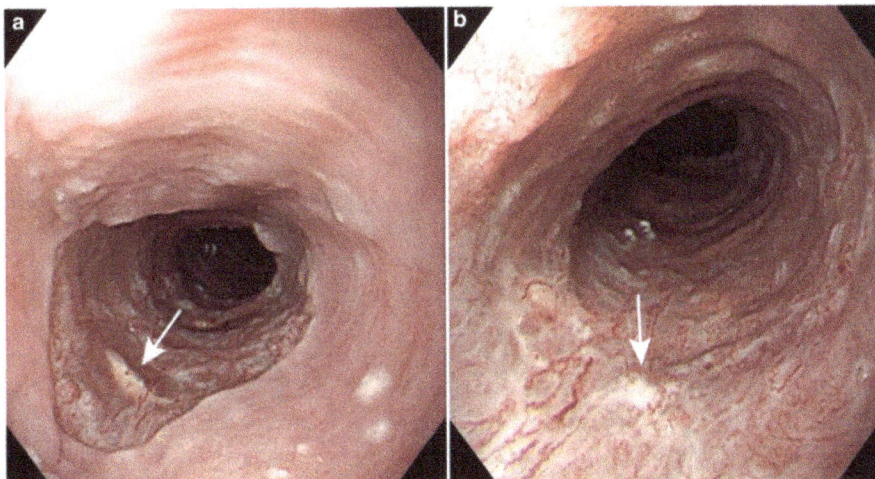

Figure 2 Endoscopic view 6 days after endoscopic submucosal dissection. Some injected triamcinolone is evident in the ulcer (white arrows). The right picture (a) is a magnification of the left picture (b).

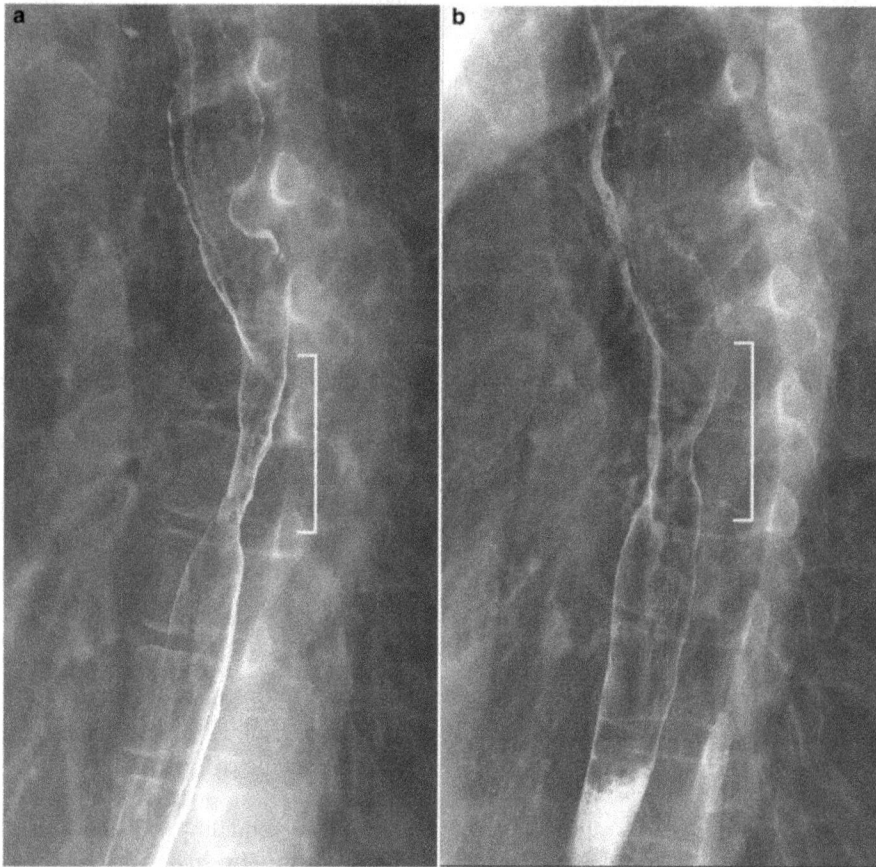

Figure 3 Esophageal stenosis assessed by esophagography. The white lines indicate the stricture caused by resection. The stricture had substantially improved 1 month later. The left esophagogram **(a)** was taken 2 months after endoscopic submucosal dissection (ESD); the right esophagogram **(b)** was taken 3 months after ESD.

reduced the mean number of dilatation sessions per patient from 12.5 to 6.1, suggesting that steroid injection may partially relieve esophageal stenoses. No steroid-related adverse events were observed, and the perforation rate during dilatation procedures was similar in the treated and control groups (1.0% *versus* 0.5%, respectively). These results suggest that a single prophylactic dose of steroid administered after ESD is safe and well tolerated. The mean minimum diameter of stenotic lumens immediately before the first dilatation treatment was significantly greater in the treated group than controls (11.0 *versus* 7.1 mm, respectively). The differences observed in duration of dilatation therapy were not statistically significant. Our trial is the first to demonstrate the partial but significant prophylactic effect of steroid injection on stricture formation in this clinical setting.

Hanaoka and colleagues previously stated that a randomized controlled trial comparing a single injection of steroid at the time of dilatation therapy may not be ethically acceptable, as the efficacy of steroid injection therapy is well recognized [10]. Furthermore, they stated that it would be better justified for a future controlled trial to

compare multiple steroid injections with systemic steroids or a different steroid injection regime. However, previous studies – including theirs – had excluded patients with circumferential defects from their trial, as these patients are known to develop extremely severe strictures [8,19]. Moreover, patients with WCMDs have been reported to require as many as 32 dilatation sessions [19], highlighting the challenges faced by clinicians in these cases. Although we are encountering more patients with circumferential mucosal defects in our clinical practice, the best way of managing them has not been determined. The results from our *post hoc* analysis confirm that patients with WCMDs are more likely to develop strictures, require more dilatation sessions and longer duration of treatment, but that they benefited most from a single prophylactic steroid injection after ESD. In patients with WCMDs and esophageal diameters of approximately 7 mm, prophylactic steroid treatment almost halved the number of dilatation sessions needed and the overall duration of treatment. This in itself is a clinically important finding, not least because a reduced incidence of esophageal perforation would be likely to

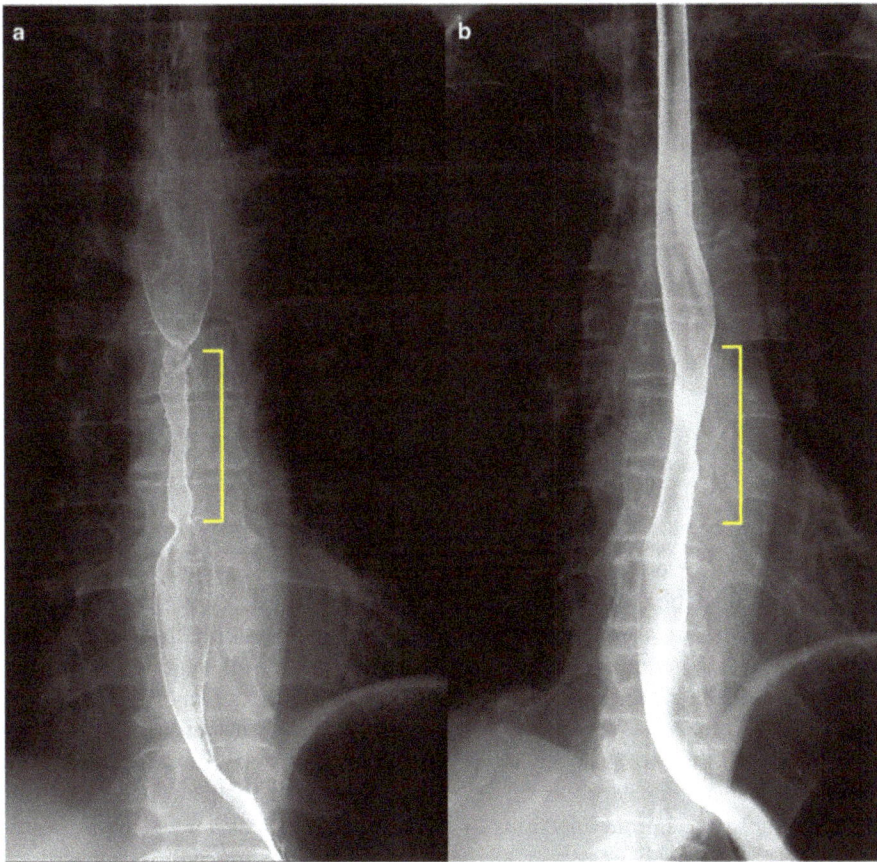

Figure 4 Barium esophagography 1 month after endoscopic submucosal dissection. The yellow lines indicate the narrow lumens owing to resection. **a**. Patient allocated to the control group, who developed a severe esophageal stricture that required 13 sessions of dilatation therapy. **b**. Patient allocated to the treatment group, who did not require dilatation.

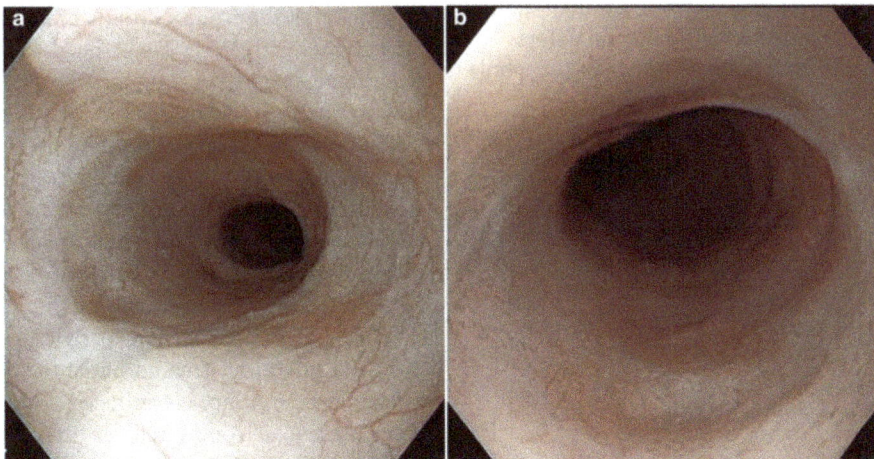

Figure 5 Typical endoscopic view 1 month after endoscopic submucosal dissection. Severe stenosis of the esophagus did not develop. The right picture **(a)** is a magnification of the left picture **(b)**.

Table 3 Characteristics of dilatation procedures undertaken in the treatment and control groups

Treatment vs. Control	Treatment group	Control group	p-value
	n = 16	n = 16	
Frequency of stricture, n (%)	10 (62.5)	14 (87.5)	0.22
Required dilatation sessions, n mean ± SD (range)	6.1 ± 6.2 (0–17)	12.5 ± 10.1 (0–40)	0.038
Perforation by dilatations, n per session (%)	1/97 (1.0)	1/200 (0.5)	0.55
Minimum diameter of strictured region, mm mean ± SD (range)	11.0 ± 4.6 (5.4-21.8)	7.1 ± 2.9 (5.1-12.8)	0.008
Duration of dilatation therapy, months mean ± SD (range)	3.5 ± 4.0 (0–13)	6.1 ± 5.0 (0–20)	0.11

Abbreviation: SD, standard deviation.

Table 5 Subgroup analysis of patients with mucosal defects involving the whole esophageal circumference

Treatment vs. Control in the WCMD	Treatment subgroup	Control subgroup	p-value
	n = 5	n = 5	
Frequency of stricture, n (%)	5 (100)	5 (100)	0.99
Required dilatation sessions, n mean ± SD (range)	10.4 ± 3.5 (6–15)	22.2 ± 10.6 (13–40)	0.046
Perforation by dilatations, n per session (%)	0/52 (0)	1/111 (0.9)	0.99
Minimum diameter of stenotic region, mm mean ± SD (range)	7.7 ± 1.7 (5.4-9.6)	6.7 ± 3.4 (5.1-12.7)	0.58
Duration for dilatations, month mean ± SD (range)	6.2 ± 4.4 (2–13)	10.0 ± 5.7 (6–20)	0.27

Abbreviations: WCMD, whole circumferential mucosal defect; NWCMD, non-WCMD; SD, standard deviation.

reduce morbidity and mortality. As it is well recognized that patients are at a lower risk of esophageal perforation if they undergo fewer dilatation treatments [3], prophylactic steroid injection might also improve patient safety, although as perforation rates are so low a large surveillance study would be needed to detect a difference.

Our findings also concur with those of previous studies, which showed that patients with smaller mucosal defects also benefited from endoscopic steroid injections to prevent post-ESD strictures. Our study may not have been adequately powered to detect these smaller – but nonetheless clinically relevant – differences in the frequency of stricture formation. Our results should be further confirmed by a large well-powered randomized controlled trial, which should also examine whether multiple steroid injections, administered during dilatation

Table 4 *Post hoc* analysis of characteristics of dilatation procedures undertaken in those with mucosal defects involving the whole circumference or less than the whole circumference of the esophagus

WCMD vs. NWCMD	WCMD group	NWCMD group	p-value
	n = 10	n = 22	
Frequency of stricture, n (%)	10 (100)	14 (63.6)	0.035
Required dilatation sessions, n mean ± SD (range)	16.3 ± 9.7 (6–40)	6.1 ± 6.4 (0–20)	0.013
Perforation by dilatations, n per session (%)	1/163 (0.6)	1/134 (0.7)	0.93
Minimum diameter of stenotic region, mm mean ± SD (range)	7.2 ± 2.6 (5.1-12.7)	9.9 ± 4.7 (5.3-21.8)	0.10
Duration of dilatations, months mean ± SD (range)	8.1 ± 5.2 (2–20)	3.3 ± 3.5 (0–20)	0.047

Abbreviations: WCMD, whole circumferential mucosal defect; NWCMD, non-WCMD; SD, standard deviation.

treatments, might benefit those patients that go on to develop esophageal stenoses.

A course of oral prednisolone has been reported to be an effective means of preventing strictures [8]. Endoscopic steroid injection is preferable to oral prednisolone in patients with diabetes mellitus, those who experience immediate or delayed adverse events after ESD, or those who require additional treatment for submucosal invasion. The systemic side effects of a locally injected steroid would likely be negligible compared with those of a systemic steroid. Histopathological analysis of excised ESD specimens showed that seven patients had tumors invading the submucosa beyond 200 μm and thus required additional therapy. Oral prednisolone would likely increase the risks associated with surgery, making it an obstacle to immediate surgical intervention. It has previously been reported that oral steroid therapy led to only three patients with WCMDs requiring a mean 0.7 sessions of dilatation therapy [8]. Thus, it remains unclear whether locally or systemically administered steroid is superior for patients with WCMDs. A head-to-head comparative study may establish a standard prophylaxis for esophageal stenosis caused by ESD.

The estimated sample size of 16 patients per group was determined by a power calculation based on expected stricture rates of 13% and 60% with and without steroid injection, respectively, informed by previously published data on esophageal peptic strictures [13]. These assumptions are now supported by another study [10], which showed that the proportion of strictures caused by ESD was 10% in steroid-treated patients and 66% in an historical control group. Nevertheless, our study might have been inadequately powered, as the stricture rates were 62.5% in the treatment group and 87.5% in the control group, a likely consequence of including 10 patients (31.3%) with circumferential mucosal defects. Furthermore,

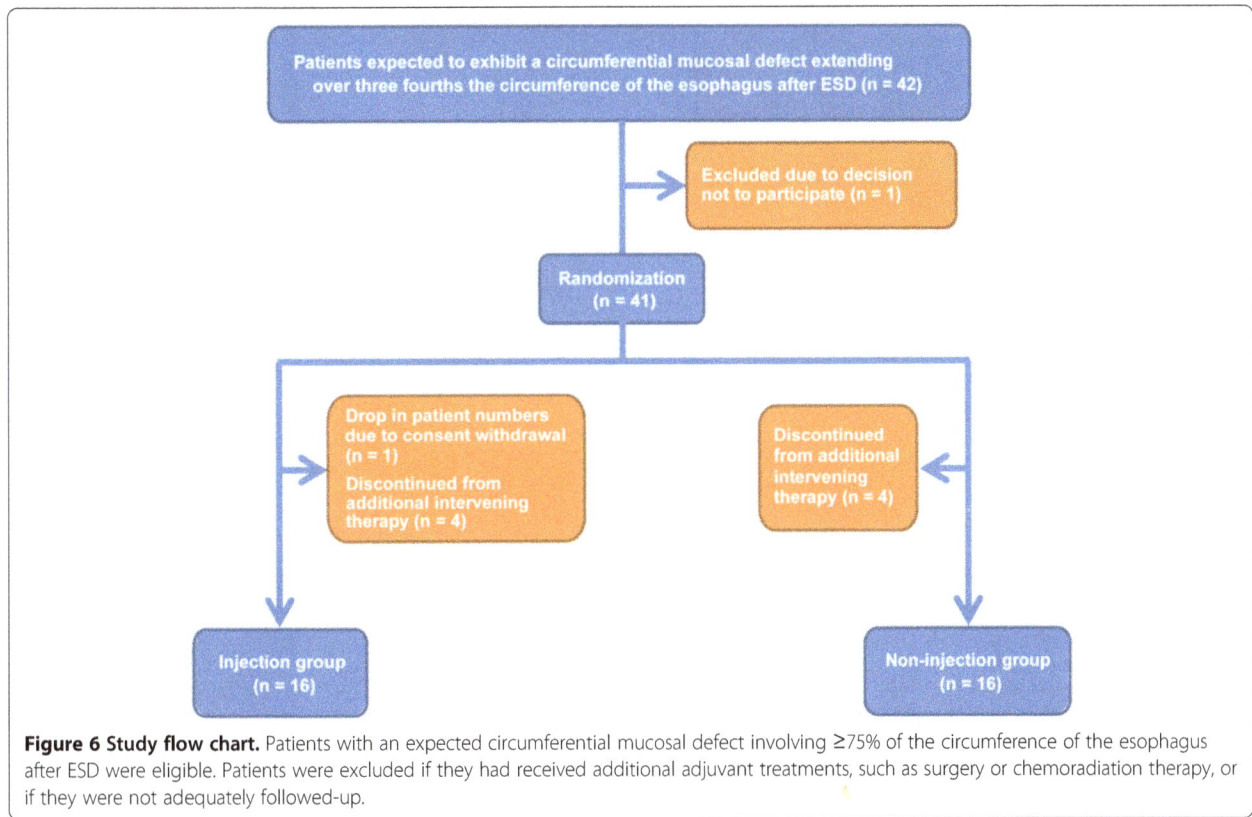

Figure 6 Study flow chart. Patients with an expected circumferential mucosal defect involving ≥75% of the circumference of the esophagus after ESD were eligible. Patients were excluded if they had received additional adjuvant treatments, such as surgery or chemoradiation therapy, or if they were not adequately followed-up.

the mean numbers of dilatation sessions required in our study were higher than in previous reports [10], again likely a consequence of the relatively high proportion of patients with circumferential lesions. The patients in our study with NWCMDs underwent a similar mean number of dilatation sessions to a broadly comparable group of patients in a previous report [9]. Our study has other limitations. First, it was an open-label design conducted by a single endoscopy specialist in a single specialist center. Second, concealment was based only on pseudo-randomization. Finally, the primary outcome measure was not significantly different between the groups, and some of our conclusions of therapeutic benefit are based on *post hoc* or subgroup analysis.

Conclusion
In summary, prophylactic endoscopic steroid injection can relieve the severity of esophageal stenoses following extensive ESD. Future studies should attempt to optimize steroid injection therapy to establish the best means of preventing stricture formation in patients at risk of developing esophageal stenosis. As it is well recognized that patients are at a lower risk of esophageal perforation if they undergo fewer dilatation treatments [3], prophylactic steroid injection might also improve patient safety, although as perforation rates are so low

a large surveillance study would be needed to detect a difference.

Competing interests
The authors declare that they have no competing interests.

Authors' contributions
HT carried out the endoscopic therapeutic maneuvers, and participated in the conception and design of the study. YA performed statistical analyses, and participated in drafting of the manuscript. SO carried out the endoscopic therapeutic maneuvers. JK participated in helping endoscopic maneuvers. KH participated in data acquisition. HT participated in the interpretation of data sequence alignment. YS participated in the conception and design of the study and performed critical revision of the manuscript. MH conceived of the study, and participated in its design and coordination and helped to draft the manuscript. All authors read and approved the final manuscript.

Acknowledgments
We thank Assistant Professor Y Hamamoto of the Division of Gastroenterology and Hepatology, Keio University School of Medicine, Japan, for providing valuable advice on the clinical trial, and Assistant Professor M Nojima of the Division of Advanced Medicine Promotion, The Advanced Clinical Research Center, The Institute of Medical Science, The University of Tokyo, for registration with the UMIN-CTR.

Author details
[1]Department of Gastroenterology, Keiyukai Daini Hospital, Hondori-13, Shiroishi-ku, Sapporo 003-0027, Japan. [2]Department of Gastroenterology, Rheumatology, and Clinical Immunology, Sapporo Medical University, S-1, W-16, Chuo-ku, Sapporo 060-8543, Japan. [3]Department of Gastroenterology, Keiyukai Sapporo Hospital, Hondori-14, Shiroishi-ku, Sapporo 003-0027, Japan. [4]Department of Surgery, Keiyukai Sapporo Hospital, Hondori-14, Shiroishi-ku, Sapporo 003-0027, Japan.

References

1. Takahashi H, Arimura Y, Masao H, Okahara S, Tanuma T, Kodaira J, et al. Endoscopic submucosal dissection is superior to conventional endoscopic resection as a curative treatment for early squamous cell carcinoma of the esophagus (with video). Gastrointest Endosc. 2010;72:255–64. 264.e1–2.

2. Katada C, Muto M, Manabe T, Boku N, Ohtsu A, Yoshida S. Esophageal stenosis after endoscopic mucosal resection of superficial esophageal lesions. Gastrointest Endosc. 2003;57:165–9.

3. Takahashi H, Arimura Y, Okahara S, Uchida S, Ishigaki S, Tsukagoshi H, et al. Risk of perforation during dilation for esophageal strictures after endoscopic resection in patients with early squamous cell carcinoma. Endoscopy. 2011;43:184–9.

4. Ohki T, Yamato M, Ota M, Takagi R, Murakami D, Kondo M, et al. Prevention of esophageal stricture after endoscopic submucosal dissection using tissue-engineered cell sheets. Gastroenterology. 2012;143:582–8. e1–2.

5. Ezoe Y, Muto M, Horimatsu T, Morita S, Miyamoto S, Mochizuki S, et al. Efficacy of preventive endoscopic balloon dilation for esophageal stricture after endoscopic resection. J Clin Gastroenterol. 2011;45:222–7.

6. Thomas T, Abrams KR, Subramanian V, Mannath J, Ragunath K. Esophageal stents for benign refractory strictures: a meta-analysis. Endoscopy. 2011;43:386–93.

7. Repici A, Vleggaar FP, Hassan C, van Boeckel PG, Romeo F, Pagano N, et al. Efficacy and safety of biodegradable stents for refractory benign esophageal strictures: the BEST (Biodegradable Esophageal Stent) study. Gastrointest Endosc. 2010;72:927–34.

8. Yamaguchi N, Isomoto H, Nakayama T, Hayashi T, Nishiyama H, Ohnita K, et al. Usefulness of oral prednisolone in the treatment of esophageal stricture after endoscopic submucosal dissection for superficial esophageal squamous cell carcinoma. Gastrointest Endosc. 2011;73:1115–21.

9. Hashimoto S, Kobayashi M, Takeuchi M, Sato Y, Narisawa R, Aoyagi Y. The efficacy of endoscopic triamcinolone injection for the prevention of esophageal stricture after endoscopic submucosal dissection. Gastrointest Endosc. 2011;74:1389–93.

10. Hanaoka N, Ishihara R, Takeuchi Y, Uedo N, Higashino K, Ohta T, et al. Intralesional steroid injection to prevent stricture after endoscopic submucosal dissection for esophageal cancer: a controlled prospective study. Endoscopy. 2012;44:1007–11.

11. Altintas E, Kacar S, Tunc B, Sezgin O, Parlak E, Altiparmak E, et al. Intralesional steroid injection in benign esophageal strictures resistant to bougie dilation. J Gastroenterol Hepatol. 2004;19:1388–91.

12. Kochhar R, Makharia GK. Usefulness of intralesional triamcinolone in treatment of benign esophageal strictures. Gastrointest Endosc. 2002;56:829–34.

13. Ramage JJI, Rumalla A, Baron TH, Pochron NL, Zinsmeister AR, Murray JA, et al. A prospective, randomized, double-blind, placebo-controlled trial of endoscopic steroid injection therapy for recalcitrant esophageal peptic strictures. Am J Gastroenterol. 2005;100:2419–25.

14. Muto M, Hironaka S, Nakane M, Boku N, Ohtsu A, Yoshida S. Association of multiple Lugol-voiding lesions with synchronous and metachronous esophageal squamous cell carcinoma in patients with head and neck cancer. Gastrointest Endosc. 2002;56:517–21.

15. Japan Esophageal Society. Japanese Classification of Esophageal Cancer, tenth edition: part I. Esophagus. 2009;6:1–25.

16. Kochman ML, McClave SA, Boyce HW. The refractory and the recurrent esophageal stricture: a definition. Gastrointest Endosc. 2005;62:474–5.

17. Hernandez LV, Jacobson JW, Harris MS, Hernandez LJ. Comparison among the perforation rates of Maloney, balloon, and savary dilation of esophageal strictures. Gastrointest Endosc. 2000;51(4 Pt 1):460–2.

18. Ihaka R, Gentleman R. R: A Language for Data Analysis and Graphics. J Comput Graph Stat. 1996;5:299–314.

19. Isomoto H, Yamaguchi N, Nakayama T, Hayashi T, Nishiyama H, Ohnita K, et al. Management of esophageal stricture after complete circular endoscopic submucosal dissection for superficial esophageal squamous cell carcinoma. BMC Gastroenterol. 2011;11:46.

4

Intra-esophageal whitish mass – a challenging diagnosis

Lidia Ciobanu[1*], Oliviu Pascu[1], Marcel Tantau[1], Oana Pinzariu[2], Bogdan Furnea[3], Emil Botan[4] and Marian Taulescu[5]

Abstract

Background: Whitish intraluminal esophageal masses might represent the endoscopic feature of a bezoar or a pedunculated tumor, most likely a fibrovascular polyp, without exclusion of other mesenchymal tumors (leiomyoma, lipoma, gastrointestinal stromal tumor, leiomyosarcoma, granular cell tumor). If a process of dystrophic calcification is also encountered the differential diagnosis can be a challenge even after histological analysis, as it is highlighted by our case.

Case presentation: A 65-year-old female whom took lactate calcium tablets for 5 years presented with progressive dysphagia. A whitish esophageal mass with an appearance of a pharmacobezoar was detected at esophagoscopy. A pedunculated tumor was considered in the differential diagnosis, but the imagistic studies ruled out a pedicle. This intraluminal esophageal mass highly suggestive for a pharmacobezoar was endoscopically removed. The challenge of correct diagnosis was raised by histological examination performed after immersion into trichloracetic acid for decalcification. The identification of hyaline fibrous tissue, with numerous crystalline basophils deposits of minerals, rare fibrocytes and very few vessels brought in discussion a mesenchymal originating mass, most likely a fibrovascular polyp, even the pedicle was not detected.

Conclusion: Based on our challenging and difficult to diagnose case we proposed an uncommon evolution: auto-amputation and calcification of an esophageal mesenchymal originating tumor (most likely a fibrovascular polyp).

Background

Esophageal intra-luminal whitish mass might represent the endoscopic appearance of a bezoar or a fibrovascular polyp, without exclusion of other mesenchymal tumors with intraluminal polypoid aspect (leiomyosarcoma, gastrointestinal stromal tumor, leiomyoma).

Bezoars, retained concretions of indigestible foreign materials that accumulate and conglomerate are rarely seen in the esophagus. Esophageal pharmaco-bezoars are associated with structural or functional abnormalities of the esophagus in addition to specific medication: antihypertensive calcium blockers [1], clomipramine [2] or glucomannan (polysaccharide) [3]. Esophageal bezoars were reported in patients with enteral feeding, most of them also receiving sucralphate or aluminum hydroxide antacids, medication known to cause bezoars [4].

The pedunculated esophageal masses are frequently represented by fibrovascular polyps, considered tumor-like lesions [5, 6]. This lesion, unique to esophagus, developed from the upper esophagus; may be due to redundant folds that get pulled down by force of swallowing [7, 8]. It is defined as a polyp composed of a core of fibrous or fibro-adipose connective tissue and blood vessels covered by thickened but otherwise normal squamous epithelium [5, 6]. It is also called fibroma, fibrolipoma, fibromyxoma and may actually be an acquired malformation or hamartoma [7, 8]; it is not included in the mesenchymal tumors of the esophagus by World Health Organisation [9]. Auto-amputation of polypoid lesions in the gastrointestinal tract is rare phenomenon, and it presumably occurs due to ischemic necrosis of the polyp by peristalsis-induced torsion or tension [10], being described for gastric polyps [11] and colonic lypoma [10, 12], not described for fibrovascular polyps of the esophagus.

The mesenchymal tumors (leiomyoma, lipoma, gastrointestinal stromal tumor, leiomiosarcoma, granular cell tumor, haemangioma) are defined as a group of

* Correspondence: ciobanulidia@yahoo.com
[1]Regional Institute of Gastroenterology and Hepatology, University of Medicine and Pharmacy, Croitorilor Street 19-21, Cluj-Napoca 400162, Romania

nonepithelial tumors with variable histogenesis, including smooth muscle, stromal (Cajal) cells, fibroblastic/myofibroblastic, endothelial origin [9]. They develop as intramural nodules, frequently detected as submucosal lesions at endoscopy. They have different patterns of growth: leiomyoma frequently develop intramurally with mediastinal extension, but leiomyosarcoma might present as polypoid intraluminal masses [9, 13].

We present a challenging diagnosis regarding an intraluminal esophageal whitish mass, initially supposed to be a bezoar based on macroscopic appearance with the lack of a pedicle, but not sustained by histological analysis. The presence of hyaline fibrous tissue, with numerous crystalline basophils deposits of minerals, rare fibrocytes and very few vessels brought in discussion a mesenchymal originating mass, most likely a fibrovascular polyp, with an uncommon evolution: autoamputation and calcification.

Case presentation

A 65-year old female was admitted with progressive dysphagia for 2 months and 5 kg weight loss. Her past medical history was significant for osteoporosis treated with calcium lactate tablets, daily, for 5 years. Upper gastrointestinal endoscopy described a 4 cm whitish firm mass in the middle esophagus (Fig. 1) and a semicircumferential deep ulcer with irregular borders on the opposite mucosa (Fig. 2). During endoscopy a pedicle was not identify by handling a polipectomy snare around the esophageal mass. Upper gastrointestinal series with gastrografin (Fig. 3) revealed an ovoid lacunar image at the distal part of the esophagus esophageal, inhomogeneous, with calcifications and smooth contours. During peristalsis the image was mobile and no pedicle was identified. The esophageal lumen was enlarged with a diverticula development at the posterior wall. Also computer tomography of

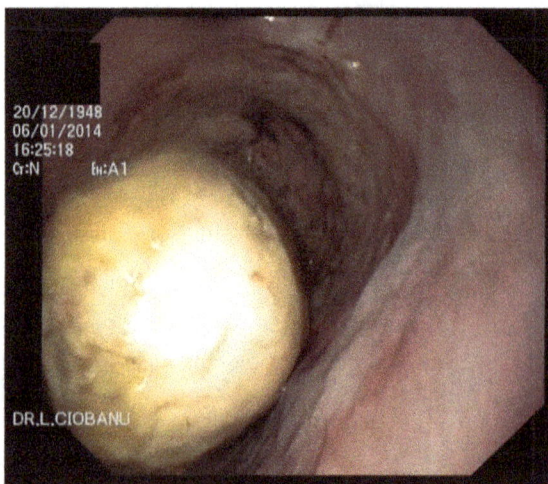

Fig. 2 Upper gastrointestinal endoscopy: a semi-circumferential deep ulcer with irregular borders on the opposite mucosa to the intraluminal mass

the thorax excluded a pedunculated tumor, describing an intra-luminal calcified esophageal mass (Fig. 4). The biopsies obtained from the esophageal ulcerated mucosa revealed inflammatory cells, without malignancy. Based on these endoscopic and imagistic results a bezoar was supposed to have been developed in an esophageal diverticula, subsequently with ulcerated mucosa.

The esophageal mass was removed with an endoscopic snare in one piece, as the fragmentation was not physically possible. The macroscopic appearance revealed a 4 cm, globular mass, heterogeneous, dense, whitish, in places with harsh yellow foci, most likely dystrophic calcification. The macroscopic examination on cross section revealed a light gray aspect (fibrous appearance) that includes multiple harsh yellow-orange structures, difficult to section (Fig. 5). This mass was immersed into trichloracetic acid for decalcification. Microscopic examination revealed hyaline fibrous tissue (Fig. 6a), stained in green in Tricrom Mason (Fig. 6b), with numerous crystalline basophils deposits of minerals, rare fibrocytes and very few vessels. The presence of capillary structures, rare fibroblasts and collagen fibers brought in discussion a mesenchymal originating mass, most likely a fibrovascular polyp. A definitive histological diagnosis was not possible, as the pedicle was not identified, but the presence of the connective tissue suggested the previous presence of a pedicle into the lesion. The long term calcium tablets intake might explain the calcification process developed into the vascular-connective tissue, revealed on histology by the numerous crystalline basophils deposits of minerals.

One month later the patient was asymptomatic. The endoscopy did not revealed an enlarged esophagus, the appearance of the esophageal mucosa was normal (without

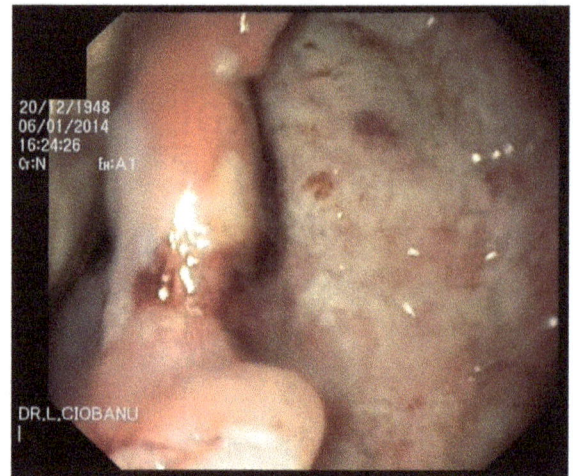

Fig. 1 Upper gastrointestinal endoscopy: a 4 cm whitish-grey firm mass present in the middle esophagus

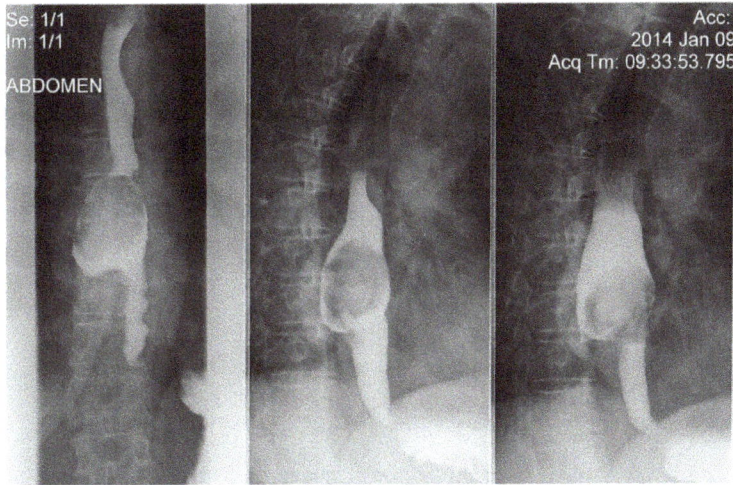

Fig. 3 Upper gastrointestinal series with gastrografin: an ovoid lacunar image at the distal part of the esophagus esophageal, inhomogeneous, with calcifications and smooth contours. The esophageal lumen was enlarge with a diverticula development at the posterior wall

ulcerations) and no diverticula was identified. No motility disturbances were found on esophageal manometry.

Based on the clinical course, the history of calcium lactate intake and histological appearance a diagnosis of an esophageal benign mesenchymal originating mass (most probably a fibrovascular polyp) auto-amputated and calcified was formulated.

Discussion

After the first endoscopy a challenging differential diagnosis process was carried out.

The intra-luminal whitish mass might have represented a bezoar developed in an esophageal diverticula with secondary ulceration of the diverticular mucosa, a fibrovascular polyp or a mesenchymal tumor (leiomyosarcoma or gastrointestinal stromal tumor) presented as a polypoid intraluminal mass with decubitus lesions on the opposite mucosa. As a pedicle was not documented on endoscopy by hadling a polypectomy snare around the mass, on X series or on computer tomography scan, a bezoar was considered. Other arguments for this initial diagnosis were the history of calcium tablets intake and the calcified mass described by imagistic studies.

The calcium lactate tablets have not been associated to a pharmacobezoar development in the literature, but calcium polystyrene sulfonate, an exchange resin used to treat hyperkalemia was reported to cause an ileum bezoar [14]. Although the paraclinical examinations did not describe a significant distal esophageal stricture, a previous diverticula could have been favored the bezoar development.

The radiological examination can frequently identify the bezoar and the associated conditions that predispose to

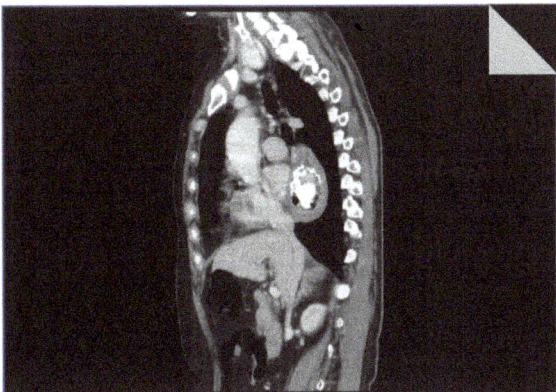

Fig. 4 CT of the thorax excluded a pedunculated tumor, describing an intra-luminal calcified esophageal mass

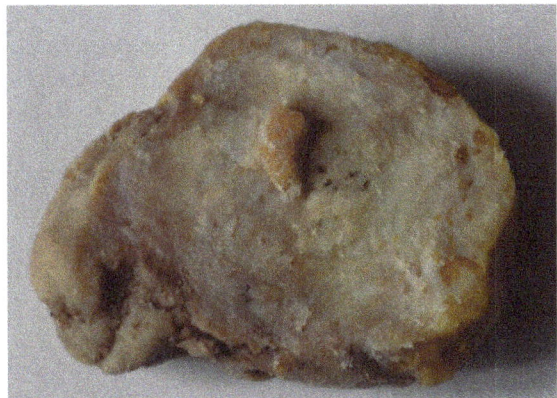

Fig. 5 The cross section macroscopic appearance: a 4 cm, globular mass, heterogeneous, whitish, in places with yellow foci, most likely dystrophic calcification

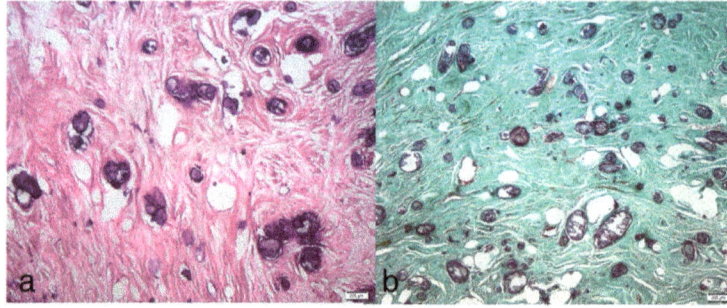

Fig. 6 Microscopic examination (200 μm) revealed an acellular hyaline fibrous tissue (**a**), stained in green in Tricrom Mason (**b**), with numerous crystalline deposits, basophiles, and very few vessels

bezoar development: epiphrenic diverticulum [15], strictures or motility disturbances like achalasia [16]. Regarding the submucosal pedunculated masses, barium studies are commonly used, but they have a low sensitivity to identify the pedicle [17–20]. The radiological correct diagnosis of fibrovascular polyp can usually be suggested by the presence of a smooth, sausage-like defect with a discrete bulbous tip [19]. The computer tomography or magnetic resonance imaging can identify in the most cases the exact site of origin of the pedicle of the fibrovascular polyps [19]. On computer tomography, the mesenchymal pedunculated tumors may appear as soft-tissue-attenuated lesions, with a paucity of fat, that expand the lumen of the esophagus [18].

The diagnostic challenge in our case continued in histological analysis. The presence of capillary structures, rare fibroblasts and collagen fibers were in favor of a connective tissue mass, most probable a fibrovascular polyp that suffered long process of calcification, argued by the numerous crystalline basophils deposits of minerals. The histological analysis excluded other mesenchymal tumors with intraluminal growth pattern (leiomyosarcoma, leiomyoma, gastrointestinal stromal tumor). The lack of adipocytes ruled out atypical lipomatous tumor that could mimick giant fibrovascular polyp of the esophagus [21].

For the differential diagnosis the most important raised question was if the vascular-connective tissue could have been found in a calcified alimentary bezoar? The connective tissue in this hypothesis must have been found at the periphery of the mass, but in our case it was homogeneous distributed into the calcified mass. For an ingested fibrous mass retained in a normal esophagus and than calcified there are no sufficient clinical and physiological arguments.

A serious contra-argument for a fibrovascular polyp is the lack of a pedicle (not identify at endoscopy, imagistic study or anatomo-pathological examination). But the presence of the vascular connective tissue described on histology is an important argument for its previous existence. In this case an auto-amputation process might be supposed.

The diverticula initially supposed to be the cause for the bezoar formation was actually secondary to mass compression. One month from the mass removal, the diverticula was not more identified at endoscopy, being another argument for an esophageal mesenchimal originating mass and a contraargument for a bezoar.

Conclusion

Based on our challenging and difficult to diagnose case we proposed a natural uncommon evolution for an esophageal mesenchymal originating mass (most likely a fibrovascular polyp): auto-amputation and calcification.

Consent

Written informed consent was obtained from the patient for publication of this Case report and any accompanying images. A copy of the written consent is available for review by the Editor of this journal.

Competing interests
The authors declare that they have no competing interests.

Authors' contributions
LC wrote the manuscript. OP1 contributed to the patient diagnosis and treatment. MT1 supervised the patient endoscopic management. OP2 and BF equally contributed to patient diagnosis and literature review. EB and MT2 made the histological analysis. All authors read and approved the final manuscript.

Acknowledgements
This paper was published under the frame of European Social Found, Human Resources Development Operational Programme 2007–2013, project number POSTDRU 159/1.5/138776: TRANSCENT.

Author details
[1]Regional Institute of Gastroenterology and Hepatology, University of Medicine and Pharmacy, Croitorilor Street 19-21, Cluj-Napoca 400162, Romania. [2]Emergency Clinic Country Hospital, Cluj-Napoca 400006, Romania. [3]Regional Institute of Gastroenterology and Hepatology, Cluj-Napoca 400162, Romania. [4]Department of Pathology, Emergency Clinic Country Hospital, Cluj-Napoca 400006, Romania. [5]Department of Pathology, Faculty of Veterinary Medicine, University of Agricultural Science and Veterinary Medicine, Cluj-Napoca 400372, Romania.

References

1. Prisant LM, Spaulding VC. Antihypertensive pharmacobezoar. J Clin Hypertens (Greenwich). 2006;8:296–8.
2. Höjer J, Personne M. Endoscopic removal of slow release clomipramine bezoars in two cases of acute poisoning. Clin Toxicol (Phila). 2008;46:317–9. doi:10.1080/15563650701378738.
3. Vanderbeek PB, Fasano C, O'Malley G, Hornstein J. Esophageal obstruction from a hygroscopic pharmacobezoar containing glucomannan. Clin Toxicol (Phila). 2007;45:80–2.
4. Marcus EL, Arnon R, Sheynkman A, Caine YG, Lysy J. Esophageal obstruction due to enteral feed bezoar: a case report and literature review. World J Gastrointest Endosc. 2010;2:352–6. doi:10.4253/wjge.v2.i10.352.
5. Stout AP, Lattes R. Tumors of the esophagus. In: Atlas of tumor pathology, section V, fascicle 20. Washington, DC: Armed Forces Institute of Pathology; 1957. p. 25–32.
6. Watanabe H, Jass JR, Sobin LH. World Health Organization: histological typing of oesophageal and gastric tumors. 2nd ed. Berlin: Springer Verlag; 1990. p. 16.
7. Choong CK, Meyers BF. Benign esophageal tumors: introduction, incidence, classification, and clinical features. Semin Thorac Cardiovasc Surg. 2003;151:3–8.
8. Lee SY, Chan WH, Sivanandan R, Lim DT, Wong WK. Recurrent giant fibrovascular polyp of the esophagus. World J Gastroenterol. 2009;15:3697–700.
9. Miettinen M, Fletcher CDM, Kingblom LG, Tsui WMS. Mesenchymal tumours of th esophagus. In: Bosman FT, Carneiro F, Hruban RH, Theise ND, editors. WHO classification of tumours of the digestive system. Lyon: IARC; 2010. p. 35–7.
10. Jeong HK, Cho SB, Seo TJ, Lee KR, Lee WS, Kim HS, et al. Autoamputation of a giant colonic lipoma. Gut Liver. 2011;5(3):380–2.
11. Nakajima T, Kamano T, Watanabe K, Meguro H, Shibasaki K. A gastric hyperplastic polyp observed endoscopically before and after autoamputation. Endoscopy. 2003;35(12):1069–71.
12. Radhi JM. Lipoma of the colon: self amputation. Am J Gastroenterol. 1993;88:1981–2.
13. Hatch 3rd GF, Wertheimer-Hatch L, Hatch KF, Davis GB, Blanchard DK, Foster Jr RS, et al. Tumors of the esophagus. World J Surg. 2000;24(4):401–11.
14. Lai TP, Yang CW, Siaop FY, Yen HH. Calcium polystyrene sulfonate bezoar in the ileum: diagnosis and treatment with double-balloon endoscopy. Endoscopy. 2013;45 Suppl 2 UCTN:E378–9. doi:10.1055/s-0033-1344835.
15. Chen YC, Tsai MC, Chen TY, Lin CC. Esophageal bezoar in a patient with esophageal epiphrenic diverticulum. Endoscopy. 2013;45 Suppl 2 UCTN:E193–4. doi:10.1055/s-0033-1344127.
16. Kim KH, Choi SC, Seo GS, Kim YS, Choi CS, Im CJ. Esophageal bezoar in a patient with achalasia: case report and literature review. Gut Liver. 2010;4:106–9. doi:10.5009/gnl.2010.4.1.106.
17. Jang KM, Lee KS, Lee SJ, Kim EA, Kim TS, Han D, et al. The spectrum of benign esophageal lesions: imaging findings. Korean J Radiol. 2002;3:199–210.
18. Chourmouzi D, Drevelegas A. Giant fibrovascular polyp of the oesophagus: a case report and review of the literature. J Med Case Rep. 2008;2:337. doi:10.1186/1752-1947-2-337.
19. Yannopoulos P, Manes K. Giant fibrovascular polyp of the esophagus - imaging techniques can localize, preoperatively, the origin of the stalk and designate the way of surgical approach: a case report. Cases J. 2009;2:6854. doi:10.4076/1757-1626-2-6854.
20. Madeira FP, Justo JW, Wietzycoski CR, Burttet LM, Kruel CD, da Rosa AP. Giant fibrovascular polyp of the esophagus: a diagnostic challenge. Arq Bras Cir Dig. 2013;26:71–3.
21. Boni A, Lisovsky M, Dal Cin P, Rosenberg AE, Srivastava A. Atypical lipomatous tumor mimicking giant fibrovascular polyp of the esophagus: report of a case and a critical review of literature. Hum Pathol. 2013;44:1165–70.

5

Successful resection of a leiomyoma causing pseudoachalasia at the esophagogastric junction by tunnel endoscopy

Bin Deng[1], Xue-Feng Gao[1], Yun-Yun Sun[1], Yuan-Zhi Wang[1], Da-Cheng Wu[1], Wei-Ming Xiao[1], Jian Wu[1] and Yan-Bing Ding[1,2*]

Abstract

Background: Pseudoachalasia is a rare disorder whose presentation strongly resembles idiopathic achalasia.

Case presentation: Here, we present a case of a 42-year-old female patient with esophageal leiomyoma who was initially diagnosed with achalasia. On endoscopical investigation, however, it became apparent that she had pseudoachalasia as consequence of a leiomyoma at the esophagogastric junction (EGJ). The condition was successfully treated through submucosal tunneling endoscopic resection.

Conclusion: This case suggests that submucosal tunneling endoscopic resection is a therapeutic u option for the treatment of pseudoachalasia caused by leiomyoma of EGJ.

Keywords: Pseudoachalasia, Esophagogastric junction, Leiomyoma

Background

Achalasia is the most common functional gastrointestinal disorder. It is characterized by aberrant upper gastrointestinal motility due to loss of peristalsis in the lower two-thirds of the esophagus and impaired relaxation of the lower esophageal sphincter [1, 2]. Achalasia can sometimes be difficult to distinguish from pseudoachalasia, a term that covers a spectrum of disorders that can mimic the clinical and investigational presentation of idiopathic achalasia [3]. In the herein presented case, general clinical assessment as well as endoscopic, manometric, and radiologic studies suggested a diagnosis of achalasia, and as a consequence the patient was scheduled to undergo peroral endoscopic myotomy (POEM). However, on performing the endoscopy for POEM, a leiomyoma originating from the muscularis propria (MP) layer and located at

the esophagogastric junction was found. A revised diagnosis of pseudoachalasia was made. As a consequence the patient was subsequently treated with submucosal tunneling endoscopic resection (STER).

Case presentation

A 42-year-old female patient was referred to the Department of Gastroenterology at the Second Clinical College of Yangzhou University, for long-standing complaints of solid and liquid dysphagia accompanied by episodes of regurgitation. She underwent two upper digestive endoscopies, on which the presence of food residues in the esophageal lumen and rebound passage through the gastroesophageal junction was observed. Gastroesophageal contrast radiography showed slight dilatation of the esophagus, an absence of primary peristalsis but presence of aperistaltic waves, and a narrow distal esophagus with a 'bird's beak' aspect (Fig. 1). A CT scan was performed, but was unremarkable and did not reveal any esophageal lesion. Esophageal manometry demonstrated a hypertensive lower esophageal sphincter pressure in conjunction with incomplete relaxation and isobaric aperistaltic pressurizations, all consistent with

* Correspondence: chinadbin@126.com
[1]Department of Gastroenterology, the Second Clinical College of Yangzhou University, Yangzhou, Jiangsu 225001, China
[2]Department of Gastroenterology, Yangzhou No. 1 People's Hospital, 368# of HanJiang middle road, Yangzhou, Jiangsu 225001, China

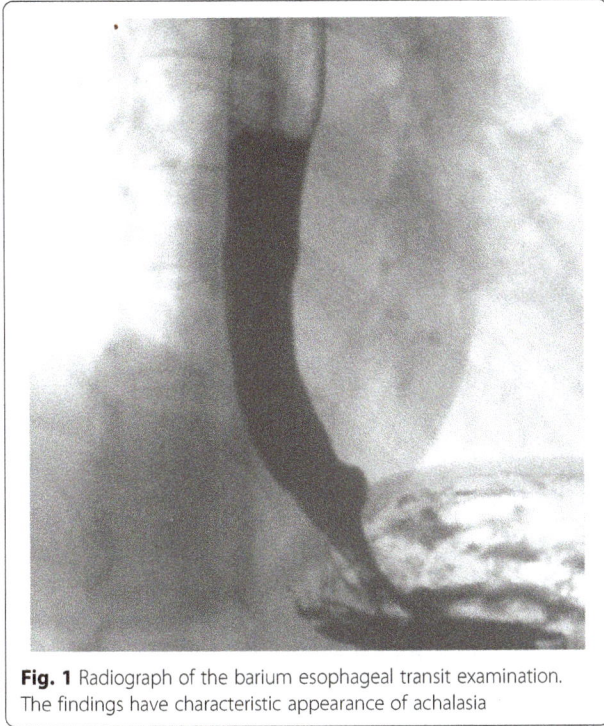

Fig. 1 Radiograph of the barium esophageal transit examination. The findings have characteristic appearance of achalasia

type II achalasia (Fig. 2). The patient was counseled regarding the diagnosis of achalasia and scheduled for POEM. Informed patient consent was obtained before the procedure. The patient was intubated and brought under general anesthesia. Subsequently, upper digestive endoscopy was performed by using a conventional endoscope. Carbon dioxide insufflation was used throughout the procedure. At the esophageal mucosa, 10 cm proximal to the gastroesophageal junction, a 2 cm longitudinal mucosal

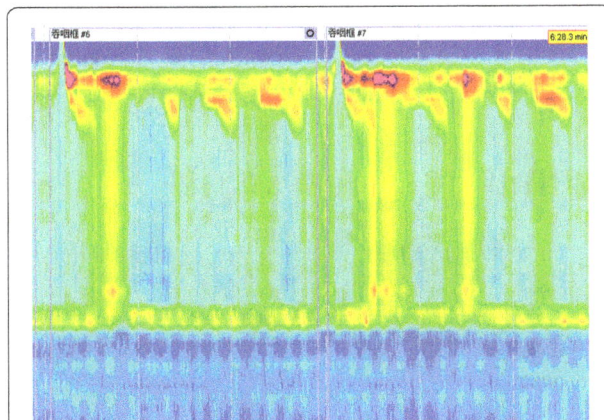

Fig. 2 Esophageal high-resolution manometry of our patient. The results show that lower esophageal sphincter pressure is reduced, with concomitant relaxation and passage of lower esophageal sphincter seen upon swallowing. The results are concordant with achalasia type II

incision was made using a Hook knife to serve as the entry point for the tunnel in the planned POEM procedure. The mucosa was then separated from muscular layer starting at beginning of the tunnel and the endoscope was then used to enlarge the submucosal tunnel by further separation of mucosa and muscularis. When the channel reached the proximity of the esophagogastric junction, however, a white band of potential tumor tissue became apparent. On encountering this structure, it was decided to resect the putative tumor by separating it from the surrounding muscular layer under direct endoscopic view using an insulated-tip knife. The then mobilized tumor was excised out of the tunnel using a snare through the mucosal entry. The endoscope was then withdrawn from the submucosal tunnel and was capable of passing the gastroesophageal junction without apparent difficulty, thus the myotomy was aborted. Several metal clips were employed to close the mucosal incision (Fig. 3). Subsequent histological evaluation combined with relevant immunohistochemistry produced a definitive diagnosis of leiomyoma (Fig. 4). Now, 10 months postoperatively the patient is largely asymptomatic.

Conclusions

Achalasia is a primary esophageal motility disorder, which manifests itself through dysphagia to liquids and solid foods. Support for a diagnosis of achalasia can be obtained by endoscopic and radiological studies, but the mainstay of the diagnostic process consists of the manometric findings. Classically, three characteristic manometric features are present in achalasia: an elevated resting lower esophageal sphincter pressure, incomplete lower esophageal sphincter relaxation, and esophageal aperistalsis [4]. Pseudoachalasia is characterized by achalasia-like symptoms caused by secondary etiologies. Clinical, radiological, and endoscopic findings closely resemble those of achalasia, but the treatment and associated prognosis are markedly different [5]. Hence, correct discrimination between achalasia and pseudoachalasia is important, but it is frequently complicated by the absence of specific pseudoachalasia-specific symptoms or findings and the relative rarity of pseudoachalasia. In our patient, the overall clinical, endoscopic, and radiographic findings clearly favored achalasia, especially in view of the concordant manometric classic type II achalasia pattern observed. Why the pseudoachalasia presented with this manometry remains unresolved and highlights the challenges that could be encountered when trying to make the correct diagnosis in this context. However, the observation of the lower esophageal leiomyoma made a differential diagnosis of pseudoachalasia more likely. Leiomyoma is the main type of submucosal tumor (SMTs) in the esophagus and its presence may manifests itself in dysphagia [6]. Interestingly, achalasia misdiagnosis in SMT-mediated dysphagia has been reported multiple times in previous studies [7, 8] and

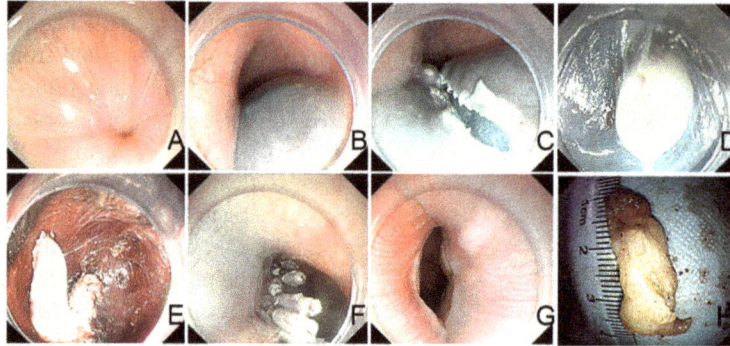

Fig. 3 Illustration of the endoscopic technique. **a** Endoscopic view of esophagogastric junction before endoscopic therapy. **b** Submucosal injection of diluted indigo carmine. **c** A 2-cm longitudinal mucosal incision was made approximately 10 cm proximal to the gastroesophageal junction. **d** Appearance of the exposed tumor in the submucosal tunnel. **e** Impression of the endoscopic view during the tumor resection. **f** Mucosal entry incision sealed with several clips. **g** Endoscopic view of the esophagogastric junction after endoscopic therapy. **h** Resected tumor specimen measuring 3.0 cm

thus this alternate diagnosis should always be in the differential diagnosis even when achalasia-concordant manometry is available. Moreover, clues to distinguish achalasia from pseudoachalasia can result from endoscopic ultrasound (EUS) [9], thus this case supports the use of EUS investigation upon this type of clinical presentation. The present case management did not involve EUS before endoscopic surgery, but in retrospect this would have been desirable.

POEM is a novel endoscopic technique for the treatment of achalasia. Since Inoue et al. [10] reported its safety and effectiveness in humans, many groups have reported similar results with minimal complications [11, 12]. Based on POEM, Xu et al. [13] developed a new endoscopic technique named STER for treating SMTS originating from the muscularis propria in the esophagus. It has already been reported that STER is also safe, effective, and feasible with respect to SMTs

at the esophagogastric junction, combining the possibility for accurate histopathologic evaluation of the lesion with its curative treatment [14]. The successful application of STER in the present study supports this notion. As both POEM and STER are in essence endoscopic tunneling techniques, they share most of technical procedures. For the present case, this was a fortunate coincidence since POEM was initiated while STER was needed to be performed, and thus secondary surgery could be avoided. It is clear, however, from this case and the body of available literature that STER might be an option for the treatment of pseudoachalasia caused by leiomyoma of EGJ.

Consent

Written informed consent was obtained from the patient for publication of this case report and any

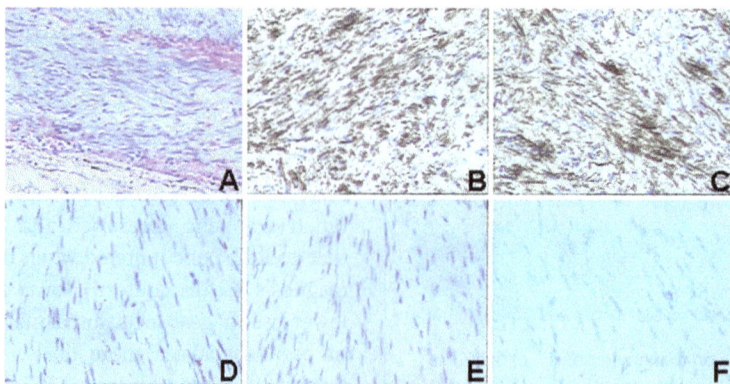

Fig. 4 Histological evaluation reveals the typical morphology of leiomyoma. Histopathological changes of the tissues determined by H&E staining (**a**), Expression of SMA (**b**), Desmin (**c**), CD34 (**d**), CD117 (**e**), and Dog-1 (**f**) as assessed by immunohistochemistry. Magnification × 200. Also note the apparently complete resection achieved

accompanying images. A copy of the written consent is available for review by the Editor in Chief of this journal. This study was reviewed and approved by the Institutional Review Board of Second Clinical College of Yangzhou University.

Abbreviations
EGJ: Esophagogastric junction; POEM: Peroral endoscopic myotomy; MP: Muscularis propria; STER: Submucosal tunneling endoscopic resection; SMT: Submucosal tumor; EUS: Endoscopic ultrasound.

Competing interests
The authors declare that they have no competing interests.

Authors' contributions
BD, XFG, YYS, YZW, DCW, WMX, and JW carried out the clinical diagnosis, provided the clinical details and participated in designing the report. BD and YBD drafted the manuscript. All authors have read and approved the final manuscript.

Authors' information
Not applicable.

Acknowledgments
This study was supported by the Yangzhou Science and Technology Commission (YZ2012125).

References
1. Sadowski DC, Ackah F, Jiang B, Svenson LW. Achalasia: incidence, prevalence and survival. A population-based study. Neurogastroenterol Motil. 2010;22:e256–61.
2. Pohl D, Tutuian R. Achalasia: an overview of diagnosis and treatment. J Gastrointestin Liver Dis. 2007;16:297–303.
3. Liu W, Fackler W, Rice TW, Richter JE, Achkar E, Goldblum JR. The pathogenesis of pseudoachalasia: a clinicopathologic study of 13 cases of a rare entity. Am J Surg Pathol. 2002;26:784–8.
4. Goldenberg SP, Burrell M, Fette GG, Vos C, Traube M. Classic and vigorous achalasia: a comparison of manometric, radiographic, and clinical findings. Gastroenterology. 1991;101:743–8.
5. Kahrilas PJ, Kishk SM, Helm JF, Dodds WJ, Harig JM, Hogan WJ. Comparison of pseudoachalasia and achalasia. Am J Med. 1987;82:439–46.
6. Nishida T, Kawai N, Yamaguchi S, Nishida Y. Submucosal tumors: comprehensive guide for the diagnosis and therapy of gastrointestinal submucosal tumors. Dig Endosc. 2013;25:479–89.
7. Mohamed A. Education and imaging. Gastrointestinal: pseudoachalasia caused by a lower esophageal stromal tumor. J Gastroenterol Hepatol. 2009;24:1152.
8. Carbonari A, Frota M, Colaiacovo R, Rossini L, Nakamura R. Esophageal duplication cyst causing megaesophagus in a young woman presenting with dysphagia. Endoscopy. 2014;46(Suppl 1 UCTN):E201–2.
9. Krishnan K, Lin CY, Keswani R, Pandolfino JE, Kahrilas PJ, Komanduri S. Endoscopic ultrasound as an adjunctive evaluation in patients with esophageal motor disorders subtyped by high-resolution manometry. Neurogastroenterol Motil. 2014;26:1172–8.
10. Inoue H, Minami H, Kobayashi Y, Sato Y, Kaga M, Suzuki M, et al. Peroral endoscopic myotomy (POEM) for esophageal achalasia. Endoscopy. 2010;42:265–71.
11. Von Renteln D, Fuchs KH, Fockens P, Bauerfeind P, Vassiliou MC, Werner YB, et al. Peroral endoscopic myotomy for the treatment of achalasia: an international prospective multicenter study. Gastroenterology. 2013;145:309–11. e1-3.
12. Ren Z, Zhong Y, Zhou P, Xu M, Cai M, Li L, et al. Perioperative management and treatment for complications during and after peroral endoscopic myotomy (POEM) for esophageal achalasia (EA) (data from 119 cases). Surg Endosc. 2012;26:3267–72.
13. Xu MD, Cai MY, Zhou PH, Qin XY, Zhong YS, Chen WF, et al. Submucosal tunneling endoscopic resection: a new technique for treating upper GI submucosal tumors originating from the muscularis propria layer (with videos). Gastrointest Endosc. 2012;75:195–9.
14. Zhou DJ, Dai ZB, Wells MM, Yu DL, Zhang J, Zhang L. Submucosal tunneling and endoscopic resection of submucosal tumors at the esophagogastric junction. World J Gastroenterol. 2015;21:578–83.

6

Physical activity is associated with reduced risk of esophageal cancer, particularly esophageal adenocarcinoma

Siddharth Singh[1], Swapna Devanna[1], Jithinraj Edakkanambeth Varayil[1], Mohammad Hassan Murad[2,3] and Prasad G Iyer[1*]

Abstract

Background: Physical activity has been inversely associated with risk of several cancers. We performed a systematic review and meta-analysis to evaluate the association between physical activity and risk of esophageal cancer (esophageal adenocarcinoma [EAC] and/or esophageal squamous cell carcinoma [ESCC]).

Methods: We conducted a comprehensive search of bibliographic databases and conference proceedings from inception through February 2013 for observational studies that examined associations between recreational and/or occupational physical activity and esophageal cancer risk. Summary adjusted odds ratio (OR) estimates with 95% confidence intervals (CI) were estimated using the random-effects model.

Results: The analysis included 9 studies (4 cohort, 5 case–control) reporting 1,871 cases of esophageal cancer among 1,381,844 patients. Meta-analysis demonstrated that the risk of esophageal cancer was 29% lower among the most physically active compared to the least physically active subjects (OR, 0.71; 95% CI, 0.57-0.89), with moderate heterogeneity ($I^2 = 47\%$). On histology-specific analysis, physical activity was associated with a 32% decreased risk of EAC (4 studies, 503 cases of EAC; OR, 0.68; 95% CI, 0.55-0.85) with minimal heterogeneity ($I^2 = 0\%$). There were only 3 studies reporting the association between physical activity and risk of ESCC with conflicting results, and the meta-analysis demonstrated a null association (OR, 1.10; 95% CI, 0.21-5.64). The results were consistent across study design, geographic location and study quality, with a non-significant trend towards a dose–response relationship.

Conclusions: Meta-analysis of published observational studies indicates that physical activity may be associated with reduced risk of esophageal adenocarcinoma. Lifestyle interventions focusing on increasing physical activity may decrease the global burden of EAC.

Keywords: Esophageal cancer, Physical activity, Exercise, Prevention, Barrett's esophagus

Background

Esophageal cancer is the 6th most common cancer worldwide, and carries a high mortality after diagnosis following the onset of symptoms [1]. While the incidence of esophageal squamous cell cancer (ESCC) is declining in the United States, the incidence of esophageal adenocarcinoma (EAC) has increased more than 6-fold in the last three decades [2]; this has been partly attributed to the obesity epidemic. Obesity, in particular central adiposity, has been implicated in a spectrum of reflux-related esophageal diseases including erosive esophagitis, Barrett's esophagus (BE) and EAC [3]. Routine endoscopic surveillance of patients with BE and endoscopic eradication therapy for a subset of patients with high-grade dysplasia are recommended [4]. However, this strategy is expensive and limited by suboptimal adherence and access.

* Correspondence: iyer.prasad@mayo.edu
[1]Division of Gastroenterology and Hepatology, Department of Internal Medicine, Mayo Clinic, 200 First Street SW, Rochester 55905MN, USA

Chemopreventive strategies using aspirin, statins or proton-pump inhibitors require a large number of patients be treated to prevent a single cancer, making it difficult to ascertain risk-benefit ratio and cost-effectiveness [3,5,6].

For non-tobacco users, diet and physical activity are the most important modifiable determinants of cancer risk [7]. Physical activity has been associated with a reduced incidence and mortality from certain cancers, including proximal and distal colorectal cancer [8], gastric cancer [9], breast and endometrial cancers [7,10]. The protective effect of physical activity against cancer is possibly mediated by counteracting the adverse carcinogenic effects of obesity, improving insulin sensitivity and decreasing systemic inflammation leading to favorable immunomodulation [11,12]. There have been several studies reporting an inverse association between physical activity and risk of esophageal cancer [13,14], but results have been inconsistent [15,16]. Several systematic reviews on physical activity and cancer prevention have not addressed esophageal cancer risk [7,17].

To better understand the relationship between physical activity and esophageal cancer risk, in particular, the risk of EAC, we performed a systematic review with meta-analysis of all studies that investigated the association between physical activity and risk of esophageal cancer in adults.

Methods

This systematic review is reported according to the Preferred Reporting Items for Systematic reviews and Meta-Analyses (PRISMA) guidelines [18]. The process followed *a priori* established protocol (available upon request).

Search strategy and selection criteria

A systematic literature search of PubMed (1966 through February 1, 2013), Embase (1988 through February 1, 2013) and Web of Science (1993 through February 1, 2013) databases was conducted to identify all relevant studies on the relationship between physical activity and risk of esophageal cancer. Studies considered in this meta-analysis were observational studies or randomized controlled trials (RCTs) that met the following inclusion criteria: (1) evaluated and clearly defined physical activity (recreational or occupational), (2) reported risk of esophageal cancer (EAC and/or ESCC) and (3) reported relative risk (RR) or odds ratio (OR) with 95% confidence intervals (CI) of the association between physical activity and esophageal cancer risk, or provided data for their calculation. A combination of key words was used in the search: (exercise OR physical activity OR walking OR motor activity) AND (esophagus) AND (cancer OR neoplasm OR carcinoma). Expansion of the search to combination of physical activity and cancer did not result in

identification of any additional articles. Then, per the protocol-defined study inclusion and exclusion criteria, two authors (S.S. and J.E.V.), independently reviewed the title and abstract of studies identified in the search to exclude studies that did not investigate the association between physical activity and the risk of esophageal cancer. The full text of the remaining articles was examined to determine whether it contained relevant information. Next, the bibliographies of the selected articles, as well as review articles on the topics were manually searched for additional articles. We also searched conference proceedings of major gastroenterology (Digestive Diseases Week, United European Gastroenterology Week, American College of Gastroenterology annual meeting) and oncology conferences (American Society of Clinical Oncology annual meeting and Gastrointestinal Research Forum; European Society of Medical Oncology annual meeting and World Congress on Gastrointestinal Cancer) from 2005–2012 for studies that had been published only in the abstract form. Inclusion was not otherwise restricted by study size, language or publication type. Studies that examined only the association between physical activity and cancer-related mortality were excluded. When there were multiple publications from the same population, only data from the most comprehensive report were included. The flow diagram summarizing study identification and selection is shown in Figure 1.

Data abstraction

After study identification, data on study and patient characteristics, exposure and outcome assessment, potential confounding variables and estimates of association were independently abstracted onto a standardized form by two authors (S.S. and S.D.). The following data were collected from each study: (a) study and patient characteristics: primary author, time period of study/year of publication, country of the population studied, age, sex, body mass index; (b) physical activity measurement: physical activity domain assessed (recreational and/or occupational) and instrument used for measurement (whether valid and reliable); (c) esophageal cancer ascertainment: histology-specific relationship (EAC and ESCC), method of outcome ascertainment (self-report, cancer registry with or without independent validation); (d) potential confounding variables accounted for: age, sex, obesity, race/ethnicity, cigarette smoking, alcohol intake, family history of esophageal cancer, other medication use (aspirin/non-steroidal anti-inflammatory drugs [NSAIDs], statins, proton-pump inhibitors) and (e) estimates of association between physical activity and esophageal cancer risk: adjusted RR or OR and 95% confidence interval (CI).

If a study combined the two physical activity domains (recreational and occupational) into a single measure, then the effect estimate for the combined measure result

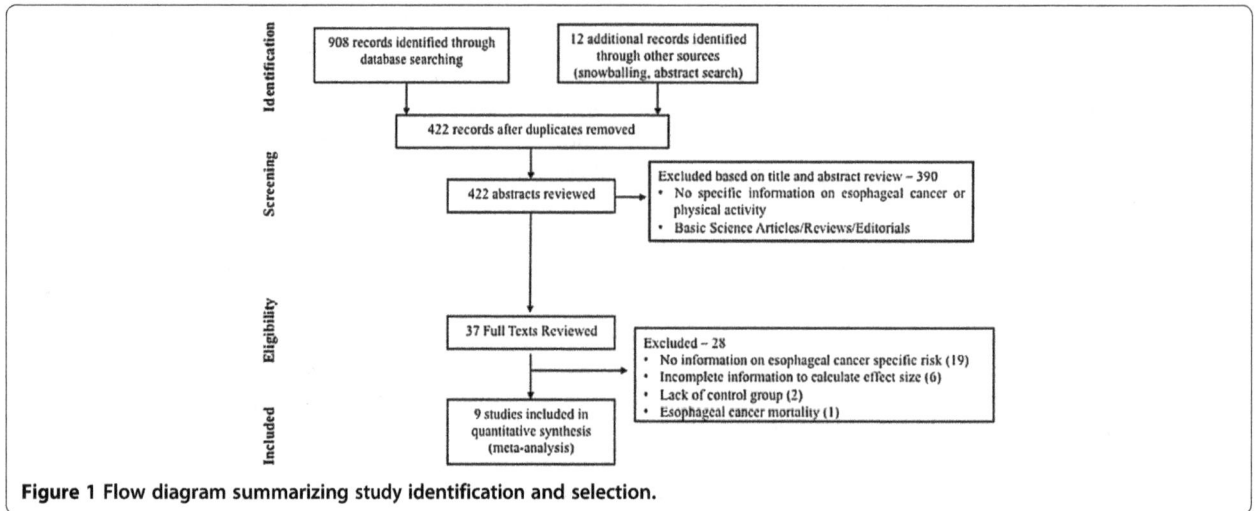

Figure 1 Flow diagram summarizing study identification and selection.

was used for the primary meta-analysis. If a study reported the effect estimates for two or more domains of physical activity separately, then we pooled the results into a single measure using fixed effects model of meta-analysis. If a study reported the effect of physical activity at multiple periods or ages and over the lifetime, we used the lifetime result. For all studies, we used the result that compared the most active group with the least active group (reference group). For studies in which the most active group was used as the reference group, we inverted the effect size and 95% CI. To estimate the dose–response relationship, using the least active group as reference, we measured the association between the middle tertile/quartile and reference as well as the association between the highest tertile/quartile and reference, and analyzed whether the difference between these estimates was significantly different. Conflicts in data abstraction were resolved by consensus, referring back to the original article.

Quality assessment

The risk of bias in included studies was assessed by two authors independently (S.S. and J.E.V.), using the methodology suggested by Boyle et al. [8]. Briefly, we used a three-item checklist to identify whether studies were at low or high risk of bias, based on: (a) study design – low risk of bias if studies were cohort or population-based case–control studies, and high risk of bias if hospital-based case–control or exclusively cancer registry-based; (b) instrument used to measure physical activity – low risk of bias if instrument was reliable as shown in index study or related study, and high risk of bias if not reported; (c) key variables adjusted or accounted for: age, sex and obesity. If a study adjusted, matched or accounted for the potential confounding effect of age, sex and obesity in their analysis, then those studies were considered to be at low risk of bias, otherwise they were considered to

be at high risk of bias. Overall, if a study was deemed to be at low-risk of bias across all these domains, then it was considered a high-quality study; if the study was at high-risk of bias across one or more of the three domains, then it was considered low-quality study [8]. The overall agreement between the two reviewers for the final determination of each study was excellent (Cohen's κ = 0.86), and disagreements were resolved by consensus.

Outcomes assessed
Primary outcome

The primary analysis focused on assessing the association between physical activity and the risk of (a) overall esophageal cancer, as well as by (b) histological subtypes – EAC and ESCC.

Subgroup analysis

A priori hypotheses to examine robustness of association and explain potential heterogeneity in the direction and magnitude of effect among different observational studies included location of study (Western population v. Asian population), study design (case–control v. cohort) and study quality (high v. low). In addition, we measured the impact of recreational and occupational activity domains separately, since the former is the modifiable aspect of energy expenditure.

Statistical analysis

We used the random-effects model described by DerSimonian and Laird to calculate pooled OR and 95% CI [19]. Since outcomes were relatively rare, OR were considered approximations of RR. Adjusted OR reported in studies was used for analysis to account for confounding variables. We assessed heterogeneity between study-specific estimates using the inconsistency index [20]. To estimate what proportion of total variation across studies was due to heterogeneity rather than chance, I^2 statistic was calculated. In this, a value of <30%, 30%-60%, 61%-75% and >75% were suggestive of low, moderate, substantial and considerable heterogeneity, respectively [21]. Once heterogeneity was noted, between-study sources of heterogeneity were investigated using subgroup analyses by stratifying original estimates according to study characteristics (as described above). In this analysis also, a p-value for differences between subgroups of <0.10 was considered statistically significant (i.e., a value of p < 0.10 suggested that stratifying based on that particular study characteristic partly explained the heterogeneity observed in the analysis). Given the small number of studies identified in our analysis, statistical tests for assessing publications bias were not performed [22]. All p-values were two tailed. For all tests (except for heterogeneity), p < 0.05 was considered statistically significant. All calculations and graphs were performed using Comprehensive Meta-Analysis (CMA) version 2 (Biostat, Englewood, NJ).

Results
Study flow
From 422 unique studies identified using the search strategy, 9 studies met the inclusion criteria [13-16,23-27]. These studies reported on the association between physical activity and 1,871 cases of esophageal cancer among 1,381,844 patients. During the peer review process, with an updated search till May 1, 2014, an additional hospital case–control study from India was identified with 704 cases of ESCC [28]. No relevant RCTs were identified. The coefficient of agreement between the two reviewers for study selection was excellent (Cohen's κ = 0.82). Six studies on dietary or socioeconomic risk factors for cancer mentioned assessing physical activity as a covariate but did not specifically measure or report association between physical activity and esophageal cancer per se [29-34]; four of these studies were published more than 15 years ago and hence, data was not accessible; additional data could not be obtained from contacting authors of two recent studies and hence, these were excluded. Two studies did not have an appropriate control group [35,36]. In a Dutch cohort, de Jonge and colleagues compared the mean physical activity levels in patients with EAC, ESCC and gastric cardia adenocarcinoma, but there was no referent population to allow calculation of a risk estimate [35]. The same group compared differences in physical activity levels in patients with BE with and without EAC and did not observe any significant differences, but an estimate of EAC risk among the most physically active to the least physically active was not possible [36]. One study reported the association between physical activity and mortality from esophageal cancer, and was excluded [37].

Characteristics and quality of included studies
Baseline characteristics
The characteristics of these studies are shown in Table 1. The earliest cohort study recruited patients starting in 1978 and latest completed recruitment in 2007, with mean reported follow-up ranging from 6 to 18.8 years. Seven studies were performed in the Western population (5 in North America, 2 in Europe) [13-16,23,25,26] and two studies were performed in Asian population [24,27]. Four studies were performed exclusively in men [13,23-25]. In three studies, recreational (with or without household) physical activity was the only measured domain [16,23,24]; in three studies, only occupational physical activity was inferred based on the job-title [14,26,27]. Physical activity was assessed using self-administered questionnaire in most of the studies, and was based on a combination of intensity, duration and frequency of recreational physical activity. Of the nine studies, three reported exclusively on risk of EAC [14,15,26], and one reported exclusively on the risk of ESCC [27]; four studies reported on risk of esophageal cancer with no separate information on risk by histological-subtype [13,23-25].

Quality assessment
Four observational studies (all cohort studies) were at low-risk of bias based on study design, exposure ascertainment and adjusting for key confounding variables, and were deemed to be of high quality (Table 2) [15,16,23,24]. The included studies variably accounted for other potential confounders: smoking (8/9), obesity (7/9), alcohol use (5/9) and family history of esophageal cancer (3/9); none of the studies adjusted for gastroesophageal reflux symptoms. Socioeconomic status, which appears to have inverse association with physical activity was accounted for in 5/9 studies. For outcome ascertainment, most studies relied on record linkage through the cancer registry (with or without review of death certificates and pathology databases), or review of medical records. In all these studies, a temporal relation between exposure and outcomes was established – physical activity preceded esophageal cancer by at least 1 year, and usually longer periods.

Physical activity and risk of esophageal cancer
Overall risk of esophageal cancer
Of the nine studies identified, four reported a statistically significant inverse association between overall physical activity and esophageal cancer risk [13,14,26,27]. On meta-analysis, risk of esophageal cancer was 29% lower among the most physically active people as compared with the least physically active people (OR, 0.71; 95% CI, 0.57-0.89) (Figure 2). There was moderate heterogeneity observed across studies ($I^2 = 47\%$).

Table 1 Baseline characteristics of the included studies

First Author, Year of Publication	Study Setting; Location	Time Period; Follow-up	Total no. of participants	No. of esophageal cancer cases (EAC/ESCC)	Physical activity domain	Physical activity measurement; valid/reliable	Outcome measurement	Variables adjusted for
Cohort Studies								
Huerta, 2010 [15]	Popula`tion-based; Europe (European Prospective Investigation into Cancer and Nutrition); 25-70y old men and women	Recruitment: 1992–2000; F/U: 8.8y	420,449	Total: 85 EAC: 85 ESCC: NA	Recreational + Occupational (separate also)	Self-administered questionnaire; Yes	Central Cancer Registries; health insurance records, cancer and pathology hospital registries, active follow-up	1,2,3,5,6,7,8
Leitzmann, 2009 [16]	Population-based; USA (NIH-AARP Diet and Health Study); 50-71y old men and women	Recruitment: 1995–1996; F/U: 8y	487,732	Total: 523 EAC: 149 ESCC: 374	Recreational	Self-administered questionnaire; Yes	Central Cancer Registry	1,2,3,4,5,6,7,8,9
Wannamethee, 2001 [23]	Population-based; England (British Regional Heart Study); 40–59 y old men	Recruitment: 1978–1980; F/U 18.8y	7,588	Total: 65 EAC: NR ESCC: NR	Recreational	Self-administered questionnaire; Yes	Central Cancer Registry, death certificates, postal follow-up	1,2,3,5,6,9
Yun, 2008 [24]	Population-based; Korea (National Health Examination Program); >40y old men	Recruitment: 1996; F/U 6y	444,963	Total: 293 EAC: NR ESCC: NR	Recreational	Self-administered questionnaire; Yes	Central Cancer registry	1,2,3,4,5,6,7,10
Case–control Studies								
Balbuena, 2008 [26]	Hospital-based; Canada	2002-2004	327	Total: 57 EAC: 57 ESCC: NA	NR	NR	NR	NR
Brownson, 1991 [25]	Cancer Registry; USA; >20y men	1984-1989	17,147 (all cancer patients)	Total: 237 EAC: NR ESCC: NR	Occupational	Job-title based; No	Central Cancer Registry	1,2,3,5
Etemadi, 2012 [27]	Hospital-based; Iran	2003-2007	871	Total: 300 EAC: NA ESCC: 300	Occupational	Self-administered questionnaire; No	Gastroenterology Clinic, based on histological validation	1,2,5,8,9
Parent, 2010 [13]	Population-based; Canada; 35-70y old men	1979-1985	784	Total: 99 EAC: NR ESCC: NR	Recreational + Occupational (separate also)	Interviewer-administered questionnaire; No	Central Cancer Registry, with independent validation	1,2,3,4,5,6,7,9
Vigen, 2006 [14]	Population-based; USA; 30-74y old men and women	1992-1997	1,983	Total: 212 EAC: 212 ESCC: NA	Occupational	Job-title based; No	Central Cancer Surveillance Program	1,2,3,4,5,9
Dar 2013* [28]	Hospital-based; India	2008-2012	2,367	Total: 703 EAC: NA ESCC: 703	Occupational	Job-title based; No	Hospital oncology clinic, based on histological validation	1,2,4,5,6,7,9

*additional study identified during the peer review process with an updated search (1-Age, 2-Sex, 3-Obesity (BMI, Weight), 4-Race/Ethnicity, 5- Smoking, 6-Alcohol, 7-Dietary factors, 8-Family history of esophageal cancer, 9-Education and Socioeconomic status, 10-Diabetes) [Abbreviations: *EAC*-Esophageal adenocarcinoma; *ESCC*-Esophageal squamous cell carcinoma; *F/U*-Follow-up; *NA*-Not applicable; *NR*-Not reported].

Table 2 Quality assessment of included studies

	Bias in study design	Bias in instrument to measure physical activity	Bias in accounting for confounding variables	Overall quality of study
Cohort studies				
Huerta [15]	Low	Low	Low	High
Leitzmann [16]	Low	Low	Low	High
Wannamethee [23]	Low	Low	Low	High
Yun [24]	Low	Low	Low	High
Case–control Studies				
Balbuena [26]	High	High	High	Low
Brownson [25]	High	High	Low	Low
Etemadi [27]	High	High	High	Low
Parent [13]	Low	High	Low	Low
Vigen [14]	Low	High	Low	Low

Briefly, we used a three-item checklist to identify whether studies were at low or high risk of bias, based on: (a) study design – low risk of bias if cohort or population-based case–control studies, and high risk of bias if hospital-based case–control or exclusively cancer registry-based; (b) instrument used to measure physical activity – low risk of bias if instrument valid and reliable as shown in index study or related study, and high risk of bias if not reported; (c) key variables adjusted or accounted for: if a study adjusted, matched or accounted for the potential confounding effect of age, sex and obesity in their analysis, then those studies were considered to be at low risk of bias, otherwise they were considered to be at high risk of bias. Overall, if a study was deemed to be at low-risk of bias across all these domains, then it was considered a high-quality study, otherwise it was considered a low-quality study.

Risk of esophageal adenocarcinoma
Of the four studies identified [14-16,26], two reported a statistically significant inverse association between physical activity and EAC risk [14,26]. On meta-analysis, risk of EAC was 32% lower among the most physically active people as compared with the least physically active people (OR, 0.68; 95% CI, 0.55-0.85) (Figure 3). There was minimal heterogeneity observed across studies ($I^2 = 0\%$).

Risk of esophageal squamous cell carcinoma
Only two studies reported the association between physical activity and risk of ESCC [16,27]. One of them, performed in Iran, observed a strong inverse association [27], whereas the other, performed in the United States, reported a null association [16]. During the peer review process, another low quality, case–control study published after data of search was identified. This study performed in India reported a 5-fold higher risk of

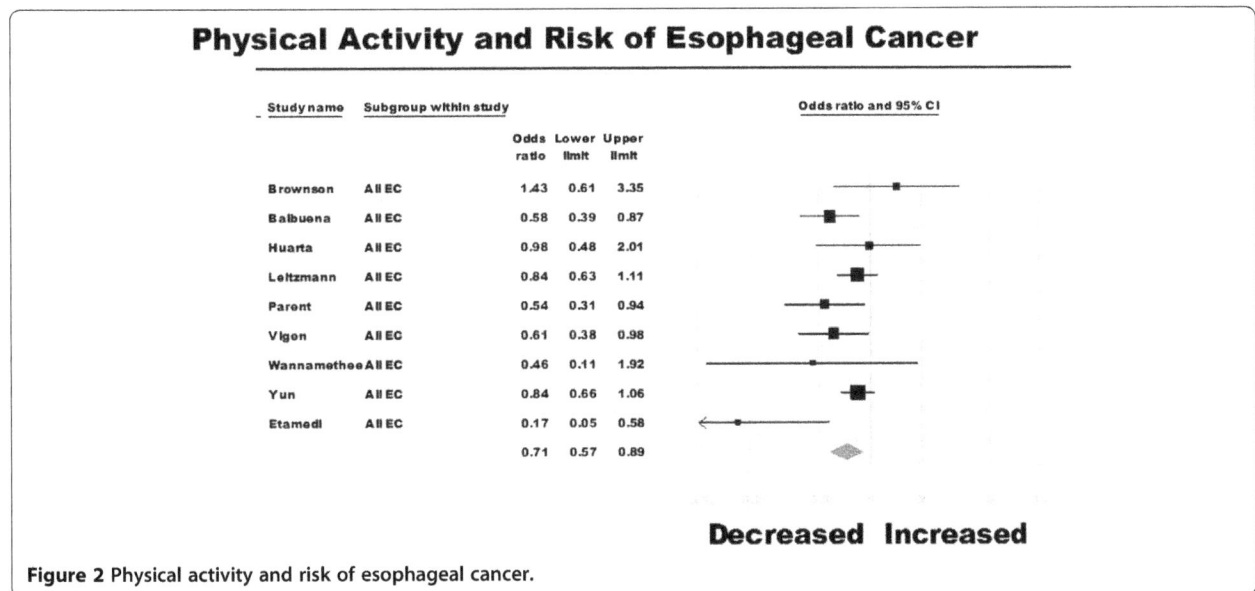
Figure 2 Physical activity and risk of esophageal cancer.

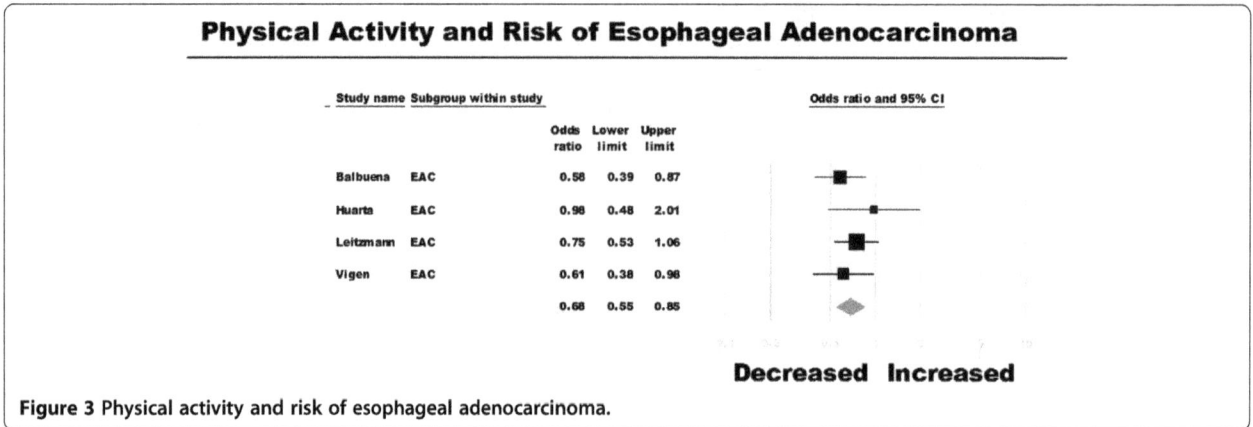

Figure 3 Physical activity and risk of esophageal adenocarcinoma.

ESCC in patients with the highest level of occupational physical activity. On meta-analysis, there was no association between physical activity and risk of ESCC (OR, 1.10; 95% CI, 0.21-5.64), albeit with considerable heterogeneity (I^2 = 95%).

Subgroup and sensitivity analyses
Subgroup analysis
On sub-group analysis, the association between physical activity and risk of esophageal cancer was stable across case–control and cohort studies, and across Western and Asian population (Table 3). On analysis by domain of physical activity, recreational physical activity, the potentially modifiable component of physical activity, was associated with a decreased risk of esophageal cancer (OR, 0.79; 95% CI, 0.67-0.93; I^2 = 0%).

Dose–response relationship
A non-significant trend towards an inverse dose response relationship between physical activity and esophageal cancer risk was observed. Using the least active group as reference, people in the middle tertile or 2nd quartile of physical activity had a non-statistically

significant 12% lower risk of esophageal cancer (5 studies; OR, 0.88; 95% CI, 0.70-1.10; I^2 = 19%) [14-16,23,25]. In comparison, the most physically active people (highest tertile of physical activity or 4th quartile) had a 24% lower risk of esophageal cancer (5 studies; OR, 0.76; 95% CI, 0.60-0.97; I^2 = 0%).

High-quality studies
On restricting analysis to the four high-quality studies [15,16,23,24], we observed that physical activity is associated with a 16% lower risk of esophageal cancer, though this association did not reach pre-specified statistical significance (OR, 0.84; 95% CI, 0.71-1.00; p = 0.05). The results were consistent across studies (I^2 = 0%).

Sensitivity analysis
To assess whether any one study had a dominant effect on the summary OR, each study was excluded and its effect on the main summary estimate was evaluated. While no study significantly affected the summary estimate, exclusion of the study by Etemadi and colleagues on the association between physical activity

Table 3 Sub-group analyses, as well as dose–response relationship, on the association of physical activity and esophageal cancer risk

Groups	Categories	No. of Studies	Adjusted OR	95% CI	Heterogeneity within groups (I^2)	P-difference between groups
Study Design	Case–control	5	0.59	0.40-0.88	51	0.11
	Cohort	4	0.84	0.71-1.00	0	
Study Location	Asian	2	0.43	0.09-2.00	84	0.51
	Western	7	0.72	0.58-0.89	18	
Study Quality	High	4	0.84	0.71-1.00	0	0.11
	Low	5	0.59	0.40-0.88	51	
Dose–response	Middle tertile[a]	5	0.88	0.70-1.10	19	0.41
	Highest tertile[a]	5	0.76	0.60-0.97	0	

[a]using least active people as reference category [Abbreviations: *EAC*-Esophageal adenocarcinoma; *ESCC*-Esophageal squamous cell carcinoma].

and risk of ESCC resulted in resolution of the previously observed marked heterogeneity in the analysis. The favorable and strong effect sizes observed in this single study were causing heterogeneity in the strength, but not the direction, of overall association. On analysis after excluding this study, the summary estimate remained significant (OR, 0.76; 95% CI, 0.64-0.89) and minimal heterogeneity was observed in the analysis (I^2 = 15%).

Given the small number of studies identified in our analysis, statistical tests for assessing publications bias were not performed.

Discussion

Based on the evidence derived from this systematic review and meta-analysis of published studies, increasing physical activity is associated with a 29% lower risk of esophageal cancer, after adjustment for important confounders including age, obesity and other risk factors for esophageal cancer. After exclusion of one study, which was responsible for heterogeneity, a 24% reduction in risk of esophageal cancer with increasing physical activity was a more conservative and consistent estimate. Specifically, the risk reduction was primarily seen in risk of EAC (32% lower risk amongst the most physically active people than the least active people), which has been strongly associated with obesity-associated chronic inflammation. We did not observe a significant association between physical activity and risk of ESCC, though the number of studies was small (3 studies). The analysis was considerably limited due to the conflicting observations from two of the included studies, with one showing a strong inverse association (OR, 0.16) and another showing a strong direct association (higher risk of ESCC with increasing occupational physical activity) (OR, 5.65). The results were stable across cohort and case–control studies in both Asian and Western population. Importantly, recreational physical activity, the potentially modifiable component of energy expenditure, was independently associated with reduced risk of esophageal cancer, with a trend towards a dose–response relationship.

With the high incidence and poor prognosis associated with esophageal cancer, cost-effective strategies aimed at preventing esophageal cancer are highly desirable. While chemopreventive strategies are attractive, currently, their cost-effectiveness and risk-benefit ratio is difficult to ascertain. This EAC risk modification observed with physical activity is comparable to the 30-40% risk reduction seen with aspirin/NSAID and statin use [3,5]. Moreover, this point estimate for EAC risk reduction with physical activity is comparable to the more established 21%, 24% and 27% reduction in risk for gastric [9], colorectal [38] and endometrial cancer [10], respectively. Previous systematic reviews have summarized evidence from

epidemiological studies on the association between physical activity and gastrointestinal cancer prevention and mortality [26,39]. However, in those reviews, only a single electronic database was searched resulting in some missed studies; there was no quality appraisal of current literature on this topic. A quantitative synthesis of the literature to calculate a summary estimate was not performed for the overall association or for sub-groups. In its 2007 report on the role of food, nutrition and physical activity, the World Cancer Research Fund and American Institute of Cancer Research did not make any statement on the role of physical activity in decreasing esophageal cancer risk [7].

Physical activity can modify the risk of cancer through several proposed mechanisms. Metabolic syndrome and insulin resistance have been associated with increased risk of cancer, particular EAC [40-43]. This is mediated by adipokines and cytokines released by metabolically active visceral fat, which result in chronic hyperinsulinemia and increase risk of insulin-like growth factor-mediated carcinogenesis [44]. Exercise decreases visceral fat, lowering the level of carcinogenic adipocytokines, improves insulin sensitivity and reduces fasting insulin and C-peptide levels, and may decrease insulin-like growth factor-1 [12]. Physical activity has been shown to decrease chronic inflammation in intervention trials decreasing interleukin-6 and tumor necrosis factor-α, independent of weight loss [12]. Additionally, exercise has been shown to have immunomodulatory effects, improving innate and acquired immune response, promoting tumor surveillance [12,45]. Studies have also shown that aerobic exercise can decrease oxidative stress and enhance DNA repair mechanisms, decreasing carcinogenesis [45]. Physically active individuals also have higher sunlight exposure and consequently, increased vitamin D levels, which may modify cell proliferation cascades [46].

Strengths and limitations

The strengths of this analysis include (a) comprehensive assessment of the association between physical activity and overall and histological-subtype specific risk of esophageal cancer; (b) analyses accounting for the effect of potential confounders particularly age, obesity and other risk factors for esophageal cancer such as smoking and alcohol use, in summarizing risk estimates by using the maximally adjusted point estimates from each study; (c) incorporating the effect of both recreational and occupational physical activity, independently on esophageal cancer risk; (d) assessment of a dose–response relationship; (e) sensitivity analyses based on study quality and (f) inclusion of all available studies and not restricting analysis based on study design, publication type or language, and hence, being at low risk for selection or publication bias.

There are several limitations in our study. First, the meta-analysis included only observational studies. No randomized controlled trials have been performed to explore this association. Despite adjusting for numerous covariates, it is not possible to eliminate the potential of residual confounding. It is possible that the observed decreased risk of esophageal cancer seen in more physically active people may relate to a 'healthy user' bias [47]. Physically active people may be more compliant with preventive health measures, as compared to patients who are not physically active. Physically inactive, and potentially poorly compliant, patients may have other unhealthy lifestyle practices predisposing them to esophageal cancer. While most of the studies accounted for some such lifestyle factors such as obesity, smoking and alcohol use, socioeconomic status was not consistently accounted for. Socioeconomic status interacts with both exposure (level of physical activity) and outcome (risk of esophageal cancer), and may have contributed to unmeasured confounding. Additionally, none of the studies adjusted for the presence of reflux symptoms or erosive esophagitis. Moderate, but not intense, physical activity has been associated with decrease in reflux symptoms in obese subjects, but not in non-obese subjects [48,49]. Hence, what is perceived as a physical activity-mediated effect may indeed represent a sum of events and interactions, which modify esophageal cancer risk in these physically active people. That said, an independent protective association was also observed on restricting analysis to high quality studies. Second, we could not assess for publication bias due to the small number of studies on this topic. Six studies on dietary or socioeconomic risk factors for cancer measured physical activity as a covariate, but did not measure the association between physical activity and esophageal cancer; one study measured the association but did not provide sufficient data on effect size, suggesting the presence of reporting and probable publication bias [31]. Third, moderate heterogeneity was observed in the overall analysis, which was primarily attributable to a single study, which showed a strong inverse association between physical activity and risk of ESCC [27]. Fourth, no credible inference can be drawn on the association between physical activity and risk of ESCC, due to the small number of low quality studies with markedly conflicting results. The timing, intensity and domain of physical activity may influence its association with health outcomes, but a detailed assessment of all these factors was not reported in individual studies. Another potential limitation that particularly applies to case–control studies evaluating cancer risk is recall bias, especially since most of these studies used a self-administered questionnaire to measure physical activity. However, on sub-group analysis, pooled analysis of prospective cohort studies reported a similar association between physical activity and esophageal cancer risk, and there was no significant difference in risk estimates between case–control and cohort studies.

Conclusions

Based on this systematic review and meta-analysis of all observational studies, we observed that the risk of esophageal cancer, in particular EAC, may be lower among the most physically active people as compared with the least physically active people. Hence, EAC risk reduction may be an additional benefit to a myriad of health benefits with being physically active, which include cardiovascular, metabolic and psychological wellbeing. Currently, it is unclear what is the ideal type, intensity, frequency and time period of physical activity that may modify cancer risk. An ongoing, 24-week randomized controlled trial of moderate-intensity aerobic and resistance training in overweight males with BE to estimate its effect on risk of progression to EAC may help shed more light on this topic [50]. For now, in the absence of interventional studies of physical activity on cancer risk, the American Cancer Society recommends "adopting a physically active lifestyle" and suggests that "adults engage in at least 150 minutes of moderate intensity or 75 minutes of vigorous intensity activity each week, or an equivalent combination, preferably spread throughout the week" [51].

Abbreviations
BE: Barrett's esophagus; CI: Confidence intervals; EAC: Esophageal adenocarcinoma; ESCC: Esophageal squamous cell cancer; OR: Odds ratio.

Competing interests
The authors declare that they have no competing interests.

Authors' contributions
SS and PGI were involved in study concept and design; SS, SD and JEV were involved in acquisition of data; SS, MHM and PGI were involved in statistical analysis and interpretation of data; SS and SD were involved in drafting of the manuscript; JEV, MHM and PGI were involved critical revision of the manuscript for important intellectual content. All authors read and approved the final manuscript.

Author details
[1]Division of Gastroenterology and Hepatology, Department of Internal Medicine, Mayo Clinic, 200 First Street SW, Rochester 55905MN, USA. [2]Department of Preventive Medicine, Mayo Clinic, Rochester, USA. [3]Knowledge and Evaluation Research Unit, Mayo Clinic, Rochester, MN, USA.

References
1.   Jemal A, Bray F, Center MM, Ferlay J, Ward E, Forman D: **Global cancer statistics.** *CA Cancer J Clin* 2011, **61**(2):69–90.
2.   Lagergren J, Lagergren P: **Recent developments in esophageal adenocarcinoma.** *CA Cancer J Clin* 2013, **63**(4):232–248.
3.   Singh S, Singh AG, Singh PP, Murad MH, Iyer PG: **Statins are associated with reduced risk of Esophageal Cancer, particularly in patients with Barrett's Esophagus: a systematic review and meta-analysis.** *Clin Gastroenterol Hepatol* 2013, **11**(6):620–629.
4.   Spechler SJ, Sharma P, Souza RF, Inadomi JM, Shaheen NJ: **American Gastroenterological Association technical review on the management of Barrett's esophagus.** *Gastroenterology* 2011, **140**(3):e18–e52. quiz e13.

5. Liao LM, Vaughan TL, Corley DA, Cook MB, Casson AG, Kamangar F, Abnet CC, Risch HA, Giffen C, Freedman ND, Chow WH, Sadeghi S, Pandeya N, Whiteman DC, Murray LJ, Bernstein L, Gammon MD, Wu AH: Nonsteroidal anti-inflammatory drug use reduces risk of adenocarcinomas of the esophagus and esophagogastric junction in a pooled analysis. Gastroenterology 2012, 142(3):442–452. e445; quiz e422-443.

6. Nguyen DM, El-Serag HB, Henderson L, Stein D, Bhattacharyya A, Sampliner RE: Medication usage and the risk of neoplasia in patients with Barrett's esophagus. Clin Gastroenterol Hepatol 2009, 7(12):1299–1304.

7. Research WCRFAIfC: Food, Nutrition, Physical Activity, and the Prevention of Cancer: A Global Perspective. Washington, DC: American Institute for Cancer Research; 2007.

8. Boyle T, Keegel T, Bull F, Heyworth J, Fritschi L: Physical activity and risks of proximal and distal colon cancers: a systematic review and meta-analysis. J Natl Cancer Inst 2012, 104(20):1548–1561.

9. Singh PP, Singh S: Statins are associated with reduced risk of gastric cancer: a systematic review and meta-analysis. Ann Oncol 2013, 24(9):1721–1730.

10. Moore SC, Gierach GL, Schatzkin A, Matthews CE: Physical activity, sedentary behaviours, and the prevention of endometrial cancer. Br J Cancer 2010, 103(7):933–938.

11. Na HK, Oliynyk S: Effects of physical activity on cancer prevention. Ann N Y Acad Sci 2011, 1229:176–183.

12. McTiernan A: Mechanisms linking physical activity with cancer. Nat Rev Cancer 2008, 8(3):205–211.

13. Parent ME, Rousseau MC, El-Zein M, Latreille B, Desy M, Siemiatycki J: Occupational and recreational physical activity during adult life and the risk of cancer among men. Cancer Epidemiol 2011, 35(2):151–159.

14. Vigen C, Bernstein L, Wu AH: Occupational physical activity and risk of adenocarcinomas of the esophagus and stomach. Int J Cancer 2006, 118(4):1004–1009.

15. Huerta JM, Navarro C, Chirlaque MD, Tormo MJ, Steindorf K, Buckland G, Carneiro F, Johnsen NF, Overvad K, Stegger J, Tjønneland A, Boutron-Ruault MC, Clavel-Chapelon F, Morois S, Boeing H, Kaaks R, Rohrmann S, Vigl M, Lagiou P, Trichopoulos D, Trichopoulou A, Bas Bueno-de-Mesquita H, Monninkhof EM, Numans ME, Peeters PH, Mattiello A, Pala V, Palli D, Tumino R, Vineis P: Prospective study of physical activity and risk of primary adenocarcinomas of the oesophagus and stomach in the EPIC (European Prospective Investigation into Cancer and nutrition) cohort. Cancer Causes Control 2010, 21(5):657–669.

16. Leitzmann MF, Koebnick C, Freedman ND, Park Y, Ballard-Barbash R, Hollenbeck A, Schatzkin A, Abnet CC: Physical activity and esophageal and gastric carcinoma in a large prospective study. Am J Prev Med 2009, 36(2):112–119.

17. Thune I, Furberg AS: Physical activity and cancer risk: dose–response and cancer, all sites and site-specific. Med Sci Sports Exerc 2001, 33(6 Suppl):S530–S550. discussion S609-510.

18. Moher D, Liberati A, Tetzlaff J, Altman DG: Preferred reporting items for systematic reviews and meta-analyses: the PRISMA statement. Ann Intern Med 2009, 151(4):264–269. W264.

19. DerSimonian R, Laird N: Meta-analysis in clinical trials. Control Clin Trials 1986, 7(3):177–188.

20. Higgins JP, Thompson SG, Deeks JJ, Altman DG: Measuring inconsistency in meta-analyses. BMJ 2003, 327(7414):557–560.

21. Guyatt GH, Oxman AD, Kunz R, Woodcock J, Brozek J, Helfand M, Alonso-Coello P, Glasziou P, Jaeschke R, Akl EA, Akl EA, Norris S, Vist G, Dahm P, Shukla VK, Higgins J, Falck-Ytter Y, Schünemann HJ, GRADE Working Group: GRADE guidelines: 7. rating the quality of evidence–inconsistency. J Clin Epidemiol 2011, 64(12):1294–1302.

22. Sterne JA, Egger M, Smith GD: Systematic reviews in health care: investigating and dealing with publication and other biases in meta-analysis. BMJ 2001, 323(7304):101–105.

23. Wannamethee SG, Shaper AG, Walker M: Physical activity and risk of cancer in middle-aged men. Br J Cancer 2001, 85(9):1311–1316.

24. Yun YH, Lim MK, Won YJ, Park SM, Chang YJ, Oh SW, Shin SA: Dietary preference, physical activity, and cancer risk in men: national health insurance corporation study. BMC Cancer 2008, 8:366.

25. Brownson RC, Chang JC, Davis JR, Smith CA: Physical activity on the job and cancer in Missouri. Am J Public Health 1991, 81(5):639–642.

26. Balbuena L, Casson AG: Physical activity, obesity and risk for esophageal adenocarcinoma. Future Oncol 2009, 5(7):1051–1063.

27. Etemadi A, Golozar A, Kamangar F, Freedman ND, Shakeri R, Matthews C, Islami F, Boffetta P, Brennan P, Abnet CC, Malekzadeh R, Dawsey SM: Large body size and sedentary lifestyle during childhood and early adulthood and esophageal squamous cell carcinoma in a high-risk population. Ann Oncol 2012, 23(6):1593–1600.

28. Dar NA, Shah IA, Bhat GA, Makhdoomi MA, Iqbal B, Rafiq R, Nisar I, Bhat AB, Nabi S, Masood A, Shah SA, Lone MM, Zargar SA, Islami F, Boffetta P: Socioeconomic status and esophageal squamous cell carcinoma risk in Kashmir India. Cancer Sci 2013, 104(9):1231–1236.

29. Gao YT, McLaughlin JK, Blot WJ, Ji BT, Dai Q, Fraumeni JF Jr: Reduced risk of esophageal cancer associated with green tea consumption. J Natl Cancer Inst 1994, 86(11):855–858.

30. Whittemore AS, Paffenbarger RS Jr, Anderson K, Lee JE: Early precursors of site-specific cancers in college men and women. J Natl Cancer Inst 1985, 74(1):43–51.

31. Lagergren J, Bergstrom R, Nyren O: Association between body mass and adenocarcinoma of the esophagus and gastric cardia. Ann Intern Med 1999, 130(11):883–890.

32. Zhang ZF, Kurtz RC, Sun M, Karpeh M Jr, Yu GP, Gargon N, Fein JS, Georgopoulos SK, Harlap S: Adenocarcinomas of the esophagus and gastric cardia: medical conditions, tobacco, alcohol, and socioeconomic factors. Cancer Epidemiol Biomarkers Prev 1996, 5(10):761–768.

33. Jessri M, Rashidkhani B, Hajizadeh B, Gotay C: Macronutrients, vitamins and minerals intake and risk of esophageal squamous cell carcinoma: a case–control study in Iran. Nutr J 2011, 10:137.

34. Hogervorst JG, Schouten LJ, Konings EJ, Goldbohm RA, van den Brandt PA: Dietary acrylamide intake is not associated with gastrointestinal cancer risk. J Nutr 2008, 138(11):2229–2236.

35. PJ DEJ, Wolters LM, Steyerberg EW, Vand H, Kusters JG, Kuipers EJ, Siersema PD: Environmental risk factors in the development of adenocarcinoma of the oesophagus or gastric cardia: a cross-sectional study in a Dutch cohort. Aliment Pharmacol Ther 2007, 26(1):31–39.

36. de Jonge PJ, Steyerberg EW, Kuipers EJ, Honkoop P, Wolters LM, Kerkhof M, van Dekken H, Siersema PD: Risk factors for the development of esophageal adenocarcinoma in Barrett's esophagus. Am J Gastroenterol 2006, 101(7):1421–1429.

37. Sundelof M, Lagergren J, Ye W: Patient demographics and lifestyle factors influencing long-term survival of oesophageal cancer and gastric cardia cancer in a nationwide study in Sweden. Eur J Cancer 2008, 44(11):1566–1571.

38. Wolin KY, Yan Y, Colditz GA, Lee IM: Physical activity and colon cancer prevention: a meta-analysis. Br J Cancer 2009, 100(4):611–616.

39. Wolin KY, Tuchman H: Physical activity and gastrointestinal cancer prevention. Recent Results Cancer Res 2011, 186:73–100.

40. Rubenstein JH, Kao JY, Madanick RD, Zhang M, Wang M, Spacek MB, Donovan JL, Bright SD, Shaheen NJ: Association of adiponectin multimers with Barrett's oesophagus. Gut 2009, 58(12):1583–1589.

41. Singh S, Sharma AN, Murad MH, Buttar NS, El-Serag HB, Katzka DA, Iyer PG: Central adiposity is associated with increased risk of esophageal inflammation, metaplasia, and adenocarcinoma: a systematic review and meta-analysis. Clin Gastroenterol Hepatol 2013, 11(11):1399–1412.

42. Duggan C, Onstad L, Hardikar S, Blount PL, Reid BJ, Vaughan TL: Association between markers of obesity and progression from Barrett's esophagus to esophageal adenocarcinoma. Clin Gastroenterol Hepatol 2013, 11(8):934–943.

43. Garcia JM, Splenser AE, Kramer J, Alsarraj A, Fitzgerald S, Ramsey D, El-Serag HB: Circulating inflammatory Cytokines and Adipokines are associated with increased risk of Barrett's Esophagus: a case–control study. Clin Gastroenterol Hepatol 2014, 12(2):229–238.

44. Inoue M, Tsugane S: Insulin resistance and cancer: epidemiological evidence. Endocr Relat Cancer 2012, 19(5):F1–F8.

45. Friedenreich CM, Neilson HK, Lynch BM: State of the epidemiological evidence on physical activity and cancer prevention. Eur J Cancer 2010, 46(14):2593–2604.

46. Deeb KK, Trump DL, Johnson CS: Vitamin D signalling pathways in cancer: potential for anticancer therapeutics. Nat Rev Cancer 2007, 7(9):684–700.

47. Shrank WH, Patrick AR, Brookhart MA: Healthy user and related biases in observational studies of preventive interventions: a primer for physicians. J Gen Intern Med 2011, 26(5):546–550.

48. Nilsson M, Johnsen R, Ye W, Hveem K, Lagergren J: Lifestyle related risk factors in the aetiology of gastro-oesophageal reflux. Gut 2004, 53(12):1730–1735.

49. Jozkow P, Wasko-Czopnik D, Medras M, Paradowski L: **Gastroesophageal reflux disease and physical activity.** *Sports Med* 2006, **36**(5):385–391.

50. Winzer BM, Paratz JD, Reeves MM, Whiteman DC: **Exercise and the Prevention of Oesophageal Cancer (EPOC) study protocol: a randomized controlled trial of exercise versus stretching in males with Barrett's oesophagus.** *BMC Cancer* 2010, **10**:292.

51. Kushi LH, Doyle C, McCullough M, Rock CL, Demark-Wahnefried W, Bandera EV, Gapstur S, Patel AV, Andrews K, Gansler T: **American cancer society guidelines on nutrition and physical activity for cancer prevention: reducing the risk of cancer with healthy food choices and physical activity.** *CA Cancer J Clin* 2012, **62**(1):30–67.

7

Endoscopic imaging modalities for diagnosing invasion depth of superficial esophageal squamous cell carcinoma

Ryu Ishihara*, Noriko Matsuura, Noboru Hanaoka, Sachiko Yamamoto, Tomofumi Akasaka, Yoji Takeuchi, Koji Higashino, Noriya Uedo and Hiroyasu Iishi

Abstract

Background: Diagnosis of cancer invasion depth is crucial for selecting the optimal treatment strategy in patients with gastrointestinal cancers. We conducted a meta-analysis to determine the utilities of different endoscopic modalities for diagnosing invasion depth of esophageal squamous cell carcinoma (SCC).

Methods: We conducted a comprehensive search of MEDLINE, Cochrane Central, and Ichushi databases to identify studies evaluating the use of endoscopic modalities for diagnosing invasion depth of superficial esophageal SCC. We excluded case reports, review articles, and studies in which the total number of patients or lesions was <10.

Results: Fourteen studies fulfilled our criteria. Summary receiver operating characteristic curves showed that magnified endoscopy (ME) and endoscopic ultrasonography (EUS) performed better than non-ME. ME was associated with high sensitivity and a very low (0.08) negative likelihood ratio (NLR), while EUS had high specificity and a very high (17.6) positive likelihood ratio (PLR) for the diagnosis of epithelial or lamina propria cancers. NLR <0.1 provided strong evidence to rule out disease, and PLR >10 provided strong evidence of a positive diagnosis.

Conclusions: EUS and ME perform better than non-ME for diagnosing invasion depth in SCC. ME has a low NLR and is a reliable modality for confirming deep invasion of cancer, while EUS has a high PLR and can reliably confirm that the cancer is limited to the surface. Effective use of these two modalities should be considered in patients with SCC.

Keywords: Esophageal cancer, Cancer invasion depth, Endoscopy, Magnified endoscopy, Endosonography, Squamous cell carcinoma

Background

Esophageal squamous cell carcinoma (SCC) is one of the common causes of cancer-related mortality worldwide [1]. Although the overall survival of patients with esophageal SCC remains poor, it can potentially be cured by esophagectomy, endoscopic resection (ER) or chemoradiotherapy if diagnosed at an early stage [2–7]. Esophagectomy has been the mainstay of treatment for superficial esophageal SCC. However, this procedure is

only possible in patients able to tolerate the procedure, and is associated with significant mortality and substantial morbidity [8, 9]. Endoscopic therapy offers an alternative, minimally invasive option for patients with superficial esophageal SCC. Although both these treatments are applicable for superficial esophageal SCC, they differ greatly in terms of their invasiveness.

Many factors, e.g. the patient's condition, metastatic status, cancer invasion depth, and size of the lesion, must be taken into account when choosing the appropriate treatment. Among these factors, cancer invasion depth correlates well with the risk of metastasis and the curability by ER [10, 11]. Diagnosis of cancer invasion

* Correspondence: isihara-ry@mc.pref.osaka.jp
Department of Gastrointestinal Oncology, Osaka Medical Center for Cancer and Cardiovascular Diseases, 1-3-3 Nakamichi Higashinari-ku, Osaka 537-8511, Japan

depth is therefore crucial for selecting the optimal treatment strategy in patients with esophageal SCC.

Many modalities, e.g. non-magnified endoscopy (non-ME), magnified endoscopy (ME), and endoscopic ultrasound (EUS) are currently used for diagnosing the invasion depth of superficial esophageal SCC. Non-ME is a conventional diagnostic modality for invasion depth, and the diagnosis is usually based on the protrusion, depression, thickness, and hardness of the esophageal wall. However, diagnosis by non-ME is subjective and may be subject to inter-observer variability. ME allows clear observation of the microvascular architecture, which is closely associated with the development of esophageal cancer. Diagnosis of esophageal cancer invasion depth using ME was introduced in the 1990s [12, 13]. This modality requires image-enhancement and magnifying functions, but can lead to a rapid and objective diagnosis. EUS is the most popular of the three modalities, but has produced conflicting results [14, 15] regarding its utility for diagnosing superficial esophageal SCC. There is thus currently no consensus on the best modality for diagnosing invasion depth in patients with superficial esophageal SCC. We therefore conducted a meta-analysis to elucidate the utilities of these modalities for the diagnosis of esophageal cancer invasion depth.

Methods
Search strategy
We searched the MEDLINE, Cochrane Central, and Ichushi databases from January 1995 to June 2015 using the following search terms: ("esophageal cancer" OR "esophageal tumor" OR "esophageal tumor" OR "esophageal neoplasia" OR "esophageal carcinoma" OR "esophageal mucosal" OR "esophageal lamina propria") AND ("diagnosis" OR "endosonography" OR "staining and labeling" OR "iodine" OR "magnifying endoscopy OR "chromoendoscopy" OR "NBI" OR "avascular area" OR "endoscopic ultrasound" OR "imaging" OR "pathology" OR "esophagoscopy") AND ("neoplasm invasiveness" OR "[T1a and EP]" OR "M1" OR "Tis" OR "[T1a and LPM]" OR "M2" OR "T1a" OR "(T1a and MM)" OR "M3" OR "T1b" OR "[pT1a and MM]" OR "T1b" OR "SM" OR "SM1" OR "SM2" OR "SM3" OR "[T1b and SM] OR "vascular involvement" OR invasion OR "infiltration" OR "depth"). Our search was restricted to English- or Japanese-language studies of human subjects. Two reviewers (R.I. and N.M.) independently screened the titles and abstracts of all the articles according to the defined inclusion and exclusion criteria. The final complete report of all selected articles was then retrieved and reviewed by the same two reviewers (R.I. and N.M.). We also manually screened the reference lists of the selected articles for any potential related articles that were not identified by the initial search (Manual searching). Discrepancies were resolved by discussions. The

protocol for this meta-analysis was registered in PROSPERO (International Prospective Register of Systematic Reviews; number 42015024462), in accordance with the most recently published guidelines [16].

Inclusion and exclusion criteria
The study population consisted of patients with esophageal SCC based on endoscopic biopsy and endoscopic examination. The intervention was endoscopic diagnosis (non-ME, ME or EUS) of cancer invasion depth for superficial SCC. The reference standard was histologic diagnosis of cancer invasion depth by ER, or from surgically resected specimens. Acceptable study designs were retrospective or prospective studies with sufficient data to allow reconstruction of a diagnostic 2×2 table (true positive, false positive, true negative, and false negative). We excluded case reports, review articles, and studies in which the total number of patients or lesions was <10. We also excluded studies that did not provide any predefined criteria to diagnose invasion depth and studies with imaging modalities that are not used in daily practice.

Cancer invasion depth
Histologic diagnosis of cancer invasion depth was divided into six categories, based on the findings: EP (cancer limited to the epithelium); LPM (cancer invading into the lamina propria); MM (cancer invading into the muscularis mucosa); SM1 (cancer invading 0.2 mm below the lower border of the muscularis mucosa in endoscopically resected specimens and cancer invading the upper third of the submucosal layer in surgically resected specimens); SM2 (cancer invading >0.2 mm into the submucosa in endoscopically resected specimens and cancer invading the middle third of the submucosal layer in surgically resected specimens); SM3 (cancer invading the lower third of the submucosal layer in surgically resected specimens) [17].

Endoscopic diagnosis of cancer invasion depth was divided into three categories: EP/LPM, MM/SM1, and ≥ SM2, because these categories correspond well with the risk of metastasis [10] and indication of ER. Moreover, most diagnostic criteria for cancer invasion depth of esophageal SCC were developed to differentiate these three categories, and there are currently no popular non-ME or ME criteria for differentiating between mucosal and submucosal cancers.

Data abstraction
Two independent reviewers (R.I. and N.M) extracted the following data from the selected studies and added them to standardized data forms: design; country; year of publication; setting; sample size; reference standard; operating frequencies of endoscope and/or probe; number of endoscopic imaging modalities used; and numbers of

true-positive, true-negative, false-positive and false-negative values.

Study quality and potential bias were assessed according to the Quality Assessment of Diagnostic Accuracy Studies-2 (QUADAS-2) tool [18], which included four key domains: patient selection, index test, reference standard, and flow timing. Each domain was assessed for risk of bias, and the first three domains were also assessed regarding applicability. Quality assessment of the studies was performed independently by R.I. and N.M, and any disagreement was resolved by discussion.

Statistical analysis
We constructed 2×2 tables for EP/LPM and $\geq$ MM, and for EP-SM1 and $\geq$ SM2 for each study, based on comparisons between the endoscopic diagnosis and final histologic diagnosis by ER or esophagectomy. The true-positive, false-positive, true-negative, and false-negative values were then calculated based on the 2×2 tables. A summary receiver operating characteristic curve (SROC) was constructed [19]. A SROC is similar to a standard ROC, except that the SROC data are obtained from the sensitivity and specificity values in the individual studies in the meta-analysis. The area under the curve (AUC) of a SROC is an indicator of the performance of a diagnostic modality [19]. A preferred test has an AUC close to 1, and a poor test has an AUC close to 0.5 [20]. The Q* index is the point where the sensitivity and specificity are equal, which is the point closest to the ideal top-left corner of the SROC space [19].

The pooled sensitivity, specificity, PLR, NLR, and diagnostic odds ratio were estimated using a fixed-effect model (Mantel–Haenszel method). Forest plots were used to show the effect size of each study. Heterogeneity was assessed using Cochran's Q test and the I^2 measure of inconsistency [21–23]. The Cochran Q test detects heterogeneity by testing the null hypothesis that all studies in a meta-analysis have the same underlying magnitude of effect. Because this test is underpowered to detect moderate degrees of heterogeneity, a P value of <0.10 was considered suggestive of significant heterogeneity [24]. The I^2 index describes the percentage of total variation among studies attributed to heterogeneity rather than chance. A value of 0% indicates no observed heterogeneity, and larger values show increasing heterogeneity. Higgins et al. [21] suggested that I^2 indexes of 25%, 50%, and 75% represented low, moderate, and high heterogeneity, respectively. For all statistical methods, except for Cochran's Q test, P <0.05 was regarded as significant. Data were analyzed using Meta-Disc (version 1.4) and Review Manager.

Results
Literature search
A total of 359 articles were initially identified using the search strategy, and 18 additional records were identified through manual searching of references (Fig. 1). Among all the studies, 300 were excluded after preliminary review of the titles and abstracts, leaving 77 articles for detailed evaluation. Of these, 63 articles failed to meet the criteria and 14 studies were finally selected for this meta-analysis [25–38]. Only two of these were prospectively designed studies [27, 36]. All of 14 were Japanese studies and 11 of them were written in Japanese. A total of 359, 1613 and 357 patients received non-ME, ME and EUS, respectively. Details of the studies are described in Table 1 [12, 13, 39].

Meta-analysis of diagnostic accuracy
Summary ROC curves showed that ME and EUS were positioned in the upper right corner of the ROC space compared with non-ME (Fig. 2a, b). The AUC was used to summarize the overall diagnostic accuracy of each modality. Non-ME, ME, and EUS had AUC values of 0.934, 0.946, and 0.975, respectively, for differentiating between EP/LPM and $\geq$ MM, while ME and EUS had AUC values of 0.999 and 0.966, respectively, for differentiating between EP-SM1 and $\geq$ SM2.

The Forest plots of sensitivity, specificity, PLR, and NLR for each modality for differentiating between EP/LPM and $\geq$ MM, and between EP-SM1 and $\geq$ SM2 are shown in Fig. 3a–d and e–h, respectively. Point estimates with 95% confidence intervals (CIs) were plotted for each group (Fig. 3 a-h). ME had significantly higher sensitivities for

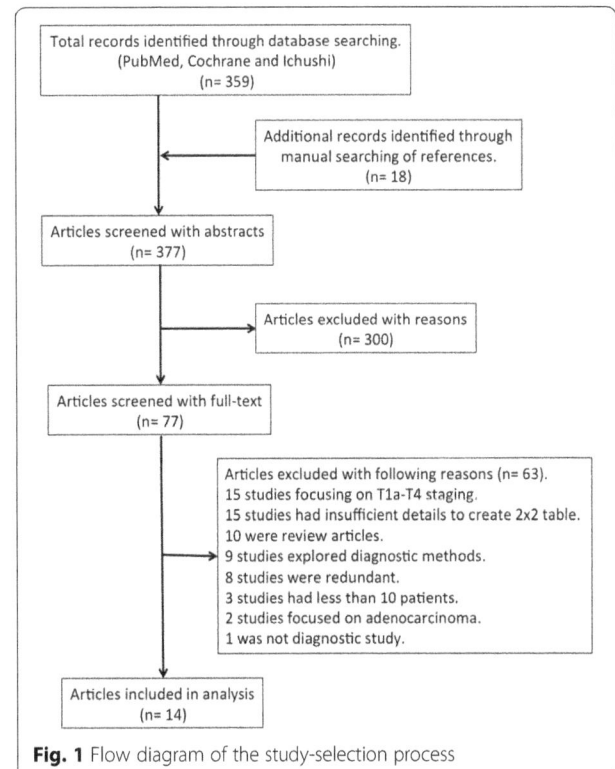

Fig. 1 Flow diagram of the study-selection process

Table 1 Characteristics of included studies

Reference number	Year	Sample size	Modality	Image enhancement	Classification	EUS method	EUS frequencies, MHz	Confirmatory study
25	1997	74	Non-ME	Non	-	-	-	Esophagectomy/ER
26	2010	236	Non-ME	Non	-	-	-	Esophagectomy/ER
27	2015	49	Non-ME/ME	NBI	Arima and Inoue	-	-	Esophagectomy/ER
28	1998	30	ME	Non	Arima	-	-	Esophagectomy/ER
29	2002	79	ME	Non	Inoue	-	-	Esophagectomy/ER
30	2006	12	ME	Non	Inoue	-	-	ER
31	2010	510	ME	FICE	Arima	-	-	Esophagectomy/ER
32	2014	220	ME	NBI	JES	-	-	ER
33	2014	249	ME	NBI	JES	-	-	ER
34	2014	464	ME	NBI	JES	-	-	Esophagectomy/ER
35	1995	40	EUS	-	-	Radial and/or mini-probe	7.5,12,20	Esophagectomy/ER
36	2006	40	EUS	-	-	Mini-probe	20	Esophagectomy/ER
37	2006	132	EUS	-	-	Radial and/or mini-probe	7.5,10,20	Esophagectomy/ER
38	2011	145	EUS	-	-	Mini-probe	20,30	Esophagectomy/ER

Non-ME non-magnified endoscopy; *ME* magnified endoscopy; *EUS* endoscopic ultrasound; *IE* Image enhancement method; *FICE* FUJI Intelligent Color Enhancement system; *NBI* Narrow band imaging system; *Arima* Arima's classification; *Inoue* Inoue's classification; *JES* Japan esophageal society classification; *ER* endoscopic resection

diagnosing EP/LPM (0.96 [95%CI: 0.91–0.96]) and EP-SM1 cancers (1.00 [95%CI: 0.99–1.00]) compared with non-ME and EUS. ME also had very low NLR for diagnosing EP/LPM (0.08 [95%CI: 0.03–0.25]) and EP-SM1 cancers (0.01 [95%CI: 0.00–0.02]). EUS showed significantly higher specificities for the diagnosis of EP/LPM (0.97 [95%CI: 0.93–0.99]) and EP-SM1 cancers (0.94 [95%CI: 0.98–0.88])

compared with non-ME and ME. EUS also had a very high PLR for diagnosing EP/LPM (17.63 [95%CI: 6.71–46.34]) and EP-SM1 cancers (11.60 [95%CI: 5.44–24.74]).

Quality and heterogeneity assessment

The qualities of the included studies evaluated according to the QUADAS-2 criteria are shown in Fig. 4. Half the

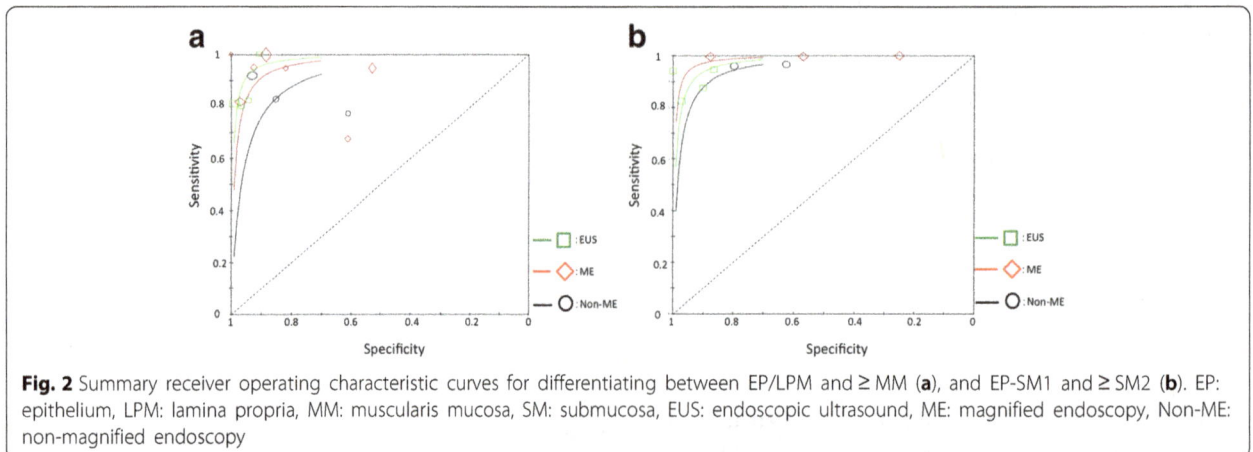

Fig. 2 Summary receiver operating characteristic curves for differentiating between EP/LPM and ≥ MM (**a**), and EP-SM1 and ≥ SM2 (**b**). EP: epithelium, LPM: lamina propria, MM: muscularis mucosa, SM: submucosa, EUS: endoscopic ultrasound, ME: magnified endoscopy, Non-ME: non-magnified endoscopy

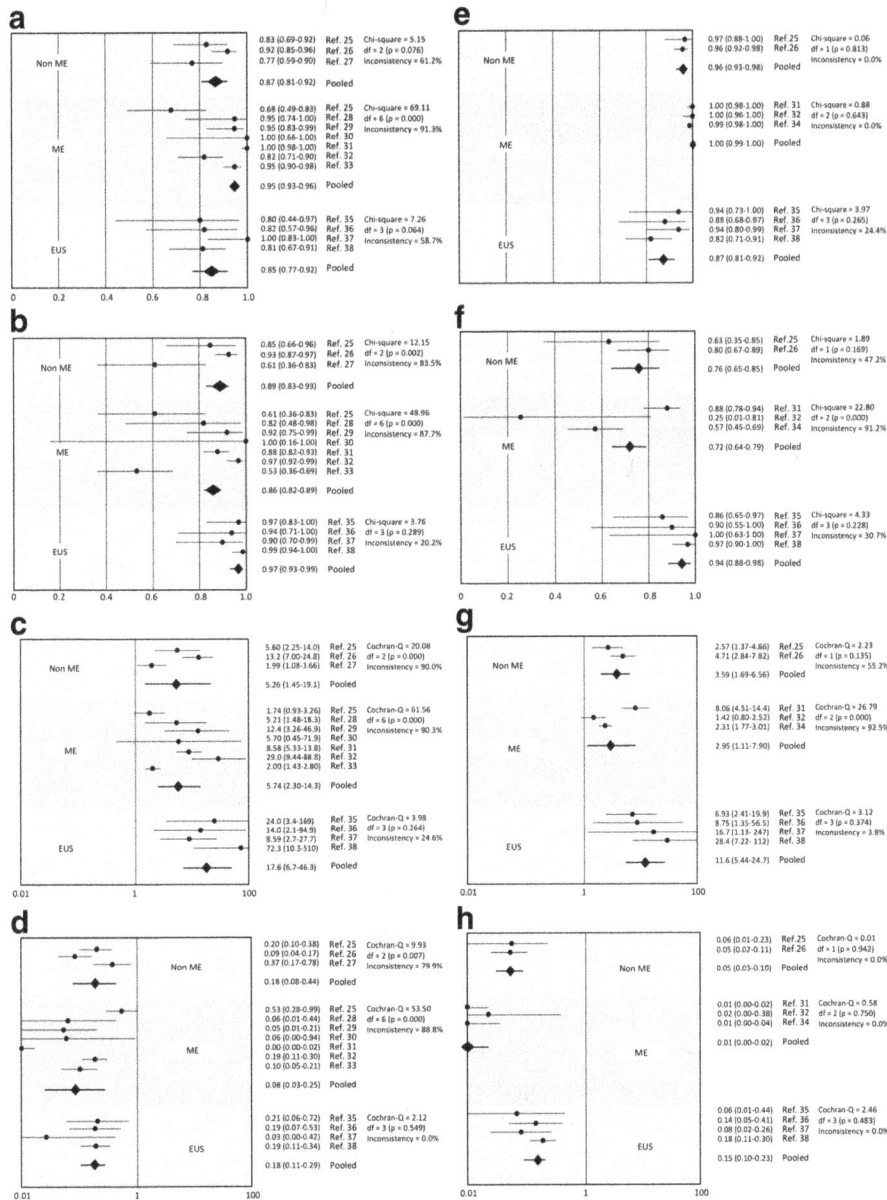

Fig. 3 a Sensitivity for differentiating between EP/LPM and ≥ MM. **b** Specificity for differentiating between EP/LPM and ≥ MM. **c** Positive likelihood ratio for differentiating between EP/LPM and ≥ MM. **d** Negative likelihood ratio for differentiating between EP/LPM and ≥ MM. **e** Sensitivity for differentiating between EP-SM1 and ≥ SM2. **f** Specificity for differentiating between EP-SM1 and ≥ SM2. **g** Positive likelihood ratio for differentiating between EP-SM1 and ≥ SM2. **h** Negative likelihood ratio for differentiating between EP-SM1 and ≥ SM2. EP: epithelium, LPM: lamina propria, MM: muscularis mucosa, SM: submucosa, EUS: endoscopic ultrasound, ME: magnified endoscopy, Non-ME: non-magnified endoscopy

studies showed risk of bias regarding "Patient selection" and "Flow and timing", mainly as a result of unclear descriptions of the patient-selection process and analysis methods. The Cochran Q test identified heterogeneities for differentiating between EP/LPM and ≥ MM by non-ME ($P = 0.076$ for sensitivity and $P = 0.002$ for specificity) and ME ($P = 0.002$ for sensitivity and $P < 0.001$ for specificity), between EP-SM1 and ≥ SM2 by ME ($P < 0.001$ for specificity). The I^2 index identified moderate to high heterogeneities for differentiating between EP/LPM and ≥ MM by non-ME (61.2% for sensitivity and 83.5% for specificity) and ME (91.3% for sensitivity and 87.7% for specificity), between EP-SM1 and ≥ SM2 by ME (91.2% for specificity). Sensitivity analysis was not performed because of the limited number of studies of each modality. However, heterogeneity for differentiating between EP/LPM and ≥ MM by non-ME was resolved by excluding one study [27], and heterogeneity for differentiating between EP-SM1 and ≥ SM2 by ME was resolved by excluding another study [31].

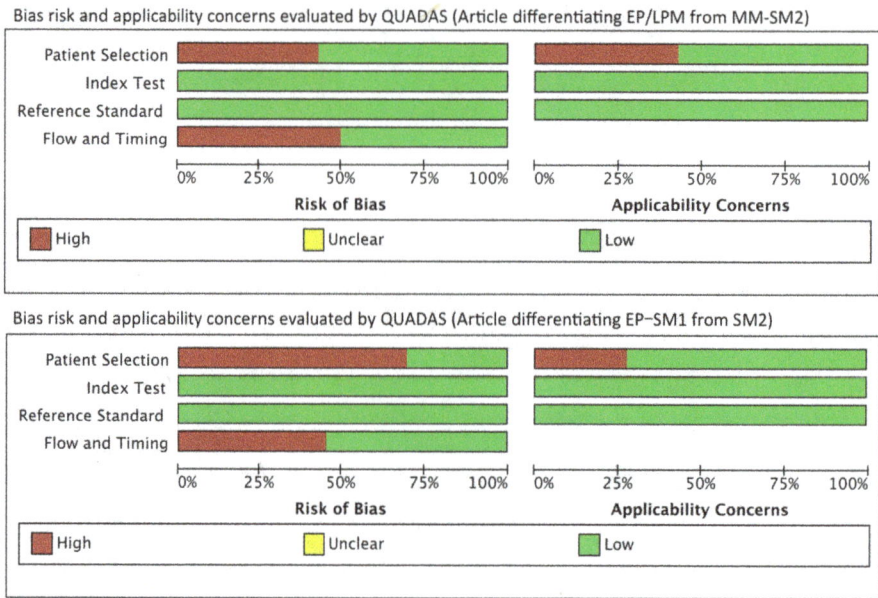

Fig. 4 Quality of the included studies evaluated according to the Quality Assessment of Diagnostic Accuracy Studies-2 (QUADAS-2) criteria. EP: epithelium, LPM: lamina propria, MM: muscularis mucosa, SM: submucosa

Discussion

The current meta-analysis analyzed the performances of non-ME, ME, and EUS for diagnosing superficial esophageal SCC. SROCs showed a trade-off between sensitivity and specificity. Given that an AUC of 1 indicated an excellent test, EUS and ME demonstrated very high diagnostic accuracies. EUS and ME had different characteristics according to our analysis. ME showed high sensitivities for the diagnosis of EP/LPM and EP-SM1 cancers and very low NLRs for the diagnosis of EP/LPM and EP-SM1 cancers. The NLR assesses the ability of the test to exclude the disease in question. An NLR <0.1 provides strong evidence to rule out the disease [40], indicating that ME is a reliable modality for confirming deep cancer invasion. EUS had high specificities and very high PLRs for the diagnosis of EP/LPM and EP-SM1 cancers. The PLR is a measure of how well the test identified the disease. A PLR >10 provides strong evidence for a positive diagnosis [40], and indicated that EUS was a reliable modality for confirming that the cancer was limited to the surface. Effective use of these two modalities to investigate these characteristics in clinical practice is important.

Although the current meta-analysis analyzed the diagnostic abilities of the individual modalities, they are usually used in combination in clinical practice. Non-ME is conducted as an initial examination in most cases, usually followed by EUS, ME, or both. However, there are currently no guidelines or consensus on how best to combine these modalities, and further studies are therefore needed to clarify the additional benefits of combinations of these modalities.

All the selected articles in the current study were reported from Japan and 11 of them were written in Japanese. This is probably because we limited the disease to SCC, and the cancer invasion depth categories to EP/LPM, MM/SM1 and ≥ SM2. This is one of the limitations of this meta-analysis and may raise some concern about generalizability of the result. This point should be confirmed by further studies outside Japan.

Classification of the invasion depth of superficial esophageal SCCs into three categories (EP/LPM, MM/SM1, and ≥ SM2) is relatively uncommon, but nevertheless practical. It can stratify the risk of metastasis [10], and is therefore closely associated with the indication for ER. According to the Japanese [41] and European [11] guidelines, ER is indicated for EP/LPM cancer, relatively indicated for MM/SM1 cancer, and not indicated for ≥ SM2 cancer. We therefore employed these categories in this meta-analysis.

There were some limitations of this meta-analysis. Non-ME and ME demonstrated heterogeneity for differentiating between EP/LPM and ≥ MM, and ME for differentiating between EP-SM1 and ≥ SM2. We were unable to perform sensitivity analyses because of the limited number of studies for each modality. However, heterogeneities for differentiating between EP/LPM and ≥ MM by non-ME [27], and between EP-SM1 and ≥ SM2 by ME were resolved by excluding one study each [31]. Most of the articles in this meta-analysis were reported from university hospitals or tertiary care hospitals, which specialize in cancer treatment. However, the two studies excluded above were unique; the former was conducted in secondary care general hospitals, and the latter was conducted by one investigator with special expertise in the diagnosis of esophageal SCC [31]. Another limitation of this meta-analysis was the low quality of the studies evaluated by QUADAS-2. Half of the studies had issues of bias regarding "Patient selection" and "Flow and timing", which may have derived from the patient-selection and analysis processes. These problems cannot be resolved by a retrospective study style, and well-designed prospective studies are required to allow a better meta-analysis to be performed to provide stronger evidence.

Conclusion

EUS and ME are preferable to non-ME for diagnosing invasion depth in esophageal SCC. ME demonstrated very low NLR, and is thus a reliable modality for confirming deep cancer invasion, while EUS showed a high PLR, and is thus a suitable modality for confirming that a cancer is limited to the surface. Combined use of these two modalities should thus be considered for determining cancer invasion depth in patients with esophageal SCC.

Abbreviations
AUC: Area under the curve; CI: Confidence interval; EUS: Endoscopic ultrasonography; ME: Magnified endoscopy; NLR: Negative likelihood ratio; PLR: Positive likelihood ratio; QUADAS-2: Quality Assessment of Diagnostic Accuracy Studies-2; SCC: Squamous cell carcinoma; SROC: Summary receiver operating characteristic curve

Acknowledgements
This meta-analysis was conducted as part of the process of creating the "Esophageal cancer diagnosis and treatment guidelines" by the Japan Esophageal Society. We greatly thank Yuko Kitagawa (Chief of the guidelines committee), Manabu Muto (member of the guidelines committee) for general advice, and Mari Sonohara for help with the literature search.

Funding
The Japan Esophageal Society supported the cost of this meta-analysis and played role in the design of the study and collection of data.

Authors' contribution
RI, NM: study design; RI, NM: data collection; RI: data analysis; RI, NH, SY, TA, YT, KH, NU, HI: interpretation of data. All authors read and approved the final manuscript.

Competing interests
The authors declare that they have no competing interests.

References
1. Parkin DM, Bray F, Ferlay J, et al. Global cancer statistics, 2002. CA Cancer J Clin. 2005;55:74–108.
2. Kodama M, Kakegawa T. Treatment of superficial cancer of the esophagus: a summary of responses to a questionnaire on superficial cancer of the esophagus in Japan. Surgery. 1998;123:432–9.
3. Ishihara R, Tanaka H, Iishi H, et al. Long-term outcome of esophageal mucosal squamous cell carcinoma without lymphovascular involvement afterendoscopic resection. Cancer. 2008;112:2166–72.
4. Katada C, Muto M, Momma K, et al. Clinical outcome after endoscopic mucosal resection for esophageal squamous cell carcinoma invading the muscularis mucosae–a multicenter retrospective cohort study. Endoscopy. 2007;39:779–83.
5. Shimizu Y, Tsukagoshi H, Fujita M, et al. Long-term outcome after endoscopic mucosal resection in patients with esophageal squamous cell carcinoma invading the muscularis mucosae or deeper. Gastrointest Endosc. 2002;56:387–90.
6. Igaki H, Kato H, Tachimori Y, et al. Clinicopathologic characteristics andsurvival of patients with clinical stage I squamous cell carcinomas of thethoracic esophagus treated with three-field lymph node dissection. Eur J Cardiothorac Surg. 2001;20:1089–94.
7. Yamamoto S, Ishihara R, Motoori M, et al. Comparison between definitive chemoradiotherapy and esophagectomy in patients with clinical stage I esophageal squamous cell carcinoma. Am J Gastroenterol. 2011;106:1048–54.
8. Birkmeyer JD, Siewers AE, Finlayson EV, et al. Hospital volume and surgical mortality in the United States. N Engl J Med. 2002;346:1128–37.
9. Chang AC, Ji H, Birkmeyer NJ, et al. Outcomes after transhiatal and transthoracic esophagectomy for cancer. Ann Thorac Surg. 2008;85:424–9.
10. Yamashina T, Ishihara R, Nagai K, et al. Long-term outcome and metastatic risk after endoscopic resection of superficial esophageal squamous cell carcinoma. Am J Gastroenterol. 2013;108:544–51.
11. Pimentel-Nunes P, Dinis-Ribeiro M, Ponchon T, et al. Endoscopic submucosal dissection: European Society of Gastrointestinal Endoscopy (ESGE) Guideline. Endoscopy. 2015;47:829–54.
12. Yoshida T, Inoue H, Usui S, et al. Narrow-band imaging system with magnifying endoscopy for superficial esophageal lesions. Gastrointest Endosc. 2004;59:288–95.
13. Arima M, Arima H, Tada M. Evaluation of microvascular pattern classification of superficial esophageal lesions by magnifying endoscopy [In Japanese]. Stomach Intest. 2007;42:589–95.
14. Pouw RE, Heldoorn N, Herrero LA, et al. Do we still need EUS in the workup of patients with early esophageal neoplasia? A retrospective analysis of 131 cases. Gastrointest Endosc. 2011;73:662–8.
15. Thosani N, Singh H, Kapadia A, et al. Diagnostic accuracy of EUS in differentiating mucosal versus submucosal invasion of superficial esophageal cancers: a systematic review and meta-analysis. Gastrointest Endosc. 2012;75:242–53.
16. Shamseer L, Moher D, Clarke M, the PRISMA-P Group. Preferred reporting items for systematic review and meta-analysis protocols (PRISMA- P) 2015: elaboration and explanation. BMJ. 2015;349:g76471.
17. Japan Esophageal Society. Japanese classification of esophageal cancer. Esophagus. 2009;7:7–22.
18. Whiting PF, Rutjes AW, Westwood ME, et al. QUADAS-2: a revised tool for the quality assessment of diagnostic accuracy studies. Ann Intern Med. 2011;155:529–36.
19. Moses LE,Shapiro D,Littenberg B. Combining independent studies of a diagnostic test into a summary ROC curve: data-analytic approaches and some additional considerations. Stat Med 1993;12:1293–316.
20. Hanley JA, Mc Neil BJ. The meaning and use of the area under a receiver operating characteristic (ROC) curve. Radiology. 1982;143:29–36.
21. Higgins JP, Thompson SG, Deeks JJ, et al. Measuring inconsistency in meta-analyses. BMJ. 2003;327:557–60.
22. Deeks JJ. Systematic reviews in health care: Systematic reviews of evaluations of diagnostic and screening tests. BMJ. 2001;323:157–62.
23. Higgins JP, Thompson SG. Quantifying heterogeneity in a meta- analysis. Stat Med. 2002;21:1539–58.
24. Thompson SG, Pocock SJ. Can meta-analyses be trusted? Lancet. 1991;338: 1127–30.
25. Chonan A, Mochizuki F, Ando M, et al. Endoscopic diagnosis of depth of invasion and classification of early esophageal cancer [In Japanese]. Rinsyo Syokakinaishikyo. 1997;12:1705–12.
26. Shimada H, Makuuchi H, Ozawa S, et al. Endoscopic estimation of tumor depth of invasion of superficial esophageal carcinoma [in Japanese]. Stomach Intest. 2010;45:1467–81.

27. Ebi M, Shimura T, Yamada T, et al. Multicenter, prospective trial of white-light imaging alone versus white-light imaging followed by magnifying endoscopy with narrow-band imaging for the real-time imaging and diagnosis of invasion depth in superficial esophageal squamous cell carcinoma. Gastrointest Endosc. 2015;81:1355–61.

28. Arima M, Arima H, Kouzu T, et al. Magnifying endoscopy for screening and diagnosing the depth of invasion of esophageal carcinoma [In Japanese]. Syokakinaishikyo. 1998;10:491–7.

29. Kumagai Y, Inoue H, Nagai K, et al. Magnifying endoscopy, stereoscopic microscopy, and the microvascular architecture of superficial esophageal carcinoma. Endoscopy. 2002;34:369–75.

30. Oshima T, Tamegai Y, Nagata N, et al. Usefulness of magnifying endoscopy determing character and invasiveness of superficial esophageal cancer [In Japanese]. Prog Dig Endosc. 2006;68:27–30.

31. Arima M, Arima H, Tada M. Diagnosis of the invasion depth of early esophageal carcinoma using magnifying endoscopy with FICE [in Japanese]. Stomach Intest. 2010;45:1515–25.

32. Fujiwara J, Momma K, Tateishi Y, et al. Endoscopic and pathological studies on type B2 blood vessels in estimation of invasion depth of superficial esophageal cancer [in Japanese]. Stomach Intest. 2014;49:174–85.

33. Dobashi A, Goda K, Kobayashi H, et al. Clinical Significance of Type B1 Vessels in the Japan Esophageal Society Classification [In Japanese]. Stomach Intest. 2014;49:153–63.

34. Ikeda H, Inoue H, Sato H, et al. Usefulness of a New classification by the Japan esophageal society to predict the depth of invasion of esophageal cancer - type B3 vessels [in Japanese]. Stomach Intest. 2014;49:186–95.

35. Simizu Y, Tsukagoshi H, Nakazato T, et al. Clinical evaluation of endoscopic ultrasonography (EUS) in the diagnosis of superficial esophageal carcinoma [In Japanese]. Rinsho Byori. 1995;43:221–6.

36. Esaki M, Matsumoto T, Moriyama T, et al. Probe EUS for the diagnosis of invasion depth in superficial esophageal cancer: a comparison between a jelly-filled method and a water-filled balloon method. Gastrointest Endosc. 2006;63:389–95.

37. Arima M, Arima H, Tada M. Clinical significance of endoscopic ultrasonogra phy versus magnifying endoscopy for estimating the depth of tumor invasion in superficial esophageal cancer [in Japanese]. Stomach Intest. 2006;41:183–96.

38. Murata Y. EUS diagnosis of the depth of superficial esophageal cancer invasion [in Japanese]. Stomach Intest. 2011;46:687–93.

39. Oyama T, Inoue H, Arima M, et al. Prediction of the invasion depth of superficial squamous cell carcinoma based on microvessel morphology: magnifying endoscopic classification of the Japan Esophageal Society. Esophagus. 2016;13:1–8.

40. Gilbert R, Logan S, Moyer VA, et al. Assessing diagnostic and screening tests: Part 1 Concepts. West J Med. 2001;174:405–9.

41. The Japan Esophageal Society. Esophageal cancer diagnosis and treatment guideline [in Japanese]. Third. ed. Tokyo: Kanehara-Shuppan; 2012

8

Esophagogastroduodenal pneumatosis with subsequent pneumoporta and intramural duodenal hematoma after endoscopic hemostas

Wei-Cheng Huang[1], Chih-Hsin Lee[2,3] and Fat-Moon Suk[1,3]*

Abstract

Background: Esophagogastroduodenal pneumatosis is the presence of air in esophagus, stomach, and duodenum simultaneously, which have never been described in the literature. Intramural duodenal hematoma (IDH) rarely occurs after endoscopic intervention. The diagnosis and treatment in both conditions are great challenge in daily practice.

Case presentation: A 70-year-old male patient, who had been taking warfarin for artificial valve replacement, developed IDH and esophagogastroduodenal pneumatosis after endoscopic hemostasis for duodenal ulcer bleeding. Initially, he had abdominal pain, gastrointestinal bleeding and hypotension. Later, he was found to have acute pancreatitis, biliary obstruction, gastric outlet obstruction and rapid decline of hemoglobin also ensued. The intramural duodenal hematoma and critical condition resolved spontaneously after conservative medical treatment.

Conclusion: Based on this case report, we suggest that intramural duodenal hematoma should be considered if a patient has the tetrad of pancreatitis, biliary obstruction, gastric outlet obstruction and rapid decline of hemoglobin after an endoscopic intervention. Those patients could be treated conservatively. But, surgery should be considered if the diseases progress or complications persist.

Keywords: Pneumatosis intestinalis, Intramural hematoma, Hemostasis, Duodenum, Endoscopy

Background

Pneumatosis intestinalis (PI), the presence of gas in the wall of the gastrointestinal tract, has been observed from esophagus to rectum. Some patients with PI carry a benign clinical course, and the gas can be absorbed spontaneously in most instances. But, PI can also lead to a fetal outcome in some patients [1]. To our knowledge, simultaneous pneumatosis of the esophagus, stomach and duodenum has never been reported.

Intramural duodenal hematoma (IDH) is a rare condition, and it occurs mostly after a blunt abdominal trauma [2]. The IDH after endoscopic intervention is even rare. Herein, we report a case of a patient who developed both esophagogastroduodenal pneumatosis and IDH after an endoscopic hemostasis for treating duodenal ulcer bleeding.

Case presentation

A 70-year-old male patient presented himself to the emergency department due to having had productive cough for one week. He has a past history of type 2 diabetes mellitus, stage III chronic kidney disease, hypertension, old pulmonary tuberculosis, and poliomyelitis. He also received a mechanical valve replacement for severe tricuspid regurgitation and has been taking warfarin for 10 years. He was admitted with the diagnosis of community-acquired pneumonia, and received amoxicillin/clavulanic acid.

On the second day after admission, the patient developed massive upper gastrointestinal bleeding with a remarkable decrease of hemoglobin from 11.1 g/dL to 7.6 g/dL. He had a profound coagulopathy with prothrombin time (PT)

* Correspondence: fmsuk@tmu.edu.tw
[1]Divisions of Gastroenterology, Wan Fang Hospital, Taipei Medical University, No. 111, Section 3, Hsing Long Road, Taipei 116, Taiwan
[3]Department of Internal Medicine, School of Medicine, College of Medicine, Taipei Medical University, Taipei, Taiwan
Full list of author information is available at the end of the article

of 43.4 s, international normalized ratio (INR) of 4.07, and activated partial thromboplastin time (aPTT) of 63.2 s. The platelet count was 252,000/µL. Warfarin was discontinued. He received blood component therapy and Vitamin K1 to correct anemia and coagulopathy. He also received intravenous esomeprazole. The panendoscopic examination showed an ulcer on the duodenal bulb with an active oozing vessel on the ulcer crater (Fig. 1-a). Hemostasis was performed with epinephrine injection and hemoclipping (Fig. 1-b).

The patient had abdominal pain, gastrointestinal bleeding and hypotension one day after the endoscopic procedure. Hemoglobin was further dropped to 5.8 g/dL, and coagulopathy was worsened with PT of 60.4 s, INR of 5.69, and aPTT of 60.1 s despite of aggressive component therapy. Total serum bilirubin level was rapidly elevated from 1.68 mg/dL to 6.00 mg/dL. Acute pancreatitis was also suspected with a lipase level of 3743 IU/L. Computed tomography of the abdomen showed a 14.4 cm × 7 cm intramural hematoma at the second portion of duodenum (Fig. 2-a). The stomach was distended which indicated gastric outlet obstruction. He also had air retention in the portal vein and wall of esophagus, stomach and bulb (Fig. 2- b to d).

The patient developed respiratory failure and shock, and he received support with mechanical ventilation. His bleeding tendency was corrected by vitamin K1 and blood component therapy. Hemodynamic instability was promptly resolved within two days. Abdominal ultrasonography taken six days later showed the finding of complete resolution of the duodenal hematoma, and was confirmed with endoscopy two weeks later (Fig. 3). But, his renal function was progressively worsened, and the patient and his family declined hemodialysis therapy. The patient died of renal failure on the 40th day after admission.

Depending on the involved site of gastrointestinal tract, clinical presentation of PI is usually nonspecific, varying from chest pain, diarrhea, constipation, abdominal pain, abdominal distension, nausea, vomiting, to gastrointestinal bleeding, or even no symptom [1, 3, 4].

Gastric pneumatosis has been described in various circumstances, including patients who have hemorrhagic radiation gastritis after Argon plasma coagulation [5], gastric ulcer [6], corrosive injury of stomach, status post endoscopy, gastric outlet obstruction, duodenal obstruction, nasogastric tube placement [3], hepatectomy with vascular reconstruction, obstructive pulmonary disease with bleb rupture [7], and high-dose dexamethasone therapy [8]. It can be divided into two categories: first, gastric emphysema, implying benign condition and usually being managed by conservative treatment; and second, emphysematous gastritis, suggesting emergent condition, and surgical intervention being critical for life-saving. Mclaughlin *et al.* have proposed to use the term gangrenous PI/nongangrenous PI instead of emphysematous gastritis/gastric emphysema, to avoid misleading [7].

IDH is also a rare condition that mostly occurs after a blunt abdominal trauma because that the duodenum has rich submucosal vascular supply and is fixed in retroperitoneum [9]. IDH has also been reported as clinical finding associated with anticoagulant therapy, blood dyscrasia, pancreatic disease, collagen vascular disease [10], and diagnostic/therapeutic endoscopy [11] such as endoscopic retrograde cholangiopancreatography with sphincterotomy and biliary stone retrieval [12]. It tends to occur in patients with liver cirrhosis, coagulopathy and hemodialysis especially [11]. IDH is usually confined from the first portion to the second portion of the duodenum due to the barrier of pylorus and ligament of Treitz. Typical symptoms of IDH include epigastric pain, vomiting, and hematochezia. Acute pancreatitis is the most frequent comorbidity in those patients [13]. Thandassery *et al.* reported a rare case in a patient who developed intramural duodenal hematoma after endoscopic retrograde cholangiopancreatogram (ERCP) with sphincterotomy and biliary stone extraction with subsequent of acute pancreatitis, biliary and gastric outlet obstruction after ERCP [12]. Our patient also had the triad of above symptoms. We

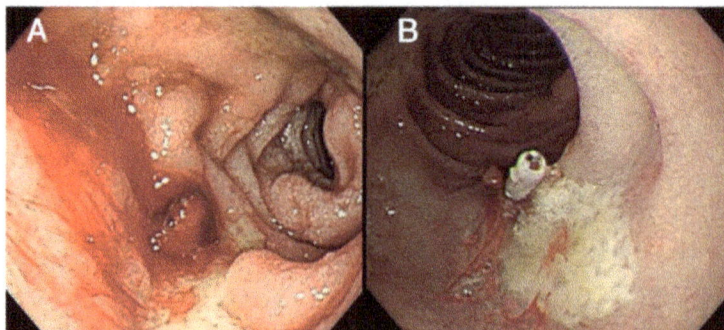

Fig. 1 a Upper gastrointestinal panendoscopy showed an exposed vessel with active oozing on the ulcer at the inferior wall of the duodenum. **b** The bleeding was stopped after hemoclipping and epinephrine injection. No immediately intramural lesion was found after the procedure

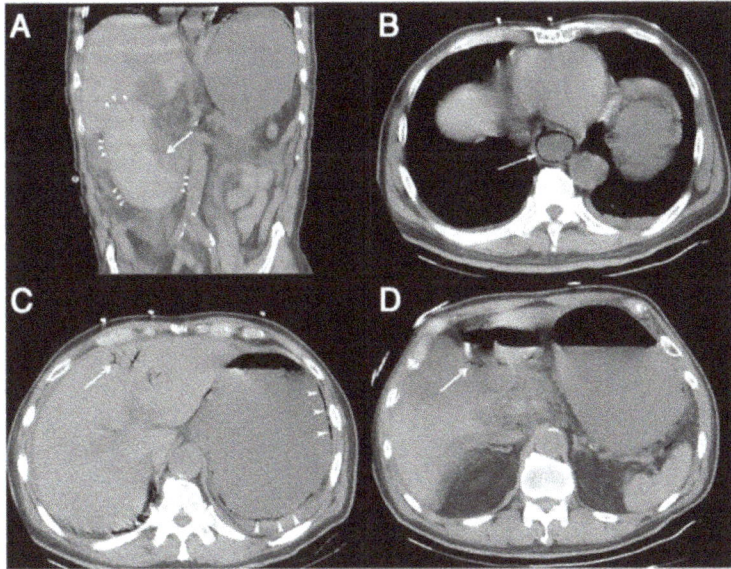

Fig. 2 Abdomen and pelvis computed tomography showed a 14.4 cm × 7 cm mass lesion (**a**, arrowhead) at the lateral side of duodenal second portion and caused lumen narrowing (**a**, arrow). The distended stomach is suggested to have gastric outlet obstruction. Pneumatosis was found at esophagus (**b**, arrow), stomach (**c**, arrowhead) and the bulb (**d**, arrow). The inflated air also entered the portal system (**c**, arrow)

also observed rapid decline of hemoglobin level in our patient and this observation has been described in other case reports [10, 14]. We suggest that the patients should be suspected to have IHD if they have the tetrad of acute pancreatitis, biliary obstruction, gastric outlet obstruction and rapid decline of hemoglobin after an endoscopic examination.

In uncomplicated cases, IDH usually resolves spontaneously with conservative treatment in 1–3 weeks [15].

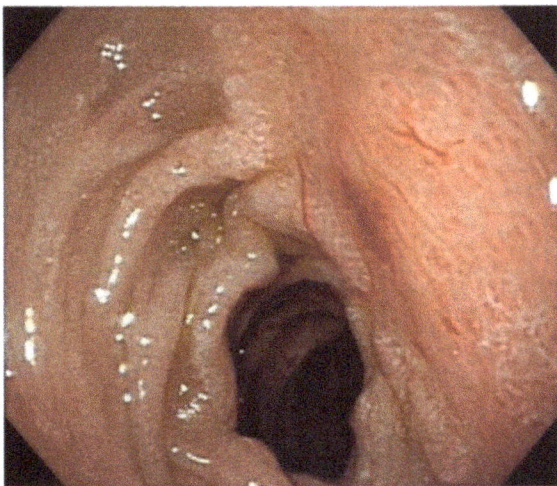

Fig. 3 Follow-up panendoscopy showed resolution of intramural duodenal hematoma, which was associated with swelling of mucosa and diminished villi on the lateral side of duodenum

Sadio *et al.* have reported a case in a patient with intramural gastric hematoma after endoscopic injection therapy, and have found that patient's hematoma disappear six days later [14]. In our patient, the IDH was spontaneously resolved under abdominal sonography six days after the endoscopy.

To our best knowledge, less than 10 cases of patients with esophageal pneumatosis have been reported [4, 16], and no esophagogastroduodenal pneumatosis has been reported. The mechanism of PI has been experimentally proved that dissection of the gas from intraluminal to the intramural compartment is due to increased intra-abdominal pressure combined with mucosal defect [1]. We hypothesize that the findings of our patient are derived from the similar mechanism. The air was inflated from the defect of the needle injection site after endoscopic hemostasis for duodenal ulcer hemorrhage, and warfarin-associated coagulopathy precipitated the formation of IDH, which further dissected the duodenal wall, leading to inflated air entering into the duodenal, gastric and esophageal wall. The inflated air finally entered the portal vein through the portal circulation system.

Traditionally, once the pneumoporta is recognized along with PI, surgical intervention is preferred due to the concern of having ischemic bowel. But, PI is a radiological finding with wide spectrum of clinical severity and outcome. Surgical or conservative treatment should be considered according to the underlying etiology [1]. In this patient, esophagogastroduodenal pneumatosis and intramural duodenal hematoma were resolved spontaneously six days later. Therefore, we suggest that conservative treatment and close clinical assessment should be considered as an initial management for patients who complicate with IDH and PI after an endoscopic procedure. But, surgery is needed for those patients if the diseases progress or complications persist.

Conclusion

Intramural hematoma and PI may be an adverse effect after endoscopic intervention, especially in patients with coagulopathy. The patient with the tetrad symptoms of acute pancreatitis, biliary obstruction, gastric outlet obstruction and rapid decline of hemoglobin after duodenal endoscopic intervention should be evaluated for the IDH. We suggest that those patients might be treated with conservative care initially, but surgical intervention is needed if the diseases progress or complications persist.

Consent

Written informed consent was obtained from the patient's wife for publication of this case report and any accompanying images. A copy of the written consent is available for review by the editors of this journal.

Abbreviations
PI: Pneumatosis intestinalis; IDH: Intramural duodenal hematoma; PT: Prothrombin time; aPTT: activated partial thromboplastin time; ERCP: Endoscopic retrograde cholangiopancreatogram.

Competing interests
The authors declare that they have no competing interests.

Authors' contributions
WC Huang collected clinical data and drafted the initial manuscript. CH Lee also helped draft the manuscript. FM Suk interpreted clinical data and improved the manuscript. All authors read the manuscript versions together and approved the final version of this manuscript.

Authors' information
Not applicable.

Acknowledgments
Not applicable.

Author details
[1]Divisions of Gastroenterology, Wan Fang Hospital, Taipei Medical University, No. 111, Section 3, Hsing Long Road, Taipei 116, Taiwan. [2]Divisions of Pulmonology, Department of Internal Medicine, Wan Fang Hospital, Taipei Medical University, Taipei, Taiwan. [3]Department of Internal Medicine, School of Medicine, College of Medicine, Taipei Medical University, Taipei, Taiwan.

References
1. St Peter SD, Abbas MA, Kelly KA. The spectrum of pneumatosis intestinalis. Arch Surg. 2003;138:68–75.
2. Hameed S, McHugh K, Shah N, Arthurs OJ. Duodenal haematoma following endoscopy as a marker of coagulopathy. Pediatr Radiol. 2014;44:392–7.
3. Zenooz NA, Robbin MR, Perez V. Gastric pneumatosis following nasogastric tube placement: a case report with literature review. Emerg Radiol. 2007;13:205–7.
4. Chelimilla H, Makker JS, Dev A. Incidental finding of esophageal pneumatosis. World J Gastrointest Endosc. 2013;5:74–8.
5. Chung YF, Koo WH. Gastric pneumatosis after endoscopic argon plasma coagulation. Ann Acad Med Singapore. 2005;34:569–70.
6. Domínguez Jiménez JL, Puente Gutiérrez JJ, Marín Moreno MA, Bernal Blanco E, Gallardo Camacho JI, Uceda VA. Gastric pneumatosis and gas in the portal venous system secondary to peptic ulcer. Gastroenterol Hepatol. 2008;31:494–6.
7. Mclaughlin SA, Nguyen JH. Conservative management of nongangrenous esophageal and gastric pneumatosis. Am Surg. 2007;73:862–4.
8. Heng Y, Schuffler MD, Haggitt RC, Rohrmann CA. Pneumatosis intestinalis: a review. Am J Gastroenterol. 1995;90:1747–58.
9. Jones WR, Hardin WJ, Davis JT, Hardy JD. Intramural hematoma of the duodenum: a review of the literature and case report. Ann Surg. 1971;173:534–44.
10. Sugai K, Kajiwara E, Mochizuki Y, Noma E, Nakashima J, Uchimura K, et al. Intramural duodenal hematoma after endoscopic therapy for a bleeding duodenal ulcer in a patient with liver cirrhosis. Intern Med. 2005;44:954–7.
11. Chung S, Park CW, Chung HW, Shin SJ, Chang YS. Intramural duodenal hematoma and hemoperitoneum after endoscopic treatment in a patient with chronic renal failure on hemodialysis: a case report. Cases J. 2009;2:9083.
12. Thandassery RB, John A, Koshy RM, Kaabi SA. Endoscopy. 2014;46 Suppl 1. Unusual Cases and Technical Notes (UCTN): E443-444.
13. Jewett Jr TC, Caldarola V, Karp MP, Allen JE, Cooney DR. Intramural hematoma of the duodenum. Arch Surg. 1988;123:54–8.
14. Sadio A, Peixoto P, Cancela E, Castanheira A, Marques V, Ministro P, et al. Intramural hematoma: a rare complication of endoscopic injection therapy for bleeding peptic ulcers. Endoscopy. 2011;43 Suppl 2:E141–2. UCTN.
15. Lukman MR, Jasmi AY, Niza SS. Massive dissecting intramural duodenal haematoma following endoscopic haemostasis of a bleeding duodenal ulcer. Asian J Surg. 2006;29:98–100.
16. Bakkali H, Aissa I, Massou S, Wartiti L, Abouelalaa K, Balkhi H, et al. Unusual complication of noninvasive ventilation: The œsogastric pneumatosis associated with a subcutaneous emphysema. Rev Pneumol Clin. 2014;70:236–9.

9

High expression of Claudin-2 in esophageal carcinoma and precancerous lesions is significantly associated with the bile salt receptors VDR and TGR5

Sohaib Abu-Farsakh[1], Tongtong Wu[2], Amy Lalonde[2], Jun Sun[3] and Zhongren Zhou[1]* (iD)

Abstract

Background: Claudins are a family of integral membrane proteins and are components of tight junctions (TJs). Many TJ proteins are known to tighten the cell structure and maintain a barrier. Claudin-2 forms gated paracellular channels and allows sodium ions and other small positively charged ions to cross between adjacent cells. Recently, we found that vitamin D receptor (VDR) enhanced Claudin-2 expression in colon and that bile salt receptors VDR and Takeda G-protein coupled receptor5 (TGR5) were highly expressed in esophageal adenocarcinoma (EAC) and precancerous lesions. Here, we examined the expression of Claudin-2 in EAC and precancerous lesions and its association with VDR and TGR5 expression.

Methods: Claudin-2 expression was examined by immunohistochemistry on tissue microarrays, containing EAC, high grade dysplasia (HGD), low grade dysplasia (LGD), Barrett's esophagus (BE), columnar cell metaplasia (CM), squamous cell carcinoma (SCC), and squamous epithelium (SE) cases. Intensity (0 to 3) and percentage were scored for each case. High expression was defined as 2–3 intensity in ≥ 10% of cells.

Results: Claudin-2 was highly expressed in 77% EAC (86/111), 38% HGD (5/13), 61% LGD (17/28), 46% BE (18/39), 45% CM (29/65), 88% SCC (23/26), and 14% SE (11/76). It was significantly more highly-expressed in EAC, SCC and glandular lesions than in SE and more in EAC than in BE and CM. A significant association was found between Claudin-2 expression and VDR and TGR5 expression. No significant association was found between expression of Claudin-2 and age, gender, grade, stage, or patients' survival time in EAC and SCC.

Conclusions: We conclude that Claudin-2 expression is significantly associated with bile acid receptors VDR and TGR5 expression. Our studies identify a novel role of a tight junction protein in the development and progression of esophageal mucosal metaplasia, dysplasia and carcinoma.

Keywords: Claudin 2, Esophageal adenocarcinoma, Barrett's esophagus, Tight junctions, VDR, TGR5

Background

The incidence of esophageal adenocarcinoma (EAC) has increased 700% in the United States over the past several decades [1]. Barrett's esophagus (BE), an intestinal-like metaplasia of the distal esophageal mucosa, is a recognized precursor lesion and risk factor for EAC. Previous studies have suggested a sequence of events leading to EAC that starts from normal esophageal squamous epithelium to reflux esophagitis, followed by BE, dysplasia, and finally EAC [2]. The development and progression of these events is hastened by inflammation, bile salts, and acid reflux from gastro-esophageal reflux disease (GERD) [3–5].

Chronic exposure to bile salts in GERD promotes injury and inflammation of the esophageal epithelium and inhibits the Notch signaling pathway [6, 7]. Bile acids induce inflammatory gene expression and modulate inflammatory responses through the bile acid receptors including farnesoid X receptor (FXR), retinoic X receptor (RXR), TGR5

* Correspondence: david_zhou@urmc.rochester.edu
[1]Department of Pathology and Laboratory Medicine, University of Rochester, Box 626601 Elmwood Ave, Rochester, NY 14642, USA

and Vitamin D receptor (VDR) [4, 8, 9]. They also alter gene expression by acting as ligands for nuclear receptors or by activating kinase signaling pathways [10, 11]. Bile acid receptors, including FXR, the Takeda G-protein-couples receptor 5 (TGR5) and VDR, have recently been identified in EAC and esophageal squamous cell carcinoma (ESCC) [4, 12–15]. We also showed that bile salts at pH of 5 destroyed intercellular junctions in squamous mucosa [16].

Claudins are a family of integral membrane proteins and are components of tight junctions (TJs) [17]. Many TJ proteins are known to tighten the cell structure and maintain a barrier [17, 18]. In contrast, Claudin-2 forms gated paracellular channels and allows sodium ions and other small positively charged ions to cross between adjacent cells [19–22]. Claudin-2 expression may be involved at early stages of transformation in inflammatory bowel disease-associated neoplasia [23]. Claudin-2 was found in various human cancers including breast, ovarian, urothelial, colorectal, prostate, and gastric cancers linking to better or worse prognosis [24–28]. Recently, we identified Claudin-2 as a target gene of VDR in colonic epithelial cells [29]. Our study has demonstrated that bile salt receptors VDR and TGR5 were highly expressed in EAC and precancerous lesions [29, 30]. However, the relationship between Claudin-2 and bile salt receptors in EAC and esophageal precancerous lesions is still unknown.

In the current study, we used immunohistochemical methods to investigate the expression of the tight junction protein Claudin-2 in EAC, esophageal precancerous lesions, and esophageal squamous cell carcinoma. The association of Claudin-2 with bile salt receptors VDR and TGR5 was also investigated.

Methods
Patients for tissue microarrays
All 111 patients with EAC used for tissue microarrays (TMAs) construction were treated with esophagectomy at the Strong Memorial Hospital/University of Rochester between 1997 and 2005 (99 male [89%], 12 female [11%]). The patient age ranged from 34 to 85 years with a mean of 64 years. The follow-up period after esophagectomy ranged from 0.3 to 142 months with a mean of 39 months.

Construction of tissue microarray
TMAs containing material from 39 cases of BE, 65 cases of columnar cell metaplasia (CM), 76 cases of squamous epithelium (SE), 28 cases of low grade dysplasia (LGD), 13 cases of high grade dysplasia (HGD), 111 cases of esophageal adenocarcinoma (EAC), and 26 cases of esophageal squamous cell carcinoma (ESCC) were constructed from representative areas of formalin-fixed specimens collected

during 1997 through 2005 at the Department of Pathology and Laboratory Medicine, University of Rochester Medical Center, Rochester, NY. Five-micron sections were cut from TMAs and stained with hematoxylin and eosin to confirm the presence of the expected tissue within each tissue core. Additional sections were cut for IHC staining. Some tissue cores in TMAs were falloff from slides during processing and were excluded from our study. The research project was approved by Research Subjects Review Board committee in University of Rochester (RSRB00028546).

Immunohistochemical staining
Tissue sections from the TMA were deparaffinized, rehydrated through graded alcohols, and washed with phosphate-buffered saline. Antigen retrieval was performed by heating sections in 10 mM citrate (pH 6.0) boiling buffer for 15 min. The tissues were permeabilized with 0.3% Triton X for 1 h at room temperature. After endogenous peroxidase activity was quenched and nonspecific binding was blocked, mouse monoclonal anti-Claudin-2 (1:200; Santa Cruz Biotechnology, Santa Cruz, CA), anti-VDR (1:100; Santa Cruz Biotechnology, Santa Cruz, CA) and anti-TGR5 antibodies (1:200; Santa Cruz Biotechnology, Santa Cruz, CA) was incubated at 4 °C overnight. Biotinylated secondary antibody (Jackson ImmunoResearch Laboratories, West Grove, PA) was allowed to incubate for 1 h. After washing, sections were incubated with avidin-biotin–peroxidase complex (Vector Laboratories, Burlingame, CA) for 1 h at room temperature. For color reaction development, slides were immersed in Vector NovaRed substrate (Vector Laboratories, Burlingame, CA) for 2 min and counterstained with Flex Hematoxylin for 2 min (Vector Laboratories, Burlingame, CA). A negative control was performed by replacing anti-VDR antibody with normal serum.

Scoring of IHC staining
All sections were reviewed independently by Z.Z. and S.A., who were blinded to all clinical and pathologic information. Discordant cases were reviewed by both investigators, and a consensus was reached. For Claudin-2 IHC stain, the percentage of positive cells was determined. The intensity of staining was graded 0, 1+, 2+, or 3+. Claudin-2 was considered to be highly expressed if 10% or more of the cells stained with an intensity score of 2+ or 3+ (Fig. 1).

Statistical analysis
All statistical tests were 2-sided. $P < 0.05$ was considered to be statistically significant. Kaplan-Meier survival estimator with log-rank test was used to analyze the patient survival rates in the Claudin-2 high expression group versus the non-high expression group. The χ2 or Fisher

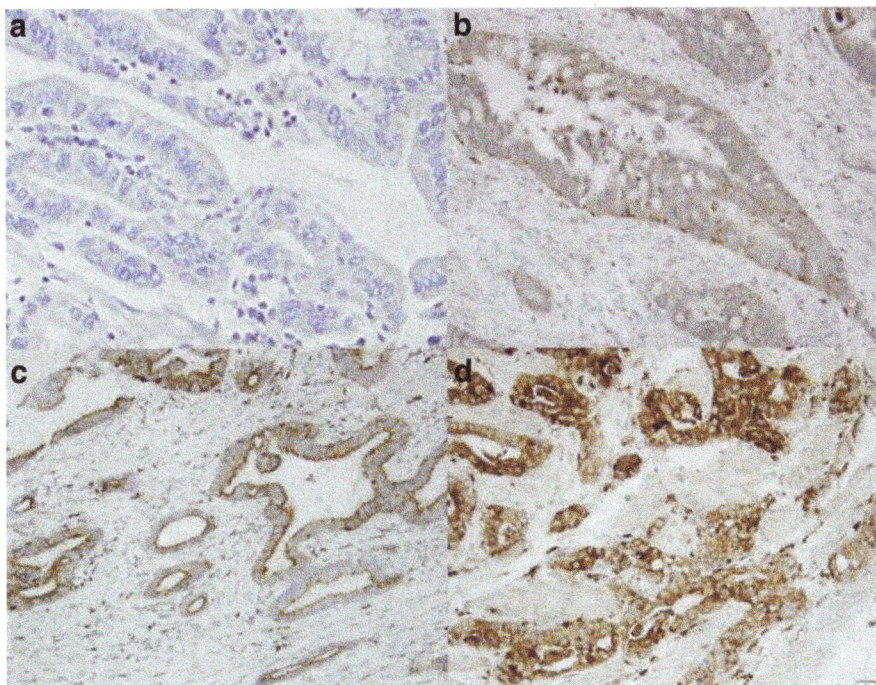

Fig. 1 Immunostain score of Claudin-2 expression in esophageal adenocarcinoma. **a** No staining (0); **b** 1+ staining, **c** 2+ staining, and **d** 3+ staining

exact tests were used to compare Claudin-2 positivity rates between EAC, HGD and LGD, BE, non–goblet cell metaplasia, and SE subcategories as appropriate. Statistical analyses were performed using SAS version 9.3 (SAS, Cary, NC).

Results

High expression of Claudin-2 in precancerous lesions, EAC, and ESCC

Claudin-2 immunostaining is located at cytoplasm and membrane, but predominantly at the cell and the basal membrane of the glands and squamous mucosa. It diffusely distributes in most of glands in columnar cell metaplasia, BE, dysplasia and EAC (Fig. 1 and Fig. 2). Claudin-2 was highly expressed in 77% EAC (86/111), 38% HGD (5/13), 61% LGD (17/28), 46% BE (18/39), 45% CM (29/65), 88% SCC (23/26), and 14% SE (11/76) (see Table 1). It is significantly more expressed in EAC than in HGD ($p = 0.0055$), BE ($p = 0.0004$) and CM ($p < 0.0001$), and significantly more expressed in both BE and CM than in SE ($p = 0.0004$ and 0.0001 respectively). It is also more expressed in SCC than in SE ($p < 0.0001$) (Fig. 3). No significant difference was found between the levels of Claudin-2 expression in CM, BE, LGD, and HGD.

Survival rate analysis in EAC cases

Kaplan-Meier analysis was used to calculate the survival curves of Claudin-2 high and non-high expression groups. Log-rank test was used to compare the effect of Claudin-2 expression in survival rates for patients with esophageal adenocarcinoma (Fig. 4). The median survival time in the Claudin-2 high expression group by immunostain was 19 months with a mean survival time of 40 months. The Claudin-2 non-high expression group had a median survival time of 20 months with a mean survival time of 33 months (censoring rate = 22%). The log-rank test failed to reveal significant differences in the survival time for the Claudin-2 high expression and non-high expression group ($p = 0.6385$; Fig. 4).

Association of high Claudin-2 expression with clinicopathologic characteristics of EAC

The association of Claudin 2 high expression with clinicopathologic features in esophageal adenocarcinoma was analyzed. None of the clinicopathologic characteristics including age, sex, TNM staging and differentiation were found to be significantly associated with Claudin-2 high expression (Table 2).

Association of high Claudin-2 expression with high TGR5 and VDR expression

VDR expression is located at both cytoplasm and cell membrane, but TGR5 predominately at cell membrane (Fig. 5) [14, 31]. TGR5 is low or moderately positive on whole layer of squamous mucosa (Fig. 5a), but VDR usually is not present on squamous mucosa and ESCC

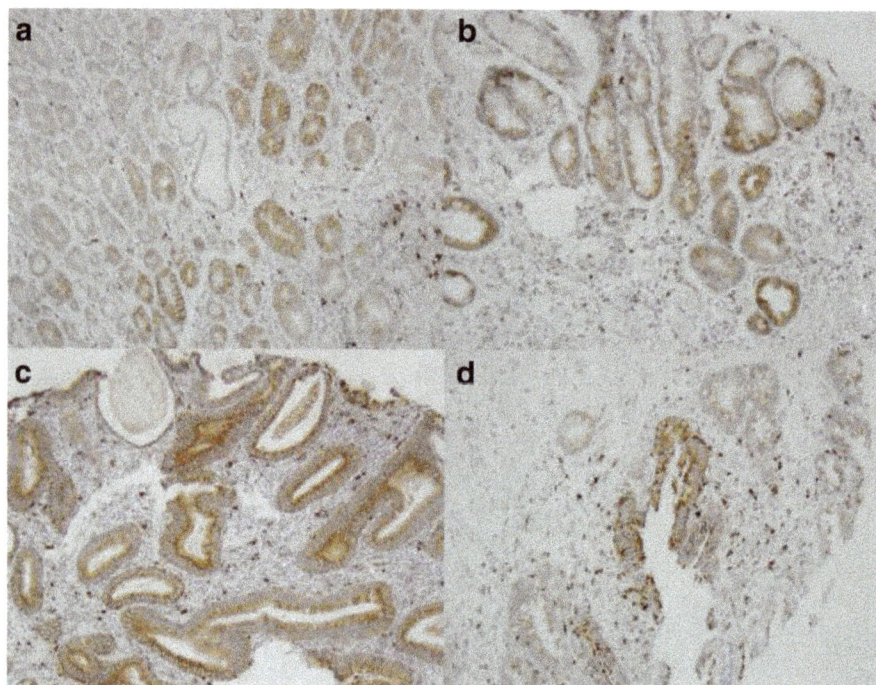

Fig. 2 Claudin-2 expression in esophageal precancerous lesions. **a** Cardiac mucosa with 2+ immunostaining; **b** Barrett's esophagus with 3+ immunostaining; **c** low grade dysplasia with diffuse 3+ immunostaining; **d** high grade dysplasia with focal 2+ immunostaining

(Fig. 5c). VDR and TGR5 expression diffusely distribute in columnar cell metaplasia, dysplasia and EAC, which is similar to the distribution of Claudin-2 (Fig. 5c and d). We further compared the expression level of Claudin-2 with TGR5 and VDR in all cases and then separately for EAC. The positive correlations of Claudin-2 high expression with TGR5 and VDR were statistically significant for the full samples ($p = 0.0051$ and 0.0046, respectively, Table 3), but Claudin-2 is not significantly associated TGR5 and VDR in EAC cases only ($p = 0.86$ and 0.65).

Discussion

In the current study, we show that tight junction protein Claudin-2 is localized to the cytoplasm and cell membrane of squamous cell and glandular cells. The proportion of cases with high Claudin-2 expression showed an upward trend from squamous mucosa to precancerous lesions to EAC. Claudin-2 was also highly expressed in esophageal squamous cell carcinoma. Claudin-2 expression positively correlated with the expression of the bile acid receptors VDR and TGR5 in esophageal tissue.

Bile acid reflux, in addition to acidic pH, is required to cause dilation of intercellular spaces in esophageal epithelium in vitro, as we showed in a previous study [16]. Another study using rat model with esophagojejunostomy and gastrectomy demonstrated that bile acids but not gastric acids induced the transition to BE [32]. We recently found that bile salt receptors VDR and TGR5 were highly expressed in esophageal adenocarcinoma (EAC) and precancerous lesions [14, 30]. The above studies might suggest that bile acids through VDR and TGR5 receptors play an important role in the dilation of

Table 1 Rate of Claudin-2 high expression in EAC and precancerous lesions and squamous cell carcinoma

Histological Type	Total (n)	High-expression (%)	Non-high expression (%)
Adenocarcinoma	111	86 (77%)	25 (23%)
High grade dysplasia	13	5 (38%)	8 (62%)
Low grade dysplasia	28	17 (61%)	11 (39%)
Barrett's esophagus	39	18 (46%)	21 (54%)
Columnar cell metaplasia	65	29 (45%)	36 (55%)
Squamous epithelium	76	11 (14%)	65 (86%)
Squamous cell carcinoma	26	23 (88%)	3 (12%)

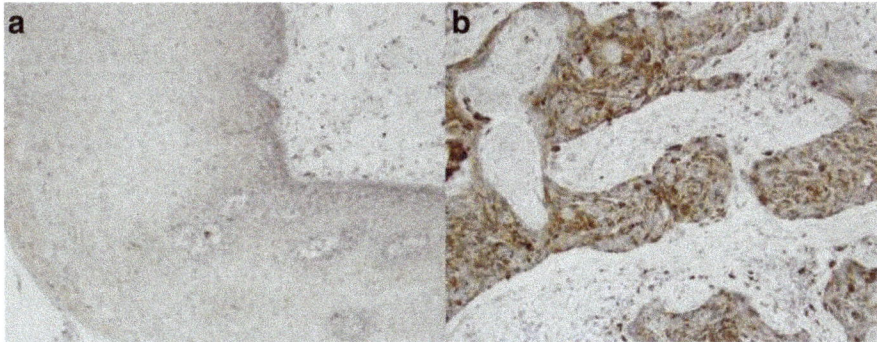

Fig. 3 Comparison of Claudin-2 expression between normal squamous epithelium and squamous cell carcinoma. **a** in normal squamous epithelium with the immunostain score is 1+; **b** in squamous cell carcinoma with the immunostain score is 3+

intercellular spaces and in the development of Barrett's esophagus.

VDR was also found to directly enhance Claudin-2 expression in intestinal epithelium [29, 33]. In addition, deoxycholic acid (DCA) and trypsin in the higher concentration of 2.5 mM can decreased the resistance of GERD patients' squamous mucosa and the claudin-3, –4 and E-cadherin expressions [18]. However, the Claudin-2 expression is found at basal and suprabasal zone of the squamous mucosa, but did not change significantly in GERD patients. We found that Claudin-2 has similar distribution in squamous mucosa compared to TGR5

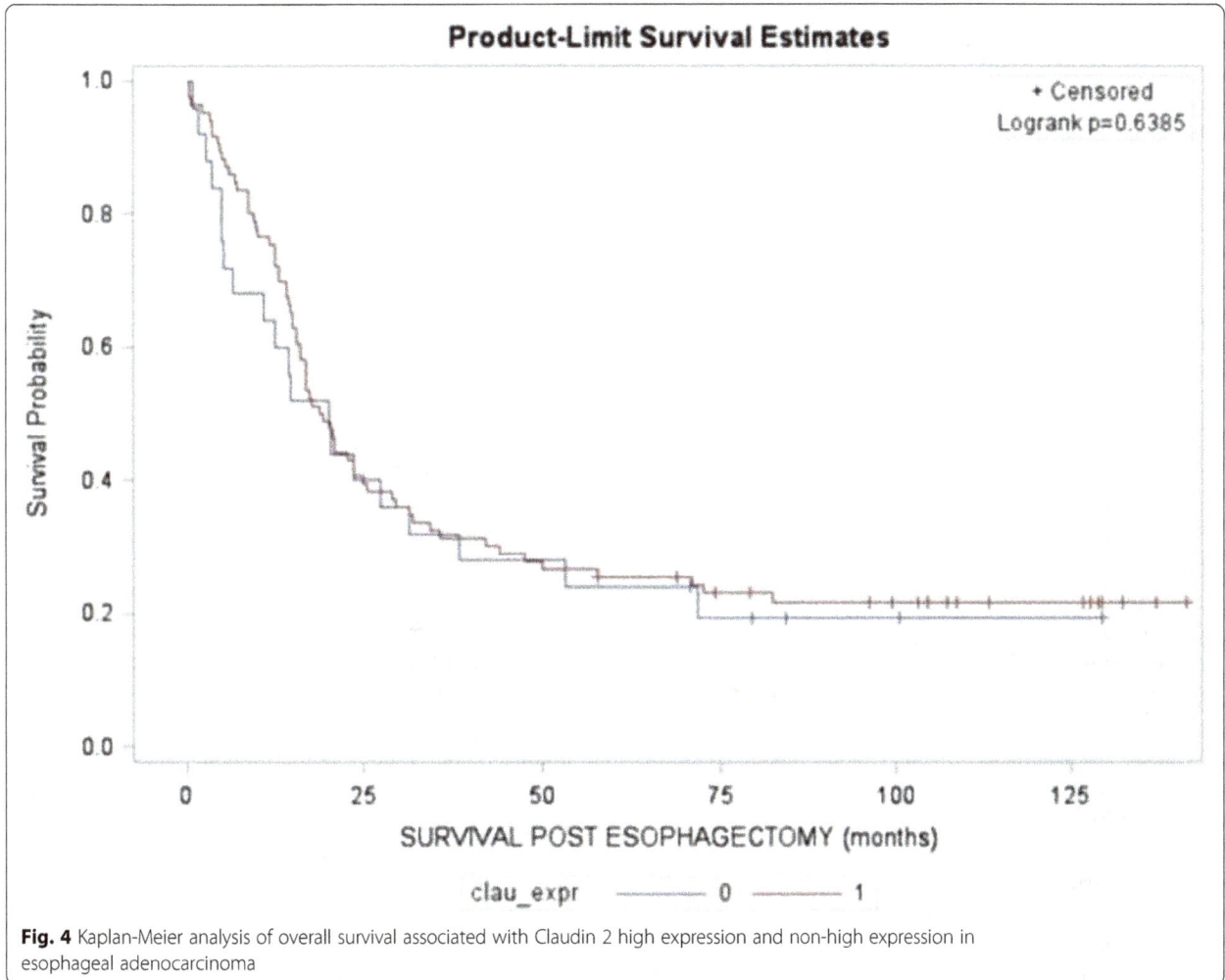

Fig. 4 Kaplan-Meier analysis of overall survival associated with Claudin 2 high expression and non-high expression in esophageal adenocarcinoma

Table 2 Examination of relationship of Claudin-2 high expression and clinicopathologic characteristics in esophageal adenocarcinoma

Covariate		High-expression	Non-high expression	P value
Age	Mean (SD)	63.9 (11.1)	63.6 (11.4)	0.9128
	Range	34 – 84	40 – 85	
Gender	Male	75	24	0.2922
	Female	11	1	
Lymph node metastasis	# (+) nodes	4.2 (5.2)	3.7 (4.5)	0.6286
Survival time		39.51 (41.55)	33.32 (35.88)	0.6385
Tumor location *Fisher's Test*	DISTAL	19	4	0.7162
	GEJ	64	21	
	Other	3	0	
Tumor location *Fisher's Test*	DISTAL	19	4	0.8078
	GEJ	64	21	
	MID	2	0	
	PROXIMAL	1	0	
TNM Stage *Fisher's Test*	1	1	0	0.6444
	2	10	1	
	3	21	8	
	4	54	16	
T stage *Fisher's Test*	1	2	0	0.4647
	2	13	1	
	3	17	6	
	4	54	18	
N stage *Fisher's Test*	0	20	6	0.7982
	1	42	13	
	2	14	5	
	3	10	1	
Differentiation (missing = 2) *Fisher's Test*	Poor	57	15	0.7075
	Moderate	23	9	
	Well	4	1	

and similar distribution in glandular cells compared to both TGR5 and VDR. In addition, Claudin-2 expression was positively correlates with the VDR and TGR5 expression. These data support our hypothesis the bile acids induce Claudin-2 expression through VDR and TGR5. Claudin-2 is a unique protein in the Claudin family and forms a cation and water selective paracellular channel in tight junctions [19, 34, 35], and its expression increases intercellular permeability which opens the gate to change the microenvironment of the esophageal epithelium and may eventually lead to columnar cell metaplasia and BE.

Based on the in vitro experiments and animal models discussed earlier, potential bile acid blocking drugs in the future might be able to reduce the expression of Claudin-2 and decrease the risk of progression to BE. However, our study utilizes an immunohistochemical method to detect the expression of Claudin-2; it has the limitation to directly prove the functional relationship between Claudin-2 and bile acid receptors. This functional relationship will be studied in future.

The rate of high expression of Claudin-2 was significantly increased from 14% in SE to 45% in columnar cell metaplasia and BE. This is consistent with the results of a previous study that found Claudin-2 overexpression in BE [36]. Mullin et al. found that leak of sucrose in the urine dramatically increased about 2 folds in esophagitis and 3 folds in BE, and that Claudin-2 expression increased 225 folds since the normal squamous epithelium showed almost no expression of Claudin-2. Some studies also showed that Claudin-1, −2, and −4 were significantly changed in GERD patients both at the transcript and protein levels compared to normal patients [18, 37]. Weimann et al. compared six immunohistochemical markers for

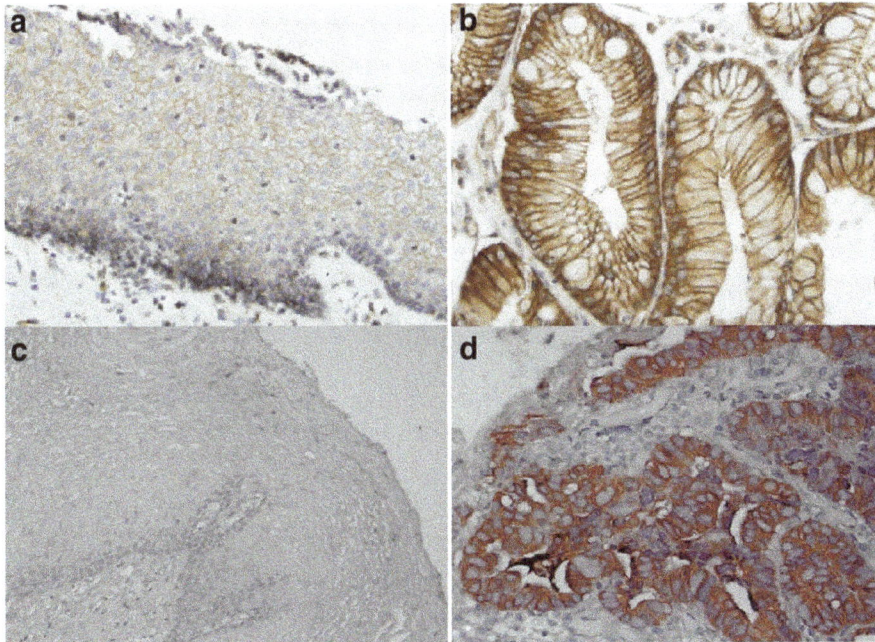

Fig. 5 TGR5 and VDR expression in esophagus. **a** TGR5 is moderately expressed in whole squamous mucosa. Focal extensive TGR5 expression is present in the basal membrane. **b** TGR5 expression is located at cell membrane and distributes the whole glands in BE case. **c** VDR is not expressed in squamous mucosa. **d** VDR expression is located at cell membrane and cytoplasm, predominately in cell membrane and distributes the whole glands in HGD case

the histologic diagnosis of neoplasia in Barrett's esophagus [38]; however, they found that Claudin-2 staining was only focal and weak and did differ significantly between normal (5%), Barrett's esophagus (2%), low- (5%) and high-grade dysplasia (7%) and EAC (16%). Our study showed that it was significantly more expressed in EAC than in HGD ($p = 0.0055$), BE ($p = 0.0004$) and CM ($p < 0.0001$), and significantly more expressed in both BE and CM than in SE ($p = 0.0004$ and 0.0001 respectively). The reason for the discordant results between their study and ours is not completely clear; however, we suggest that the antibodies used might be a possible reason. They used an anti-Claudin-2 rabbit polyclonal antibody (Panomics, Redwood City, CA, USA) and we used an anti-Claudin-2 mouse monoclonal antibody (Santa Cruz, CA, USA). In

addition, our antibodies were validated by Western Blot in a previous study [29]. Furthermore, the number of the cases in each study was different; they had a relatively small number of samples in each group.

Studies have shown that different Claudins can be over or under-expressed in various human cancers including breast, ovarian, urothelial, colorectal, prostate, and gastric cancers. Their over or under-expression has been linked to better or worse prognosis in some cancer types [24–27]. In the esophagus, Claudins-3, –4 and –7 were reported to have increased expression in esophageal adenocarcinoma [39]. In our study, we found that Claudin-2 was more highly expressed in EAC compared to precancerous lesions and normal esophageal squamous mucosa, suggesting that Claudin-2 might have a role in the development and progression of EAC. However, we did not find a significant correlation between Claudin-2 expression in EAC and patient's survival or other clinico-pathologic features. Claudin-2 was also overexpressed in ESCC; no correlation was identified between Claudin-2 expression in ESCC and patient's survival.

Table 3 Association between Claudin-2 high expression and each of TGR5 and VDR high expression across all cases

	Claudin-2 High-expression	Claudin-2 Non-high expression	P value
TGR5 High-expression	113	76	0.0051*
TGR5 Non-high expression	76	93	
VDR High-expression	117	83	0.0046*
VDR Non-high expression	52	71	

Conclusion

In summary, we conclude that Claudin-2 expression is significantly increased from normal squamous mucosa to columnar cell metaplasia, BE, low- and high-grade dysplasia to EAC. The expression of Claudin-2 positively correlates with the expression of the bile acid receptors

VDR and TGR5. This implies that bile acid reflux may induce Claudin-2 over expression and increase the risk of the development of BE. Our study provides new insights into the role of a tight junction protein and bile acid receptors in the pathogenesis of Barrett's esophagus and esophageal cancer.

Abbreviation
BE: Barrett's esophagus; CM: Columnar cell metaplasia; EAC: Esophageal adenocarcinoma; GERD: Gastroesophageal reflux disease; HGD: High grade dysplasia; IHC: Immunohistochemistry; LGD: Low grade dysplasia; SCC: Squamous cell carcinoma; SE: and squamous epithelium; TGR5: The G-protein couples bile acid receptor; TMA: Tissue microarray; TNM: Tumor node metastasis; VDR: Vitamin D receptor

Acknowledgments
We thank Qi Yang and Loralee McMahon for immunohistochemistry staining.

Funding
We would like to acknowledge the National Institutes of Health grant NIDDK R01 DK105118 to Jun Sun.

Authors' contribution
ZZ and JS: Designing the project; interpreting data, editing the paper. ZZ and SA: Scoring all IHC slides from TMA, writing the paper. WT and AL: Performing statistical analysis, writing part of the "Results" section. All authors read and approved the final manuscript.

Authors' information
SA is a third year resident; this abstract was presented in USCAP meeting in 2016.

Competing interests
All authors declare that they have no competing interest.

Author details
[1]Department of Pathology and Laboratory Medicine, University of Rochester, Box 626601 Elmwood Ave, Rochester, NY 14642, USA. [2]Department of Biostatistics and Computational Biology, University of Rochester Medical Center, 265 Crittenden Boulevard CU 420630, Rochester, NY 14642-0630, USA. [3]Department of Medicine, Division of Gastroenterology and Hepatology, University of Illinois College of Medicine, 840 South Wood Street MC 716, Chicago, IL 60612, USA.

References
1. Corley DA, Kubo A, Levin TR, Block G, Habel L, Rumore G, Quesenberry C, Buffler P. Race, ethnicity, sex and temporal differences in Barrett's oesophagus diagnosis: a large community-based study, 1994–2006. Gut. 2009;58(2):182–8.
2. Chen X, Yang CS. Esophageal adenocarcinoma: a review and perspectives on the mechanism of carcinogenesis and chemoprevention. Carcinogenesis. 2001;22(8):1119–29.
3. Quante M, Bhagat G, Abrams JA, Marache F, Good P, Lee MD, Lee Y, Friedman R, Asfaha S, Dubeykovskaya Z, et al. Bile acid and inflammation activate gastric cardia stem cells in a mouse model of Barrett-like metaplasia. Cancer Cell. 2012;21(1):36–51.
4. Hong J, Behar J, Wands J, Resnick M, Wang LJ, DeLellis RA, Lambeth D, Souza RF, Spechler SJ, Cao W. Role of a novel bile acid receptor TGR5 in the development of oesophageal adenocarcinoma. Gut. 2010;59(2):170–80.
5. Fang Y, Chen X, Bajpai M, Verma A, Das KM, Souza RF, Garman KS, Donohoe CL, O'Farrell NJ, Reynolds JV, et al. Cellular origins and molecular mechanisms of Barrett's esophagus and esophageal adenocarcinoma. Ann N Y Acad Sci. 2013;1300:187–99.
6. Matsuzaki J, Suzuki H, Tsugawa H, Watanabe M, Hossain S, Arai E, Saito Y, Sekine S, Akaike T, Kanai Y, et al. Bile acids increase levels of microRNAs 221 and 222, leading to degradation of CDX2 during esophageal carcinogenesis. Gastroenterology. 2013;145(6):1300–11.
7. Tamagawa Y, Ishimura N, Uno G, Yuki T, Kazumori H, Ishihara S, Amano Y, Kinoshita Y. Notch signaling pathway and Cdx2 expression in the development of Barrett's esophagus. Lab Invest. 2012;92(6):896–909.
8. Qin P, Borges-Marcucci LA, Evans MJ, Harnish DC. Bile acid signaling through FXR induces intracellular adhesion molecule-1 expression in mouse liver and human hepatocytes. Am J Physiol Gastrointest Liver Physiol. 2005;289(2):G267–273.
9. Fiorucci S, Cipriani S, Mencarelli A, Renga B, Distrutti E, Baldelli F. Counter-regulatory role of bile acid activated receptors in immunity and inflammation. Curr Mol Med. 2010;10(6):579–95.
10. Huang J, Huang J, Ma Y, Wang H, Yang J, Xiong T, Du L. The Cdx-2 polymorphism in the VDR gene is associated with increased risk of cancer: a meta-analysis. Mol Biol Rep. 2013;40(7):4219–25.
11. Gupta S, Stravitz RT, Dent P, Hylemon PB. Down-regulation of cholesterol 7alpha-hydroxylase (CYP7A1) gene expression by bile acids in primary rat hepatocytes is mediated by the c-Jun N-terminal kinase pathway. J Biol Chem. 2001;276(19):15816–22.
12. De Gottardi A, Dumonceau JM, Bruttin F, Vonlaufen A, Morard I, Spahr L, Rubbia-Brandt L, Frossard JL, Dinjens WN, Rabinovitch PS, et al. Expression of the bile acid receptor FXR in Barrett's esophagus and enhancement of apoptosis by guggulsterone in vitro. Mol Cancer. 2006;5:48.
13. Mimori K, Tanaka Y, Yoshinaga K, Masuda T, Yamashita K, Okamoto M, Inoue H, Mori M. Clinical significance of the overexpression of the candidate oncogene CYP24 in esophageal cancer. Ann Oncol. 2004;15(2):236–41.
14. Chunhong Pang AL, Tony E Godfrey, Jianwen Que, Jun Sun, Tongtong Wu, Zhongren Zhou: Bile salt receptor TGR5 is highly expressed in esophageal adenocarcinoma and precancerous lesions with significantly worse overall survival and gender differences. Clinical and Experimental Gastroenterology 2016, in press.
15. Pols TW, Nomura M, Harach T, Lo Sasso G, Oosterveer MH, Thomas C, Rizzo G, Gioiello A, Adorini L, Pellicciari R, et al. TGR5 activation inhibits atherosclerosis by reducing macrophage inflammation and lipid loading. Cell Metab. 2011;14(6):747–57.
16. Ghatak S, Reveiller M, Toia L, Ivanov AI, Zhou Z, Redmond EM, Godfrey TE, Peters JH. Bile Salts at Low pH Cause Dilation of Intercellular Spaces in In Vitro Stratified Primary Esophageal Cells, Possibly by Modulating Wnt Signaling. J Gastrointest Surg. 2016;20(3):500–9.
17. Gunzel D, Yu AS. Claudins and the modulation of tight junction permeability. Physiol Rev. 2013;93(2):525–69.
18. Bjorkman EV, Edebo A, Oltean M, Casselbrant A. Esophageal barrier function and tight junction expression in healthy subjects and patients with gastroesophageal reflux disease: functionality of esophageal mucosa exposed to bile salt and trypsin in vitro. Scand J Gastroenterol. 2013;48(10):1118–26.
19. Weber CR, Liang GH, Wang Y, Das S, Shen L, Yu AS, Nelson DJ, Turner JR. Claudin-2-dependent paracellular channels are dynamically gated. Elife. 2015;4:e09906.
20. Amasheh S, Meiri N, Gitter AH, Schoneberg T, Mankertz J, Schulzke JD, Fromm M. Claudin-2 expression induces cation-selective channels in tight junctions of epithelial cells. J Cell Sci. 2002;115(Pt 24):4969–76.
21. Muto S, Hata M, Taniguchi J, Tsuruoka S, Moriwaki K, Saitou M, Furuse K, Sasaki H, Fujimura A, Imai M, et al. Claudin-2-deficient mice are defective in the leaky and cation-selective paracellular permeability properties of renal proximal tubules. Proc Natl Acad Sci U S A. 2010;107(17):8011–6.
22. Mankertz J, Schulzke JD. Altered permeability in inflammatory bowel disease: pathophysiology and clinical implications. Curr Opin Gastroenterol. 2007;23(4):379–83.
23. Weber CR, Nalle SC, Tretiakova M, Rubin DT, Turner JR. Claudin-1 and claudin-2 expression is elevated in inflammatory bowel disease and may contribute to early neoplastic transformation. Lab Invest. 2008;88(10):1110 20.

24. Kwon MJ. Emerging roles of claudins in human cancer. Int J Mol Sci. 2013; 14(9):18148–80.

25. Szekely E, Torzsok P, Riesz P, Korompay A, Fintha A, Szekely T, Lotz G, Nyirady P, Romics I, Timar J, et al. Expression of claudins and their prognostic significance in noninvasive urothelial neoplasms of the human urinary bladder. J Histochem Cytochem. 2011;59(10):932–41.

26. Lu S, Singh K, Mangray S, Tavares R, Noble L, Resnick MB, Yakirevich E. Claudin expression in high-grade invasive ductal carcinoma of the breast: correlation with the molecular subtype. Mod Pathol. 2013;26(4):485–95.

27. English DP, Santin AD. Claudins overexpression in ovarian cancer: potential targets for Clostridium Perfringens Enterotoxin (CPE) based diagnosis and therapy. Int J Mol Sci. 2013;14(5):10412–37.

28. Dhawan P, Ahmad R, Chaturvedi R, Smith JJ, Midha R, Mittal MK, Krishnan M, Chen X, Eschrich S, Yeatman TJ, et al. Claudin-2 expression increases tumorigenicity of colon cancer cells: role of epidermal growth factor receptor activation. Oncogene. 2011;30(29):3234–47.

29. Zhang YG, Wu S, Lu R, Zhou D, Zhou J, Carmeliet G, Petrof E, Claud EC, Sun J. Tight junction CLDN2 gene is a direct target of the vitamin D receptor. Sci Rep. 2015;5:10642.

30. Zhou Z, Xia Y, Bandla S, Zakharov V, Wu S, Peters J, Godfrey TE, Sun J. Vitamin D receptor is highly expressed in precancerous lesions and esophageal adenocarcinoma with significant sex difference. Hum Pathol. 2014;45(8):1744–51.

31. Zhou H, Xu C, Gu M. Vitamin D receptor (VDR) gene polymorphisms and Graves' disease: a meta-analysis. Clin Endocrinol (Oxf). 2009;70(6):938–45.

32. Sun D, Wang X, Gai Z, Song X, Jia X, Tian H. Bile acids but not acidic acids induce Barrett's esophagus. Int J Clin Exp Pathol. 2015;8(2):1384–92.

33. Kuhne H, Hause G, Grundmann SM, Schutkowski A, Brandsch C, Stangl GI. Vitamin D receptor knockout mice exhibit elongated intestinal microvilli and increased ezrin expression. Nutr Res. 2016;36(2):184–92.

34. Amasheh S, Milatz S, Krug SM, Markov AG, Gunzel D, Amasheh M, Fromm M. Tight junction proteins as channel formers and barrier builders. Ann N Y Acad Sci. 2009;1165:211–9.

35. Luettig J, Rosenthal R, Barmeyer C, Schulzke JD. Claudin-2 as a mediator of leaky gut barrier during intestinal inflammation. Tissue Barriers. 2015;3(1–2): e977176.

36. Mullin JM, Valenzano MC, Trembeth S, Allegretti PD, Verrecchio JJ, Schmidt JD, Jain V, Meddings JB, Mercogliano G, Thornton JJ. Transepithelial leak in Barrett's esophagus. Dig Dis Sci. 2006;51(12):2326–36.

37. Monkemuller K, Wex T, Kuester D, Fry LC, Kandulski A, Kropf S, Roessner A, Malfertheiner P. Role of tight junction proteins in gastroesophageal reflux disease. BMC Gastroenterol. 2012;12:128.

38. Weimann A, Rieger A, Zimmermann M, Gross M, Hoffmann P, Slevogt H, Morawietz L. Comparison of six immunohistochemical markers for the histologic diagnosis of neoplasia in Barrett's esophagus. Virchows Arch. 2010;457(5):537–45.

39. Montgomery E, Mamelak AJ, Gibson M, Maitra A, Sheikh S, Amr SS, Yang S, Brock M, Forastiere A, Zhang S, et al. Overexpression of claudin proteins in esophageal adenocarcinoma and its precursor lesions. Appl Immunohistochem Mol Morphol. 2006;14(1):24–30.

10

Assessment of esophageal involvement in systemic sclerosis and morphea (localized scleroderma) by clinical, endoscopic, manometric and pH metric features

Tasleem Arif[1,3*], Qazi Masood[1], Jaswinder Singh[2] and Iffat Hassan[1]

Abstract

Background: Systemic sclerosis (SSc) is a generalized disorder of unknown etiology affecting the connective tissue of the body. It affects the skin and various internal organs. Gastrointestinal tract involvement is seen in almost 90% of the patients. Esophagus is the most frequently affected part of the gastrointestinal tract. Esophageal motility disturbance classically manifests as a reduced lower esophageal sphincter pressure (LESP) and loss of distal esophageal body peristalsis. Consequently, SSc patients may be complicated by erosive esophagitis and eventually by Barrett's esophagus and esophageal adenocarcinoma. Morphea, also known as localized scleroderma, is characterized by predominant skin involvement, with occasional involvement of subjacent muscles and usually sparing the internal organs. The involvement of esophagus in morphea has been studied very scarcely. The proposed study will investigate the esophageal involvement in the two forms of scleroderma (systemic and localized), compare the same and address any need of upper gastrointestinal evaluation in morphea (localized scleroderma) patients.

Methods: 56 and 31 newly and already diagnosed cases of SSc and morphea respectively were taken up for the study. All the patients were inquired about the dyspeptic symptoms (heartburn and/or acid regurgitation and/or dysphagia). Upper gastrointestinal endoscopy, esophageal manometry and 24-hour pH monitoring were done in 52, 47 and 41 patients of SSc; and 28, 25 and 20 patients of morphea respectively.

Results: Esophageal symptoms were present in 39 cases (69.6%) of SSc which were mild in 22 (39.3%), moderate in 14 (25%), severe in three (5.3%); while only four cases (7.1%) of morphea had esophageal symptoms all of which were mild in severity. Reflux esophagitis was seen in 17 cases (32.7%) of SSc and only two cases (7.14%) of morphea. Manometric abnormalities were seen in 32 cases (68.1%) of SSc and none in morphea. Ambulatory 24-hour esophageal pH monitoring documented abnormal reflux in 33 cases (80.5%) of SSc and no such abnormality in morphea.

Conclusion: While the esophageal involvement is frequent in SSc, no such motility disorder is seen in morphea. Meticulous upper gastrointestinal tract evaluation is justified only in SSc and not in morphea.

Keywords: Endoscopy, Esophageal manometry, Morphea, Reflux esophagitis, Systemic sclerosis

* Correspondence: dr_tasleem_arif@yahoo.com
[1]Postgraduate Department of Dermatology, STDs & Leprosy, Government Medical College, Srinagar, Jammu and Kashmir, India
[3]Postgraduate Department of Dermatology, STDs and Leprosy, Jawaharlal Nehru Medical College (JNMC), Aligarh Muslim University (AMU), Aligarh, India

Background

Systemic sclerosis (SSc) is a generalized disorder of unknown etiology affecting the connective tissue of the body. It affects the skin and various internal organs like gastrointestinal tract, lungs, heart and kidneys [1]. Gastrointestinal tract involvement is very common, affecting about 90% of the systemic sclerosis patients [2,3]. Esophagus is the most frequently affected part of the gastrointestinal tract [4]. Esophageal smooth muscle becomes atrophied and replaced by fibrous tissue leading to severe motility disturbance of distal esophagus [5,6]. Esophageal motility disturbance classically manifests as a reduced lower esophageal sphincter pressure (LESP) and loss of distal esophageal Body peristalsis [7-9]. As a consequence of this involvement, patients usually manifest with heartburn, dysphagia and regurgitation [10]. Heartburn and regurgitation are due to reflux of gastric juice across an incompetent lower esophageal sphincter (LES), whereas dysphagia may result from esophageal peptic stricture or disturbed esophageal peristalsis [11,12]. Esophageal complications like esophageal stenosis, Barrett esophagus and esophageal adenocarcinoma are more frequent in SSc than the general population [4,13-17].

Morphea, also called as localized scleroderma, predominantly involves the skin and occasionally involves subjacent muscles. However, it usually spares the internal organs. Morphea may range from small plaques to extensive disease with cosmetic and functional deformities [18]. The esophageal involvement in morphea has been studied scarcely and the data regarding this subject is meager. The present study was designed to investigate the esophageal involvement in the systemic (SSc) and localized (morphea) forms of scleroderma and to compare the same. It will also address any need of upper gastrointestinal evaluation in the morphea (localized scleroderma) patients.

Methods

This was a hospital based study carried out in the Postgraduate Department of Dermatology, Sexually Transmitted Diseases and Leprosy of Shri Maharaja Hari Singh (SMHS) Hospital (Associated teaching hospital of Government Medical College Srinagar) and the Department of Gastroenterology Sheri-Kashmir Institute of Medical Science (SKIMS) Soura. It was a prospective observational study involving the newly as well as already diagnosed patients of systemic sclerosis and morphea over a period of one and a half year (March 2011-August 2013). The study was approved by the ethical committees of the two hospitals viz., Institutional Ethics Committee (IEC) SKIMS and Ethical committee Government Medical College (EC-GMC) Srinagar. The diagnosis of systemic sclerosis was made according to the American Rheumatology Association (ARA) criteria [19]. Morphea was diagnosed

by the clinical and histopathological features after taking a standard punch biopsy of the skin.

Inclusion criteria: 1) All newly as well as already diagnosed patients of systemic sclerosis and morphea. 2) Both sexes were included. 3) Age ≥ 13 years.

Exclusion criteria: 1) Presence of pregnancy or a history of pregnancy in the last six months. 2) Age <13 years. 3) Other connective tissue disease or mixed connective tissue diseases. 4) Diabetes mellitus.

In the primary assessment, data collected included patient's age, gender, clinical characteristics of the disease (age at onset, duration), type of systemic sclerosis (diffuse or limited defined according to Le Roy classification [20]) and the presence or absence of symptoms of gastro-esophageal reflux disease (GERD) viz., heartburn, acid regurgitation and dysphagia. Each symptom was graded on a scale from 0 to 3 by intensity (0 = absent, 1 = mild, could be ignored by the patient, 2 = moderate, could not be ignored, but had no effect on daily life activities; 3 = severe or incapacitating, affecting daily life activities) and by frequency (0 = absent or less than one per month; 1 = less than 1 per week; 2 = several times per week; 3 = every day) [21]. Symptoms were then categorized as mild (score less than or equal to six), moderate (score of seven to twelve) and severe [score greater than twelve, or when one symptom was considered incapacitating every day (score = 9)]. Drugs which are known to suppress acid (Proton pump inhibitors and H2 blockers) or alter esophageal motility (anticholinergics, sedatives, antihypertensive and anti-angina drugs) were discontinued 2 weeks before inclusion. A proper consent (verbal and written) was given by the patient or his guardian before carrying out any procedure, for the participation in the study and for the consequent publication of the data which may also contain their personal details and their images. The patients were enrolled in the study only after meeting the above requirements of the consent.

Esophago-gastroduodenoscopy (EGD)

52 patients (out of total 56) of SSc and 28 patients (out of total 31) of morphea were undertaken for upper gastrointestinal endoscopy. Fibreoptic video-endoscope (Fujinon, EG-201FP, Japan) was used to look for the signs of esophagitis which was graded according to the Los Angeles classification for reflux esophagitis [22,23].

Esophageal manometry

This procedure was performed to measure lower esophageal sphincter pressure and amplitude of the body contractions of distal esophagus. Patients were instructed to wear loose clothes and avoid wearing necklace. The procedure was conducted in the supine position with the patient fasting over night. The manometric instrument used in our study (Red Tech, inc 26234 Alizaa Cnayon Dr.

Los Angeles, USA 91302) consisted of a special mutilumen (16 channel) catheter system. The catheter was connected to external pressure transducers. The catheter was continuously perfused with distilled water at a rate of 0.5 ml/min by a low compliance pneumohydraulic capillary infusion system. The catheter assembly was passed through the nose after applying xylocaine jelly locally until all recording orifices were in the stomach. The station pull-through of the lower esophageal sphincter (LES) was performed at one cm intervals. The LES pressure recorded was measured at end-expiratory variation to the mean gastric baseline pressure. At least, 10 wet swallows (10 ml water each) were administered; each separated by 30 seconds period. The amplitude of pressure wave was measured from the mean intraesophageal baseline pressure to the peak of the wave. Reference values for esophageal manometry were taken from Benjamin et al. [24].

Ambulatory 24-hour esophageal pH monitoring
This procedure was performed to objectively document abnormal reflux of gastric acidic contents into the lower esophagus and the consequent drop in lower esophageal pH. It was done after a standard esophageal motility study. Lower esophageal pH was measured with an esophageal probe (Antimony probe). The pH electrode was passed through the anesthetized nose of sitting patient into the stomach until acid pH was recorded. After that, the patient would remain supine and electrode was slowly withdrawn in the supine position. In each case a rapid pH change from acid to above pH 5 could be identified and pH electrode kept 5cms above this identified Zone (LES) already determined by manometric technique. The distance between the tip of the catheter and the nostril was recorded and kept constant for 24-hour esophageal pH study. The pH measuring unit was calibrated at 37°c using buffer solution of pH 4 and 7. The pH probe and reference electrodes were connected to a portable solid state recorder (Red Tech Medical Systems Pvt. Ltd) which is a family of portable self programmable data loggers for recording the biological variables completely based on micro processing technology. The esophageal pH measurements were stored and then transferred to a computer for analysis. The equipment used by us for pH manometry was an older version lacking the option for calculating the impedance-pH metry which is currently considered to be the gold standard for studying the gastroesophageal reflux disease. Reflux disease was considered abnormal if any of the following criteria were exceeded: 1) Percentage of total time with pH <4 (normal <5.5%); 2) Percentage of upright time with pH <4 (normal <8.2%); 3) Percentage of supine time with pH <4 (normal <3%) [8]; 4) De-Meesters Score (normal <14.7) [25]. Patients with abnormal reflux were considered as refluxers; those with upright reflux were classified as mild refluxers, supine as moderate and combined as having severe reflux.

Statistical analysis
The data collected was analyzed by using statistical package for social sciences (SPSS) Version 16.0. The following tests were also used: Chi-square test, Fischer's Exact test and Student's 't' test. A p value of < 0.05 was considered as statistically significant.

Results
Fifty six patients of SSc and 31 patients of morphea were taken up for the study. Among SSc patients, 50 (89.3%) were females and 6 (10.7%) were males with a female to male ratio of 8.3:1. The average age of the patient was 44.96 ± 13.80 years (21–80). Most of the patients 17 (30.4%) were in the age group of 50–59, followed by 40–49 (12, 21.4%) (Table 1). The average age of the onset of the disease in SSc in case of females was earlier (35.2 ± 13.3 years) than in males (42.3 ± 13.5 years) but it was statistically insignificant (p = 0.219). However, the average duration of disease in case of females was lesser (9 ± 7 years) than in males (9.3 ± 11.98) which was also statistically insignificant (p = 0.927). According to Le Roy classification, 40 (71.4%) patients belonged to limited variant of SSc (lSSc) while the remaining 16 (28.6%) patients were having the diffuse disease (dSSc).

Among 31 patients of morphea, females (24; 77.4%) outnumbered the males (7; 22.6%); the average age of the patient was 30.06 ± 10.45 years (14–58). Most of the patients were in the age group 20–29 (11; 35.5%) followed by 30–39 (10; 32.3%) and 10–19 (6; 19.4%) (Table 2). The average age of the onset of the disease in males (24.9 ± 5.96 years) was earlier than in females (28.5 ± 12.42 years) but it was not statistically significant (p = 0.463). Similarly, the mean duration of disease in case of males (2.1 ± 1.76 years) was lesser than in females (2.6 ± 2.34) which was also statistically not significant.

Table 1 Demographic profile of SSc (N = 56)

Age – group	Number	(%)
20 - 29	7	12.5%
30 - 39	10	17.9%
40 - 49	12	21.4%
50 - 59	17	30.4%
≥ 60	10	17.9%
Total	56	100%
Mean ± SD = 44.96 ± 13.80	Range = (21,80)	
SEX	**Number**	**%age**
Female	50	89.3%
Male	6	10.7%

Table 2 Demographic profile of morphea

Age-group	Number	(%)
10 - 19	6	19.4
20 - 29	11	35.5
30 - 39	10	32.3%
40 - 49	2	6.5%
50 -59	2	6.5%
Total	31	100%
Mean ± SD = 30.06 ± 10.45	*Range = (14,58)*	

SEX	Number	%age
Female	24	77.4%
Male	7	22.6%

The localized plaque type (Figure 1A) morphea was the commonest (21, 67.7%) morphological type seen followed by linear (Figure 1B) (7, 22.6%) and generalized (2, 6.5%) types. Only one (3.2%) patient of morphea Profundus was seen. However, no case of pansclerotic or en coup de sabre was encountered during our study period.

Among 56 patients of SSc, esophageal symptoms (heartburn and/or acid regurgitation and/or dysphagia) were seen in 39 (69.6%) patients; it was mild in 22 (39.3%), moderate in 14 (25%) and severe in 3 (5.3%). On the contrary, only 4 (12.9%) patients of morphea were having esophageal symptoms which were of mild severity and the difference between the two diseases was statistically significant (p < 0.001) (Table 3).

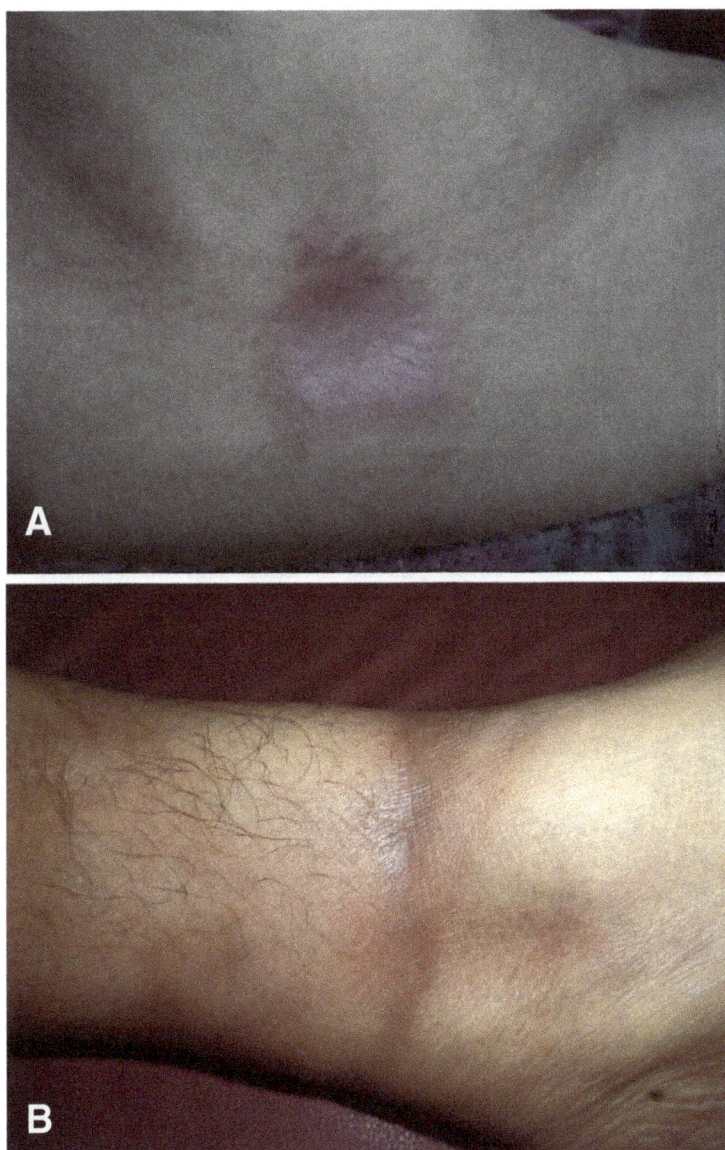

Figure 1 Clinical types of morphea. A Plaque type morphea: A brownish hyperpigmented indurated plaque over the upper chest in a 26 year old female. **B** Linear morphea: Brownish hyperpigmented indurated linear plaque encircling lower leg.

Table 3 Esophageal symptoms in SSc (N=56) and morphea (N=31)

	Mild symptoms	Moderate symptoms	Severe symptoms	Total symptomatic	P value, significance
Limited SSc (N=40)	15	9	1	25 (62.5%)	0.129 (Not Sig.)
Diffuse SSc (N=16)	7	5	2	14 (87.5%)	
Total SSc	22	14	3	39 (69.6%)	<0.001 (Sig.)
Morphea	4	0	0	04 (12.9%)	

Reflux esophagitis was seen 17 (32.7%) patients of SSc; it was grade A in 8 (15.4%), grade B in 5 (9.6%), grade C in 2 (3.8%) and grade D (Figure 2A) in only 1 (1.9%). Complicated esophagitis like stricture (Figure 2B) was seen in only 1 (1.9%) patient in our study. Only 2 (7.1%) patients of morphea had esophagitis both of which were of grade A severity and both of them had associated antral gastritis and one of them gave the history of non steroidal anti-inflammatory drug (NSAID) intake (Table 4). It should be noted here that the

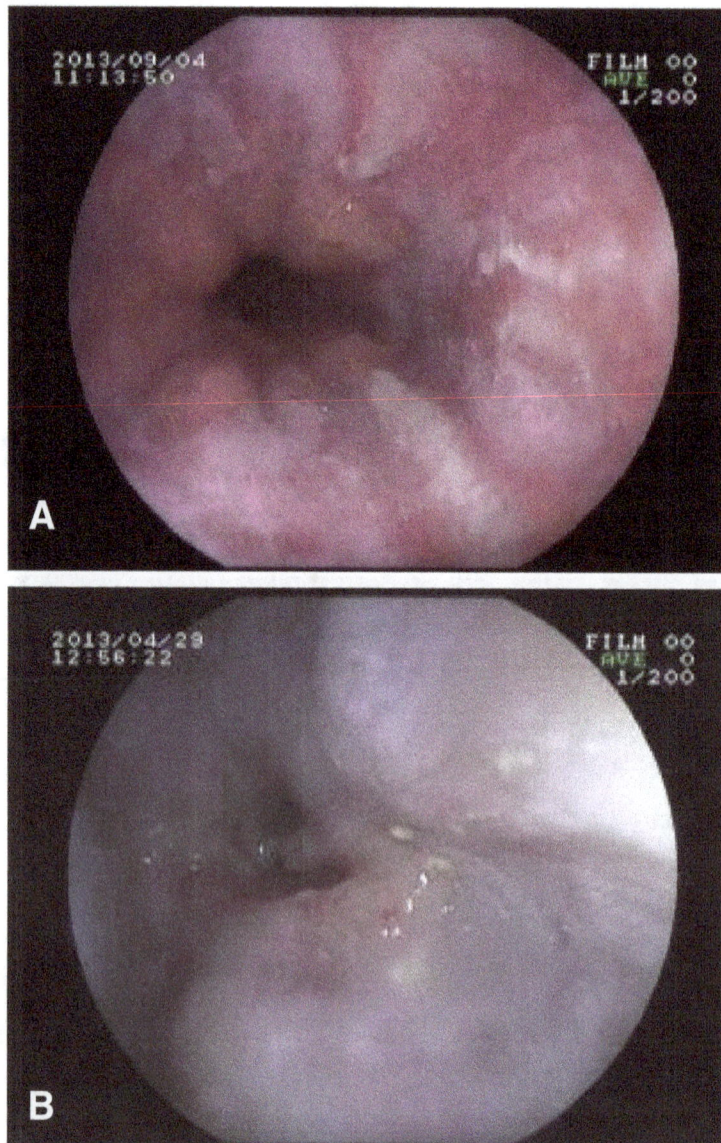

Figure 2 EGD in systemic sclerosis. A Grade D esophagitis: Circumferential involvement of lower esophagus involving more than 75% in systemic sclerosis. **B** Esophageal stricture: Narrowed lumen of the lower esophagus due to the longstanding esophagitis in systemic sclerosis.

Table 4 Reflux esophagitis in SSc and morphea

Grade	SSc (N=52)		Morphea (N=28)		P –value
	Number	%age	Number	%age	
A	8	15.4	2	7.1	
B	5	9.6	-	-	
C	2	3.8	-	-	0.022 (Sig.)
D	1	1.9	-	-	
Stricture	1	1.9	-	-	
Total Esophagitis	17/52	32.7	2/28	7.1	

prevalence of reflux esophagitis in SSc (32.7%) was more than that of morphea (7.1%) and the difference was statistically highly significant (p = 0.022).

Esophageal manometry was studied in 47 and 25 patients of SSc and morphea respectively to look for LES pressure and the contractions of distal body of esophagus. The mean LES pressure was lower (13.2 ± 11.8) in SSc as compared to morphea (31.94 ± 5.61) which was statistically significant (p = <0.001) revealing an overall low LES pressure in SSc patients. Similarly, the mean amplitude of the body of distal esophagus in SSc was less (30.1 ± 29.30) as compared to morphea (77.6 ± 9.38) and the difference was statistically significant (p < 0.001) (Table 5).

Abnormal manometry was seen in 32 (68.1%) patients of SSc. There was a low LES pressure in 25 (53.2%) patients and distal esophageal body dysmotility in 31 (66%) patients. Out of these 31 patients with esophageal motor disorder (EMD), 19 (40.4%) had hypoperistalsis while the remaining 12 (25.5%) had aperistalsis (Figure 3) (Table 6). On the other hand, none of the patients in the morphea revealed any abnormal manometry.

Forty one patients of SSc and 20 patients of morphea were studied for esophageal pH monitoring. Total reflux time percent, supine reflux time percent, upright reflux time percent and Demeesters score were abnormally high in SSc as compared to morphea patients and the difference was statistically highly significant in each of the four parameters studied. These results showed the significant involvement of esophagus in SSc in comparison to morphea (Table 7).

The abnormal reflux (Figure 4) was seen in 33 (80.5%) patients of SSc and they were considered as refluxers. Supine refluxers (15, 45.5%) were the commonest followed

Table 5 Esophageal manometry in SSc (N=47) and morphea (N=25)

Parameter	SSc (Mean, SD)	Morphea (Mean, SD)	P –value	Reference values
LES Pressure	(13.2,11.80)	(31.94, 5.61)	<0.001	10-26 mm Hg
Amplitude of contractions of distal esophagus	(30.1, 29.30)	(77.6, 9.38)	<0.001	50-110 mm Hg

by upright (13, 39.4%) and combined refluxers (5, 15.2%). However, in morphea no such abnormal reflux was demonstrated on pH monitoring (Table 8).

Discussion

In our study, females outnumbered males in both SSc and morphea patients which is in accordance with various studies [18,26]. Average age of onset of disease in the SSc patients in our study was earlier in females (fourth decade,35.2 years) than in males which was 42.3 years (5th decade). Similar observations were made by Medsger et al., who studied the epidemiology of SSc and found the peak onset of disease in females in the fourth decade and later in males [26]. The peak incidence of morphea has been estimated to be between 20 and 40 years of age in the literature [27,28]. Similar results were observed in our study as 67.8% of the morphea patients were in the age group 20–39.

Overall incidence of esophageal symptoms in SSc has been estimated between 42% and 79% [29-31]. In our study, the esophageal symptoms were present in 69.6% of the SSc patients which is well in between the range provided by the most published studies. The esophageal involvement in morphea is controversial. Weihrauch et al. studied 14 patients of morphea to assess esophageal involvement by radiography and manometry. Esophageal symptoms were found in only 3 (21.4%) patients [32]. However, in our study the esophageal symptoms were seen in 12.9% of morphea patients. The higher prevalence in the former may be due to their lower sample size. Our study showed a high prevalence of esophageal symptoms in SSc (69.9%) in comparison to the morphea patients (12.9%) which were statistically significant.

Prevalence of reflux esophagitis in SSc has averaged between 30% and 40%. In fact, it is variously reported between 3.2% and 60% [33-37]. Reflux esophagitis in our study, was seen in 32.7% of the patients which is supported by the above studies. Guariso et al. studied 14 patients of morphea for esophageal involvement in a pilot study. He found endoscopically proven esophagitis in 5 (35.7%) patients [38]. However, in our study, only 2 (7.1%) cases of esophagitis were seen revealing a less frequent involvement of esophagus in morphea compared to SSc. Moreover, both these morphea cases that had esophagitis, also had associated antral gastritis; and one of these two patients also gave the history of NSAID intake.

The overall frequency of manometric abnormalities reported in SSc has been very high ranging from 70 - 96%. Reduced LES pressure is present in more than 50% of cases; esophageal motor disorders (EMDs) in more than 60% of cases. Hypoperistalsis has been noted in 48%–81% of cases while aperistalsis in 23%–52% of patients

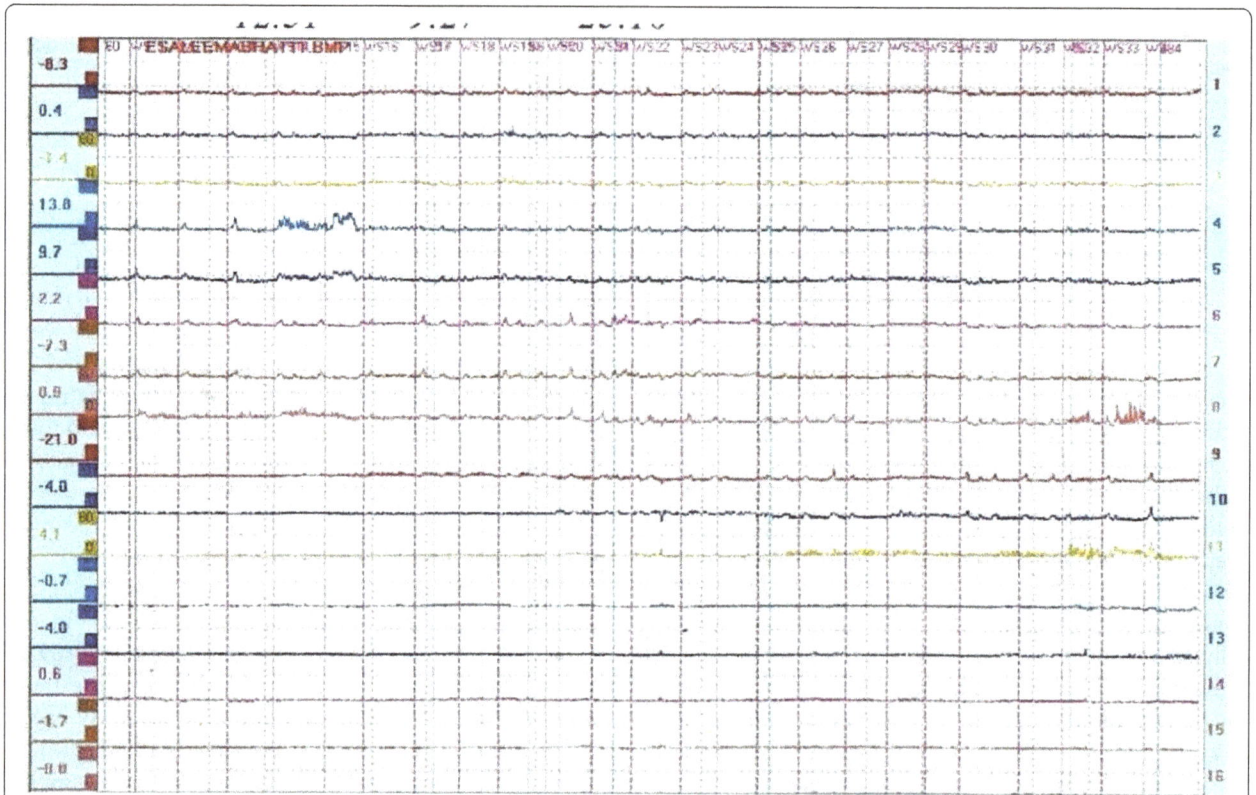

Figure 3 Esophageal manometry. Flat waves during esophageal manometry showing aperistalsis in SSc. Note that there are no appreciable esophageal body contractions.

[39]. Lahcene et al. [40] studied the prevalence and risk factors of esophageal motor disorders in systemic sclerosis and found the prevalence of esophageal motor disorders in 81% of patients and a hypotensive lower esophageal sphincter in 62% of the patients. Another study by Savarino, et al. [41] evaluated retrospectively abnormalities of esophageal motility, gastric emptying, oro-cecal transit time (OCTT) and small intestine bacterial overgrowth (SIBO) in a large cohort of SSc patients. Reduced LES pressure and ineffective esophageal motility was encountered in 70% of SSc patients [41]. In our study, the overall manometric abnormalities were seen in 68.1%; low LES pressure in 53.2%; EMDs in 66%; hypoperistalsis in 40.4% and severe aperistalsis in 25.5% cases. All our observations are in accordance with the most published studies. However, none of our morphea patients had any lower esophageal motor abnormalities which are in agreement with the study done by Weirauch et al. Thus, our study revealed a high prevalence of esophageal dysmotility in SSc patients and no such abnormality in morphea patients.

There are many causes of GERD in SSc. The reduction or absence of LES pressure is the primary facilitator of gastric acid reflux into the esophageal lumen. Esophageal dysmotility leads to impaired acid clearance and results in prolongation of esophageal exposure time to gastric acid. Delayed gastric emptying is also a promoter of GERD in SSc patients [42,43]. Currently, Impedance pH-metry is considered to be the gold standard for the diagnosis of GERD [44]. However, impedance pH-metry

Table 6 Esophageal manometry in SSc (N=47) and morphea (N=25)

Parameter	SSc Number	%age	Morphea Number	%age
Abnormal manometry	32	68.1	0	0
Low LES Pressure	25	53.2	0	0
Esophageal motor disorder(EMD)	31	66.0	0	0
-Hypoperistalsis	19	40.4	0	0
-Aperistalsis	12	25.5	0	0

Table 7 24-hour pH study in SSc and morphea

Parameter	SSc (Mean, SD)	Morphea (Mean, SD)	P –value	Reference values
Total reflux time percent	(8.5, 4.45)	(1.5, 0.85)	<0.001	<5.5%
Supine reflux time percent	(4.1, 3.80)	(0.6, 0.35)	<0.001	<3%
Upright reflux time percent	(6.1, 5.54)	(2.03, 1.22)	0.002	<8.2%
Demeesters score	(22.9, 13.9)	(3.5, 1.66)	<0.001	<14.7

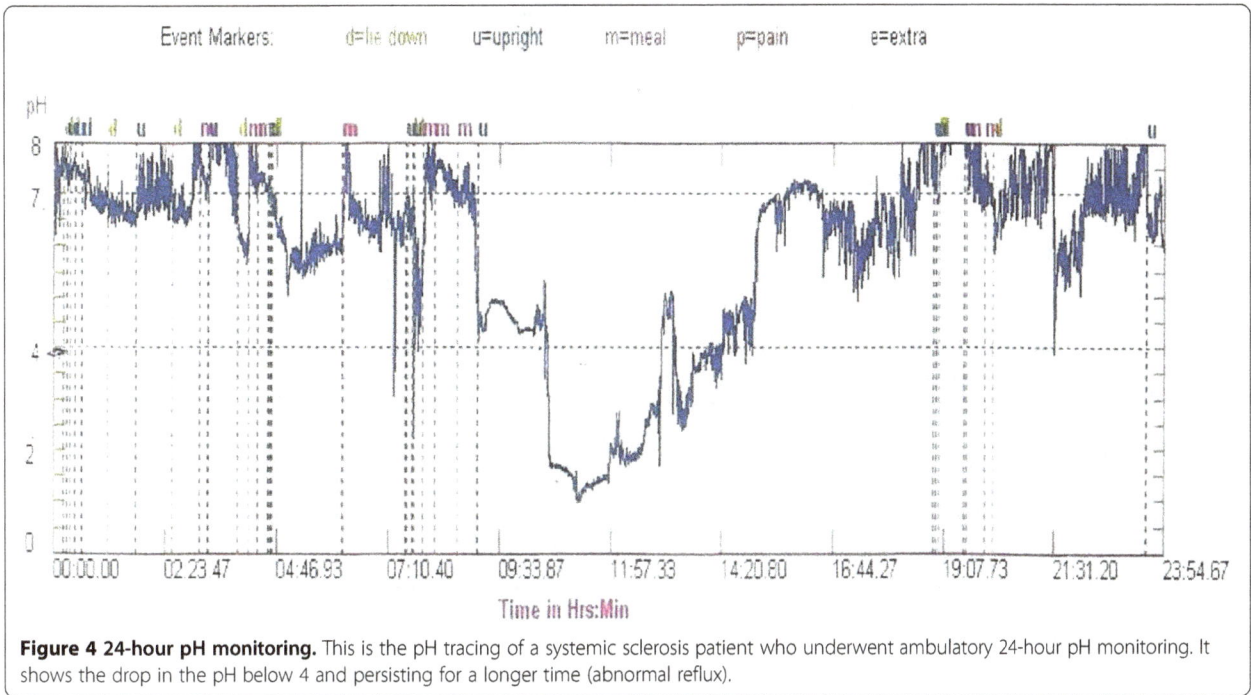

Figure 4 24-hour pH monitoring. This is the pH tracing of a systemic sclerosis patient who underwent ambulatory 24-hour pH monitoring. It shows the drop in the pH below 4 and persisting for a longer time (abnormal reflux).

was not done in our patients as our set up lacked the facility for the same. A study done by Zaninotto et al., showed reflux in 84.6% of the SSc cases; marked abnormalities in esophageal motility and in acid exposure in the distal esophagus were observed in SSc patients only [45]. Another study by Thonhofer et al. [46] investigated the upper GI-tract of patients suffering from SSc and mixed connective tissue disease (MCTD) and found dysmotility of the distal esophagus in 85% of their patients. In our study, abnormal reflux was seen in 80.5% of the cases of SSc. However, not a single case of abnormal reflux was documented in morphea patients. Hence, GERD is significant in SSc only. It should be noted that there were certain limitations in our study. Lack of controls, inability to study upper esophageal sphincter and impedance pH-metry were the limiting factors of the study.

Conclusion

Esophageal involvement in SSc is very frequent while its involvement in morphea is insignificant. Every patient of

SSc needs a meticulous upper gastrointestinal evaluation whether symptomatic or not. However, such an evaluation in morphea seems to be unjustified. It can be inferred that the referral of a SSc patient for EGD, manometry and 24-hour pH study can detect esophageal changes at the earliest and affect the future prognosis of the disease.

Abbreviations
SSc: Systemic sclerosis; LES: Lower esophageal sphincter; LESP: Lower esophageal sphincter pressure; ARA: American Rheumatology Association; GERD: Gastroesophageal reflux disease; EGD: Esophago-gastroduodenoscopy; SPSS: Statistical package for social sciences; lSSc: Limited SSc; dSSc: Diffuse SSc; NSAID: Non steroidal anti-inflammatory drug; EMD: Esophageal motor disorder.

Competing interests
The authors declare that they have no competing interests.

Authors' contributions
TA made the design of the study, collected data, performed statistical analysis and drafted the manuscript. JS carried out the endoscopy, manometry and pH-monitoring. QM and IH participated in the design of the study, coordinated and helped to draft the manuscript and made the final editing. All authors read and approved the final manuscript.

Author details
[1]Postgraduate Department of Dermatology, STDs & Leprosy, Government Medical College, Srinagar, Jammu and Kashmir, India. [2]Department of Gastroenterology, SKIMS, Soura, Srinagar, Kashmir, India. [3]Postgraduate Department of Dermatology, STDs and Leprosy, Jawaharlal Nehru Medical College (JNMC), Aligarh Muslim University (AMU), Aligarh, India.

References
1. Curzio C. Discussionil anatomico-pratiche di un raro, e stravagante morbo cutaneo in una giovane donna felicemente curato in questo grande

Table 8 24-hour pH study results in SSc (N=41) and morphea (N=20)

Parameter	SSc		Morphea	
	Number	Percent	Number	Percent
Total refluxors	33	80.5	0	0
Upright refluxors	13	39.4	0	0
Supine refluxors	15	45.5	0	0
Combined refluxors	5	15.2	0	0

ospedale degl' incurabili. Napoli, Presso Giovanni di Simone, 1753. Curzio C. An account of an extraordinary disease of the skin and its cure. Translated by R. Watson. Philosophical Trans 1754, 48:579

2. Yarze JC, Varga J, Stamfl D, Castell DO, Jimenez SA. Esophageal function in systemic sclerosis: a prospective evaluation of motility and acid reflux in 36 patients. Am J Gastroenterol. 1993;88:870–6.

3. Drane WE, Karvelis K, Johnson DA, Curran JJ, Silverman ED. Progressive systemic sclerosis: radionuclide esophageal scintigraphy and manometry. Radiology. 1986;160:73–6.

4. Poirier TJ, Ranklin GB. Gastrointestinal manifestation of progressive systemic scleroderma based on a review of 364 cases. Am J Gastroenterol. 1972;58:30–44.

5. Lock G, Pfeifer M, Straub RH, Zeuner M, Lang B, Scholmerich J, et al. Association of esophageal dysfunction and pulmonary function impairment in systemic sclerosis. Am J Gastroenterol. 1998;93:341–5.

6. Orringer MB, Dabich L, Zarafonetis CJD, Sloan H. Gastroesophageal reflux in esophageal scleroderma: diagnosis and implications. Ann Thorac Surg. 1976;22:120–30.

7. Murphy JR, McNally P, Peller P, Shay SS. Prolonged clearance is the primary abnormal reflux parameter in patients with progressive systemic sclerosis and esophagitis. Dig Dis Sci. 1992;37:833–41.

8. Petrokubi RJ, Jeffries GH. Cimetidine versus antacid in scleroderma with reflux esophagitis: a randomized double-blind controlled study. Gastroenterol. 1979;77:691–5.

9. Tang DM, Pathikonda M, Harrison M, Fisher RS, Friedenberg FK, Parkman HP. Symptoms and esophageal motility based on phenotypic findings of scleroderma. Diseases of the Esophagus. 2013;26:197–203. doi:10.1111/j.1442-2050.2012.01349.x.

10. Cohen S, Laufer I, Snape WJ, Shiau YF, Levine G, Jimenez S. The gastrointestinal manifestation of scleroderma: pathogenesis and management. Gastroenterol. 1980;79:155–66.

11. Summerling AM. Oesophageal changes in systemic sclerosis. Gut. 1966;7:402–8.

12. Turner R, Lipshutz W, Miller W, Rittenberg G, Schumacher HR, Cohen S. Esophageal dysfunction in collagen disease. Am J Med Sci. 1973;265:191–9.

13. Aubert A, Lazareth I, Vayssairat M, Fiessinger JN, Petite JP. L'oesophagite au cours de la sclérodermiesystémique. Prévalence-et-facteurs de survenue chez 46 patients. Gastroenterol Clin Biol. 1991;15:945–9.

14. Katzka DA, Reynolds JC, Saul SH, Plotkin A, Lang CA, Ouyang A, et al. Barrett's metapalasia and adenocarcinoma of the esophagus in scleroderma. Am J Med. 1987;82:46–52.

15. Wipff J, Allanore Y, Soussi T, Terris B, Abitbol V, Raymond J, et al. Prevalence of Barrett's esophagus in systemic sclerosis. Arthritis Rheum. 2005;52:2882–8.

16. Ebert EC. Esophageal disease in scleroderma. J Clin Gastroenterol. 2006;40:769–75.

17. Ntoumazios SK, Voulgari PV, Potsis K, Koutis E, Tsifetaki N, Assimakopoulos DA. Esophageal involvement in scleroderma: gastroesophageal reflux, the common problem. Semin Arthritis Rheum. 2006;36(3):173–81. Epub 2006 Oct 11.

18. Zancanaro PCQ, Isaac AR, Garcia LT, Costa IMC. Localized scleroderma in children: clinical, diagnostic and therapeutic aspects. An Bras Dermatol. 2009;84:161–72.

19. Subcommittee for Scleroderma Criteria of the American Rheumatism Association Diagnostic and Therapeutic Criteria Committee. Preliminary criteria for the classification of systemic sclerosis (scleroderma). Arthritis Rheum. 1980;23:58–90.

20. Le Roy EC, Black C, Fleischmajer R. Scleroderma (systemic sclerosis): classification, subsets and pathogenesis. J Rheumatol. 1988;15:202–5.

21. Dombal FT, Hall R. The evaluation of medical care from the clinician's point of view, what should we measure, and can we trust our measurements ? In evaluation of efficacy of medical action. Amsterdam: Elsevier-North Holland; 1979. p. 13–29.

22. Armstrong D, Bennett JR, Blum AL, Dent J, De Dombal FT, Galmiche JP, et al. The endoscopic assessment of esophagitis: a progress report on observer agreement. Gastroenterology. 1996;111:85–92.

23. Lundell L, Dent J, Bennett J, Blum A, Armstrong D, Galmiche J, et al. Endoscopic assessment of esophagitis: clinical and functional correlates and further validation of the Los Angeles classification. Gut. 1999;45:172–80.

24. Benjamin SB, Richter JE, Cordova CM, Knuff TE, Castell DO. Prospective manometric evaluation with pharmacologic provocation of patients with suspected esophageal motility dysfunction. Gastroenterology. 1983;84:893–901.

25. Mainie I, Tutuian R, Castell DO. Comparison between the combined analysis and the De Meester Score to predict response to PPI therapy. J clin Gastroenterol. 2006;40:602–5.

26. Medsger TA, Masi AT. Epidemiology of systemic sclerosis (scleroderma). Ann Intern Med. 1971;74:714–21.

27. Heite HJ. Ergebnisse häufi gkeitanalytischer Untersuchungen bei der Sklerodermie. Arch Dermatol Syphilol. 1955;200:426–33.

28. Christianson HB, Dorsey CS, Kierland RR, O'Leary PA. Localized scleroderma: a clinical study of 235 cases. Arch Dermatol. 1956;74:629–39.

29. Tuffanelli DL, Winkelman RK. Systemic scleroderma: a clinical study of 727 cases. Arch Dermatol. 1961;84:359–67.

30. Lock G, Holstege A, Lang B, Scholmerich J. Gastrointestinal manifestations of progressive systemic sclerosis. Am J Gastroenterol. 1997;92:763–71.

31. Rose S, Young MA, Reynolds JC. Gastrointestinal manifestations of scleroderma. Gastroenterol Clin North Am. 1998;27:563–94.

32. Weihrauch TR, Korting GW. Manometric assessment of oesophageal involvement in progressive systemic sclerosis, morphoea and Raynaud's disease. Brit J Dermatol. 1982;107:325–32.

33. Marie I, Ducrotté P, Denis P, Hellot MF, Levesque H. Oesophageal mucosal involvement in patients with systemic sclerosis receiving proton pump inhibitor therapy. Aliment Pharmacol Ther. 2006;24:1593–601.

34. Abu-Shakra M, Guillemin F, Lee P. Gastro-intestinal manifestations of systemic sclerosis. Semin Arthritis Rheum. 1994;24:29–39.

35. Zamost BJ, Hirschberg J, Ippolti AF, Furst DE, Clements PJ, Weinstein WN. Esophagitis in scleroderma. Prevalence and risk factors. Gastroenterology. 1987;92:412–8.

36. Hendel L. Esophageal and small intestinal manifestations of progressive systemic sclerosis. Dan Med Bull. 1994;41:371–85.

37. De Castro Parga ML, Alonso P, Garcia Porrua C, Prada JI. Esophageal mucosal lesions and scleroderma: prévalence, symptoms and risk factors. Rev Esp Enferm Dig. 1996;88:93–8.

38. Guariso G, Conte S, Galeazzi F, Vettorato MG, Martini G, Zulian F. Esophageal involvement in juvenile localized scleroderma: a pilot study. Clin Exp Rheumatol. 2007;25:786–9.

39. Lahcene M, Oumnia N, Matougui N, Boudjella M, Tebaibia A, Touchene B. Esophageal Involvement in Scleroderma: Clinical, Endoscopic, and Manometric Features. ISRN Rheumatology. 2011;2011:Article ID 325826. 5 pages, 2011. doi:10.5402/2011/325826.

40. Lahcene M, Oumnia N, Matougui N, Boudjella M, Tebaibia A, Touchene B. Esophageal dysmotility in scleroderma: a prospective study of 183 cases. Gastroenterol Clin Biol. 2009;33(6–7):466–9.

41. Savarino E, Mei F, Parodi A, Ghio M, Furnari M, Gentile A, et al. Gastrointestinal motility disorder assessment in systemic sclerosis. Rheumatology. 2013;52:1095–100.

42. Sallam H, Mcnearney TA, Chen JDZ. Systematic review: pathophysiology and management of gastrointestinal dysmotility in systemic sclerosis (scleroderma). Aliment Pharmacol Ther. 2006;23:691–712.

43. Gemignani L, Savarino V, Ghio M, Parodi A, Zentilin P, de Bortoli N, et al. Lactulose breath test to assess oro-cecal transit delay and estimate esophageal dysmotility in scleroderma patients. Semin Arthritis Rheum. 2013;42(5):522–9.

44. Pandolfino JE, Vela MF. Esophageal-reflux monitoring. Gastrointest Endosc. 2009;69(4):917–30.

45. Zaninotto G, Peserico A, Costantini M, Salvador L, Rondinone R. Oesophageal motility and lower oesophageal sphincter competence in progressive systemic sclerosis and localized scleroderma. Scand J Gastroenterol. 1989;24:95–102.

46. Thonhofer R, Siegel C, Trummer M, Graninger W. Early endoscopy in systemic sclerosis without gastrointestinal symptoms. Rheumatol Int. 2012;32:165–8.

11

Cyclin E involved in early stage carcinogenesis of esophageal adenocarcinoma by SNP DNA microarray and immunohistochemical studies

Zhongren Zhou[1][*], Santhoshi Bandla[2], Jiqing Ye[1], Yinglin Xia[3], Jianwen Que[4], James D Luketich[5], Arjun Pennathur[5], Jeffrey H Peters[2], Dongfeng Tan[6] and Tony E Godfrey[7]

Abstract

Background: Cyclin E is a cell cycle regulator which is critical for driving G1/S transition. Abnormal levels of cyclin E have been found in many cancers. However, the level changes of cyclin E in esophageal adenocarcinoma and its precancerous lesion have not been well studied. Here, we focus on the gene amplification and expression of cyclin E in these lesions, and aim to ascertain the relationship with clinicopathological characteristics.

Methods: Genomic DNA was analyzed from 116 esophageal adenocarcinoma and 26 precancerous lesion patients using Affymetrix SNP 6.0 arrays. The protein overexpression of cyclin E was also detected using immunohistochemistry from tissue microarrays containing esophageal adenocarcinoma and precancerous lesions. Patient survival and other clinical data were collected and analyzed. The intensity and percentage of the cyclin E expressing cells in tissue microarrays were scored by two pathologists. Fisher exact tests and Kaplan-Meier methods were used to analyze data.

Results: By genomic analysis, cyclin E was amplified in 19.0% of the EAC samples. By immunohistochemistry, high expression of cyclin E was observed in 2.3% of squamous mucosa tissues, 3.7% in columnar cell metaplasia, 5.8% in Barrett's esophagus, 19.0% in low grade dysplasia, 35.7% in high grade dysplasia, and 16.7% in esophageal adenocarcinoma. The differences in cyclin E high expression between neoplastic groups and non-dysplasia groups are statistically significant ($p < 0.05$). The prognosis for patients with high cyclin E expression appeared slightly better than for those with low cyclin E expression although this was not statistically significant ($p = 0.13$).

Conclusions: The expression of cyclin E significantly increases from non-dysplasia esophageal lesion to low and high grade dysplasia, suggesting that cyclin E plays an important role in the early stage of carcinogenesis. Importantly, cyclin E is also amplified and highly expressed in a subset of esophageal adenocarcinoma patients, but this increase is not associated with worse prognosis.

Keywords: Esophageal adenocarcinoma, Cyclin E, Amplification, High expression, Barrett's esophagus, SNP DNA microarray, Biomarker, Overall survival

* Correspondence: David_zhou@urmc.rochester.edu
[1]Departments of Pathology and Laboratory Medicine, University of Rochester, Rochester, 601 Elmwood Ave, Box 626, Rochester, NY 14642, USA
Full list of author information is available at the end of the article

Background

The incidence of esophageal adenocarcinoma (EAC) has increased approximately 600% in the US and other Western Countries over the last 30 years [1]. EAC tends to be diagnosed late with most patients in locally advanced or metastatic disease. Consequently, the overall prognosis for patients with EAC is very poor at approximately 15%, with 5-year overall survival. More than 50 percent of patients have either unresectable tumors or radiographically visible metastases at the time of diagnosis [2]. Identification of early biomarkers with high sensitivity and specificity will provide physicians with valuable information for surveillance, diagnosis, prognosis, and possible treatment options for esophageal adenocarcinoma. Previous studies have suggested that esophageal adenocarcinoma develops in the following order: normal esophageal epithelium, reflux esophagitis, Barrett's esophagus (BE), dysplasia, and finally esophageal adenocarcinoma [3]. During these events, a series of genetic and epigenetic aberrations contributes to the carcinogenesis, which will be potential biomarkers for early screening, surveillance and treatment of the dysplasia and adenocarcinoma.

Cyclin E, an activating subunit of cyclin dependent kinase 2 (*CDK2*), is encoded by human cyclin E1 gene (*CCNE1*) on chromosome 19q12-13. Cyclin E plays a key role to promote G1 cell cycle transition to S-phase. The oncogenic activity of cyclin E is involved in multiple functions including a regulatory network comprised CDK inhibitors, the p53 and FBW7 tumor suppressor pathways, signal transduction pathways, controlling cell cycle progression, and microRNAs [4,5]. Genetic and pharmacologic targeting of the cyclin E-CDK-2 complex resulted in marked growth inhibition of lung cancer cells [6], suggesting a potential chemotherapeutic approach for lung cancer. In breast cancer, the depletion of cyclin E by siRNA promoted apoptosis of cyclin E overexpressing cells and blocked their proliferation, transformation phenotype and tumor growth in nude mice. Liang and colleagues concluded that cyclin E may serve as a novel and effective therapeutic target [7]. In addition, the amplification and overexpression of cyclin E have been reported in a variety of cancers including breast [7,8], lung [9], ovarian [10], stomach [11,12], colorectal [13,14], bladder [15], endometrial carcinoma [16] and thyroid [17]. In the esophagus, a few studies found cyclin E amplification and overexpression in esophageal adenocarcinoma and precancerous lesion in small samples [18-21].

The cyclin E expression was first reported in low-grade dysplasia (2/21), high grade dysplasia (3/17), adenocarcinoma (5/35) and Barrett's esophagus (43%) in 60 samples by an immunohistochemistry [21,22]. Cyclin E gene amplification in esophageal adenocarcinoma was also confirmed in 13.8% (9/65) [19] and 12.6% (11 of 87) [20] in esophageal adenocarcinoma by quantitative PCR molecular analysis

[19,20]. However, the sample size of previous studies is small and the results were not consistent. In addition, the relationship between high expression of cyclin E or gene amplification and the patient survival is unknown.

In the current study, we (i) used high resolution SNP DNA microarray to study cyclin E amplification in the large scale of esophageal adenocarcinoma and precancerous lesions; (ii) used immunohistochemical method to confirm the high expression of cyclin E in a larger number of esophageal adenocarcinoma and precancerous lesions; and (iii) studied the association of cyclin E amplification and high expression with patients' overall survival and clinicopathological features.

Methods

Patients for Affymetrix SNP 6.0 analysis

Frozen tumors were obtained from 116 patients undergoing esophagectomy at the University of Pittsburgh Medical Center, Pittsburgh, PA between 2002 and 2008. Patient age ranged from 43–88 and the cohort consisted of 95 males and 21 females. Final pathologic stages were stage I (28), stage II (31), stage III (50) and stage IV (7). All tumor specimens were evaluated by a pathologist and were determined to be >70% tumor cell representation. Only 112 specimens were used for survival analysis as we excluded 4 peri-operative chemotherapy patients.

Frozen Barrett's esophagus (intestinal metaplasia: n = 26) and esophageal columnar cell metaplasia (metaplasia without goblet cells; n = 25) biopsy tissues were obtained from patients undergoing endoscopy at the University of Rochester Medical Center from 2008 to 2012. All pathologic diagnoses were evaluated by pathologists. All studies were approved by research subjects review board at University of Pittsburgh and University of Rochester.

Affymetrix SNP 6.0 analysis

Genomic DNA was isolated using the QiaAmp DNA Mini Kit (Qiagen, CA) and 600 mg was used for labeling and array hybridization at the SUNY Upstate Medical University microarray core facility (Syracuse, NY) using kits and protocols provided by Affymetrix. Data analysis was performed using Nexus 6.0 Copy Number Analysis software (Biodiscovery, Inc. CA). Log_2 DNA copy number ratios for the tumor and pre-neoplastic samples were generated in reference to a baseline file created using DNA from normal esophageal mucosa from a subset (n = 15) of the Pittsburgh patient cohort. Data was segmented using the SNP-Rank segmentation algorithm with a minimum of 8 probe sets and significance threshold of p-value of 10^{-6}. Log_2 copy number threshold for gains were set at +0.15 (~2.2 copies) while high level gains were set at +0.5 (~2.8 copies). More information on this patient cohort and a comprehensive genomic analysis of these tumors is to be published by Dulak et al [23]. Microarray data on this cohort has been submitted to the Gene Expression Omnibus (GSE36460) with an online link (http://www.ncbi.nlm.nih.gov/geo/query/acc.cgi?acc=GSE36460).

Construction of tissue microarray

Tissue microarrays, containing 34 cases of Barrett's esophagus (BE), 81 cases of columnar cell metaplasia (CCM), 86 cases of squamous epithelium (SE), 21 cases of low grade dysplasia (LGD), 14 cases of high grade dysplasia (HGD), and 117 cases of esophageal adenocarcinoma (EAC), were constructed from the representative areas of formalin-fixed specimens collected between 1997–2005 in the Department of Pathology and Laboratory Medicine, University of Rochester Medical Center/Strong Memorial Hospital, Rochester, New York. Five-micron sections were cut from tissue microarrays and were stained with H&E to confirm the presence of the expected tissue histology within each tissue core. Additional sections were cut for immunohistochemistry analysis.

Patients for tissue microarrays

All 117 patients with EAC used for the tissue microarray construction were treated with esophagectomy at Strong Memorial Hospital/University of Rochester from 1997 to 2005. These patients included 105 males and 12 females. The patients' ages ranged from 34 to 85 years (Table 1). The follow-up period after esophagectomy ranged from 0.3 to 142 months with a mean of 39 months.

Immunohistochemistry

Tissue sections from the tissue microarray were deparaffinized, rehydrated through graded alcohol, and washed with phosphate buffered saline. Antigen retrieval for cyclin E was performed by heating sections in 99°C water bath for 40 minutes. After endogenous peroxidase activity was quenched and nonspecific binding was blocked, ready-to-use mouse monoclonal antibody anti-cyclin E (Santa Cruz, CA) was incubated at room temperature for 30 minutes. The secondary antibody (Flex HRP) was allowed to incubate for 30 minutes. After washing, sections were incubated with Flex DAB Chromogen for 10 minutes and counterstained with Flex Hematoxylin

for 5 minutes. A colon adenocarcinoma with known cyclin E high expression served as positive control. Negative control was performed by replacing the anti-cyclin E antibody with the normal serum. Several tissue cores were falloff glass during this processing.

Scoring of immunohistochemistry

All sections were reviewed independently by JY and ZZ blinded to all clinical and pathologic information. Discordant cases were reviewed by both JY and ZZ and a final consensus was reached. The percentage (0-100%) of the cells with positive nuclear staining was recorded. The intensity of cyclin E nuclear staining was graded as 0, 1+, 2+, or 3+. No nuclear stain or positive nuclear stain in less than 10% was defined as 0 (Figure 1A); weakly nuclear stain in 10% or more cells was defined as 1+ (Figure 1B); relatively strong nuclear stain in 10% or more cells was defined as 2+ (Figure 1C); very strong nuclear stain in 10% or more cells was defined as 3+ (Figure 1D). Cyclin E protein was considered highly expressed if 10% or more of cells stained with a moderate to strong intensity (2+ and 3+, respectively) (Figure 1).

Statistical analysis

All the descriptive statistics in this study were presented as means. A P-value of less than 0.05 was considered statistically significant. The univariate analysis with cyclin E was conducted first and then followed with a multivariate analysis, including age, gender, and clinical covariates: lymph node metastasis and tumor stage. Chi-square and Fisher exact tests were used as appropriately to compare cyclin E positivity rates from columnar cell mucosa, dysplasia to adenocarcinoma. To evaluate the influence of high expression of cyclin E in esophageal adenocarcinoma, comparative risk analysis using the Kaplan-Meier method cooperated with the log-rank test was performed with cyclin E amplified and non-amplified groups. All the statistical analyses were conducted with SAS 9.3 software (SAS Institute Inc., Cary, NC).

Results

Genomic analysis of cyclin E amplification

Analysis of 116 EAC specimens using high density copy number microarrays revealed amplification of *CCNE1* in 19.0% (22/116) (Figure 2). In this cohort, the median overall survival of patients with *CCNE1* amplification was approximately 20 months compared with 25 months for those without amplification ($p = 0.22$). *CCNE1* amplification was not observed in Barrett's esophagus (0/26) or columnar cell metaplasia specimens (0/25).

Table 1 Distribution of patients in Age and Sex with esophageal adenocarcinoma and precancerous lesion using immunohistochemical study

Diagnosis	Total	Female	Male	Age
Adenocarcinoma	117	12	105	65
High grade dysplasia	14	2	12	67
Low grade dysplasia	21	0	21	71
Barrett's esophagus	34	4	30	67
Columnar cell metaplasia	81	7	74	64
squamous epithelium	86	19	67	65

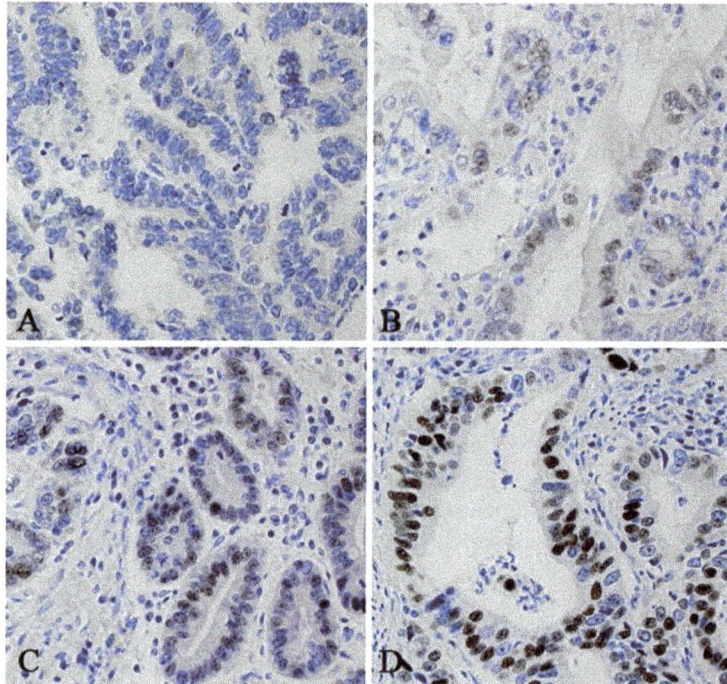

Figure 1 The intensity of cyclin E immunohistochemical study with nuclear staining. A. 0; Negative or very week intensity of cyclin E nuclear stain in one EAC sample; **B**. 1+: weak intensity of cyclin E nuclear stain in one EAC sample; **C**. 2+: moderate intensity of cyclin E nuclear stain in one EAC sample; and **D**. 3+: strong intensity of cyclin E nuclear stain in one EAC sample.

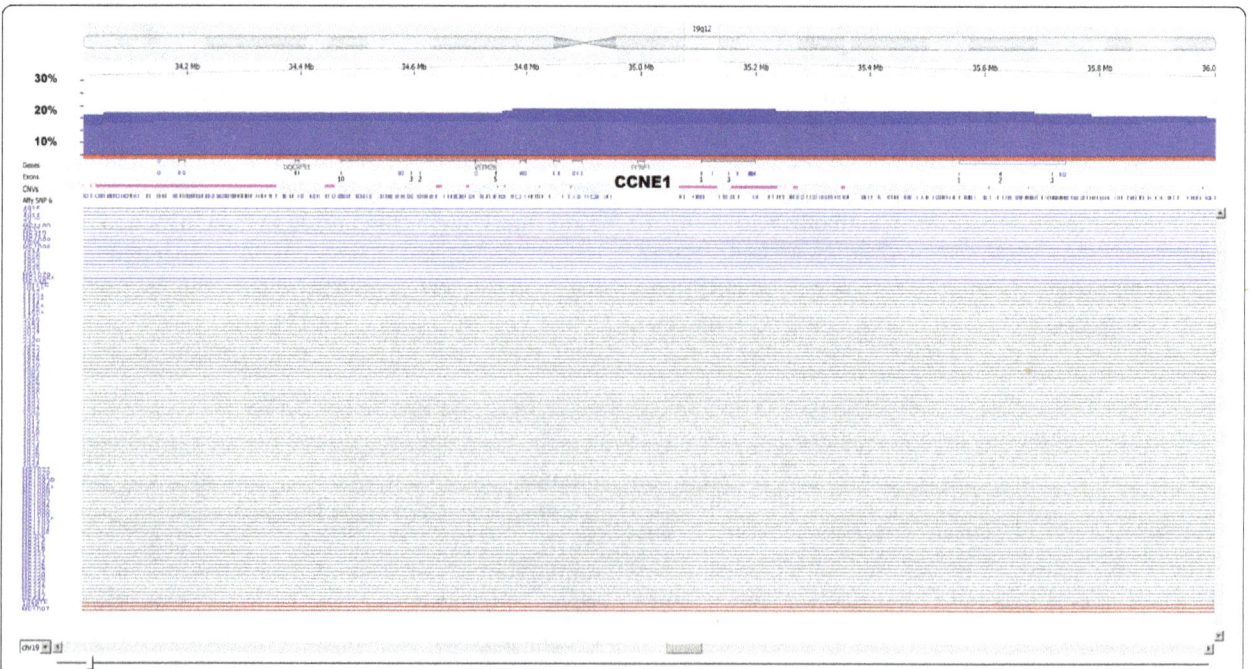

Figure 2 Frequency histogram showing amplification of the *CCNE1* locus at chromosome 19q12-13 in 116 esophageal adenocarcinoma samples using high density copy number SNP microarrays. This locus is amplified in 22/116 (19.0%) cases in this patient cohort, approximately half of which are considered high copy number amplification events.

Immunohistochemical characteristics and analysis of cyclin E expression

By immunohistochemical analysis, high expression of cyclin E was observed in 2.3% of normal squamous mucosa (2/86), 3.7% in columnar cell metaplasia (3/81), 5.8% in Barrett's esophagus (2/34), 19.0% in low grade dysplasia (4/21), and 35.7% in high grade dysplasia (5/14). In esophageal adenocarcinoma high cyclin E expression was observed in 16.7% (19/114) of cases. This was not statistically significantly different from high grade dysplasia. Qualitatively, we observed that normal squamous mucosa and columnar cell metaplasia usually have weak, focal staining whereas high grade dysplasia or adenocarcinoma have strong, diffuse staining (Table 2 and Figure 3).

Chi-square and Fisher exact tests were used to compare cyclin E percentages among all various histological groups including squamous epithelium, columnar cell mucosa, Barrett's esophagus, low- and high-grade dysplasia, and adenocarcinoma. The differences of cyclin E high expression between all neoplastic groups (including EAC, HGD and LGD) and non-dysplasia groups (including CCM and SE) are statistically significant (p < 0.05) (Table 3). No significant difference is identified among neoplastic groups. In addition, no significant difference of cyclin E high expression is identified between squamous mucosa and columnar cell metaplasia. Barrett's esophagus group is only significantly different from high grade dysplasia (Table 3).

Survival analysis of cyclin E high expression in EAC

Kaplan-Meier analysis and the log-rank test were used to calculate the effect of the cyclin E high expression in patients with EAC on survival. The mean overall survival in the cyclin E high expression group was 42 months, while that in the group without high cyclin E expression was 38 months. The log-rank test showed a trend towards better overall survival in the high-cyclin E group but this was not statistically significance ($p = 0.13$, Figure 4).

Multivariate survival analysis of clinical covariates including age, gender, histologic grade, and stage in EAC, found that age, differentiation and stage ($p < 0.05$) have strong association with patient survival, but gender ($p = 0.66$) was not significantly associated with patients' survival in EAC.

Correlation of cyclin E high expression and clinicopathological characteristics

The correlation of high cyclin E expression with clinicopathological features was analyzed. High expression of cyclin E is not associated with age, gender, stage, differentiation and lymph node metastasis (data not shown).

Discussion

In this study we found that cyclin E shows a significantly higher frequency of high expression in neoplastic lesions (low- and high-grade dysplasia or adenocarcinoma) compared to non-dysplastic tissues (Barrett's esophagus, columnar cell metaplasia and squamous epithelium). With SNP DNA microarray study, the amplification of cyclin E was also present in esophageal adenocarcinoma, but was not identified in Barrett's esophagus and columnar cell metaplasia. In addition, we found that high expression of cyclin E may be associated with better prognosis although this did not reach statistical significance.

Sarbia et al. first reported that the expression of cyclin E in esophagus tissues in small samples was present in 0 of 24 SE (0.0%), 2 of 21 LGD (9.5%), 3 of 17 HGD (17.6%), and 5 of 35 CA (14.3%) [22]. In our study, cyclin E shows similar frequency of high expression in 16.7% esophageal adenocarcinoma (19/114), but a higher frequency of expression in high grade dysplasia (35.7%) and low grade dysplasia (19.0%) compared to their study. In addition, we found that cyclin E is highly expressed with lower rates at 5.8% in Barrett's esophagus (2/34), 3.7% in columnar cell metaplasia (3/81), and 2.3% in squamous mucosa (2/86). Umansky et al. also reported the expression of cyclin E (43%), p16 (73%), p21 (88%), p27 (95%), and cyclin D1 (47%) in Barrett's esophagus, which was down-regulated by acid suppression of proton pump inhibition (PPI). However, no amplification or deletion was identified by Southern blot analysis [21]. This suggests that episodes of acid reflux might trigger proliferation and inhibit programmed cell death signaling pathways. In our study, no amplification was identified in Barrett's esophagus (0/26) and columnar cell metaplasia (0/25) by SNP DNA microarray method. However, high expression of cyclin E (5.8%) in BE is significant lower than that in Umansky's study (43%). The mechanism is unclear how cyclin E is highly expressed in BE and columnar cell metaplasia without the amplification. Cyclin E amplification was observed at 13.8% (9/65) [19] and 12.6% (11 of 87) [20] in esophageal adenocarcinoma, which is lower than our SNP DNA microarray data (19.0%).

Table 2 High expression of cyclin E in esophageal adenocarcinoma, low and high dysplasia, Barrett's esophagus, columnar cell metaplasia and squamous cells

Diagnosis	Non-/low expression (n; %)	High expression (n; %)	Total
squamous epithelium	84 (97.7)	2 (2.3)	86
Columnar cell metaplasia	78 (96.3)	3 (3.7)	81
Barrett's esophagus	32 (94.2)	2 (5.8)	34
Low grade dysplasia	17 (81.0)	4 (19.0)	21
High grade dysplasia	9 (64.3)	5 (35.7)	14
Adenocarcinoma	95 (83.3)	19 (16.7)	114

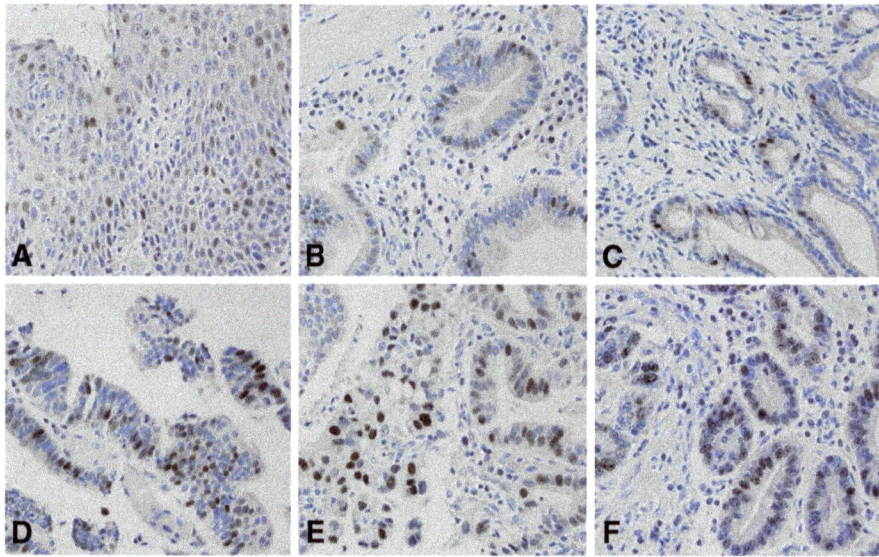

Figure 3 High expression of cyclin E in various histologic types by immunohistochemical studies. Cyclin E immunostain shows weakly nuclear stain in squamous mucosa **(A)**, columnar cell metaplasia **(B)** and Barrett's esophagus **(C)**. Cyclin E shows strong nuclear stain in low grade dysplasia **(D)**, high grade dysplasia **(E)** and adenocarcinoma **(F)**.

Cyclin E was reported to be expressed in precancerous lesion of colon adenocarcinoma [14,24,25]. Expression of cyclin E has been shown in 25% of colorectal adenomas, the most important precursor lesions of colorectal carcinoma [24]. With 1,2-dimethyl-hydrazine dihydrochloride

Table 3 Comparison of the frequency of cyclin E high expression between various groups by Fisher exact test (*p* value)

Group1	Group 2	p
SE	CCM	0.3060
SE	BE	0.2496
SE	LGD	0.0121*
SE	HGD	0.0014*
SE	AC	0.0011*
CCM	BE	0.3119
CCM	LGD	0.0277*
CCM	HGD	0.0014*
CCM	AC	0.0051*
BE	LGD	0.1158
BE	HGD	0.0153*
BE	AC	0.0890
LGD	HGD	0.1697
LGD	AC	0.2192
HGD	AC	0.0538

*The frequency of cyclin E high expression shows significantly different between these pairs.
CCM, Columnar cell metaplasia; BE, Barrett's Esophagus; LGD, Low grade dysplasia (LGD); HGD, High grade dysplasia; EAC, Esophageal adenocarcinoma; SE, Squamous epithelium.

(DMH)-induced rat colon adenocarcinoma, cyclin E expression was detected in 87.5% of the adenomas and in 92.3% of the adenocarcinomas [25]. Hur and colleagues also found that cyclin E expression both in the mRNA and protein levels was present in normal colonic mucosa, adenomas and adenocarcinomas. There was a significant difference in the degree of expression of cyclin E between normal mucosa and adenomas, but there was not a significant difference between adenomas and adenocarcinomas. They indicated that cyclin E plays an important role during the multistage process of rat colon carcinogenesis, especially at a relatively early stage [25]. In human samples, the increase of cyclin E expression also was reported in colon mucosa. The median of cyclin E expression significantly increased in normal through hyperplastic and adenomatous tissues and slightly decreased in adenocarcinoma of colon samples [14], which confirmed the finding in the rat model and proved that the expression of cyclin E promoted abnormal proliferation of cells during colorectal carcinogenesis [14]. In the esophagus, our data and previous studies also showed that the high expression of cyclin E significantly increased from non-dysplasia group (normal squamous epithelium, columnar cell metaplasia) to neoplastic group (low and high grade dysplasia). The high expression of cyclin E reached its peak in high grade dysplasia and decreased in adenocarcinoma. Our findings in the esophagus agree to the previous studies in colon. High expression of cyclin E may play an important role in early stage of carcinogenesis in esophagus and could be a potential targeted marker to early interfere with cancer progress and stratify high risk patients with precancerous lesion for close surveillance.

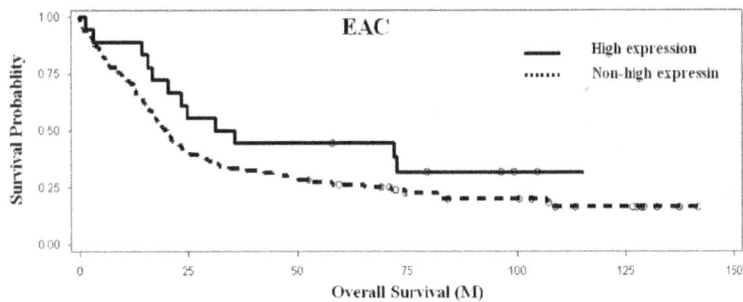

Figure 4 Kaplan-Meier analysis of overall survival associated with high cyclin E expression in esophageal adenocarcinoma. No significant association of overall survival with cyclin E high expression ($p = 0.13$) in 117 EAC patients.

Cyclin E and paired CDK 2 are important antineoplastic targets in oncology. siRNA treatment significantly reduced *CCNE1* or *cyclin E-CDK-2* complex expression and significantly inhibited cell growth in *CCNE1*-expressing cells, suggesting that *CCNE1*-targeted therapy may benefit ovarian, breast and lung cancer patients with *CCNE1* amplification [6,7,10]. In addition, cyclin E siRNA synergistically enhanced the cell killing effects of doxorubicin in cell culture and suppressed the tumor growth in mice. They concluded that cyclin E may serve as a novel and effective therapeutic target [7]. Our study showed both amplification and high expression of cyclin E in esophagus precancerous lesion and adenocarcinoma, suggesting the further study of potential effect in the inhibition of cyclin E expression for target therapy of esophageal precancerous lesion.

Amplification and high expression of cyclin E were reported to relate with poor prognosis in many different tumors [8-10,12,14-16,26]. In meta-analysis of lung non-small cell carcinoma from fourteen studies (2606 cases) [27], cyclin E over-expression was found to be a strong predictor of poor prognosis in lung carcinoma patients (HR: 1.38, 95% CI: 1.07-1.79; P = 0.014). In ovarian cancer, the amplification was identified in 18 (20%) of 88 ovarian carcinoma, which was significantly correlated with shorter disease-free survival and overall survival [10]. In gastric [11] and colorectal adenocarcinoma [28], overexpression of cyclin E was a potential prognostic markers. It is surprising to find both amplification and high expression of cyclin E in esophageal adenocarcinoma in our study were not significantly associated with patient overall survival, even with a little better overall survival rate with high expression of cyclin E. The controversial data for the prognosis was reported in the colon [29,30], ovary [31], stomach [11,12] and lung [9]. In the esophagus, similar to the cyclin E study, we recently found that HER2 amplification and expression were associated with better but not significantly better prognoses [32], which is confirmed by a Mayo clinical study [33]. They further proved that HER2 positivity was significantly

associated with a better survival. Therefore, the function of oncogene may play different roles in various organs or tumors. Furthermore, our findings needs to be confirmed by different studies since the cyclin E expression and amplification are associated with the sensitivity of methods, race of patients, location of tumors and preoperative neoadjuvant therapy.

Conclusions

The high expression of cyclin E significantly increases from non-dysplasia esophageal lesion, to low and high grade dysplasia. It implies that cyclin E may play an important role in early stage of carcinogenesis and could be a potential marker for a target therapy of precancerous lesion. In addition, the amplification and high expression of cyclin E are associated with a better prognosis, but not statistically significant.

Competing interests
The authors declare that they have no competing interests.

Authors' contributions
ZZ and TG: Designing the project; ZZ: Write the paper. ZZ, TG, JQ and DT: editing the paper and consultation for the project. ZZ and JY: Scoring all IHC slides from TMA; YX: Involving data analysis; TG and SB: Analyzing SNP DNA microarray data; JP, AP, and DT: Collecting the clinicopathological information and tissue. All authors read and approved the final manuscript.

Acknowledgements
We thank Dr. Jorge Yao for tissue microarray construction. We thank Qi Yang and Loralee McMahon for immunohistochemistry.
All studies were approved by research subjects review board at University of Pittsburgh and University of Rochester. Written informed consent was obtained from the patient for the publication of this report and any accompanying images.

Author details
[1]Departments of Pathology and Laboratory Medicine, University of Rochester, Rochester, 601 Elmwood Ave, Box 626, Rochester, NY 14642, USA. [2]Departments of Surgery, University of Rochester, Rochester, NY, USA. [3]Biostatistics and Computational Biology, University of Rochester, Rochester, NY, USA. [4]Biomedical Genetics, University of Rochester, Rochester, NY, USA. [5]Department of Cardiothoracic Surgery, University of Pittsburgh Medical Center, Pittsburgh, PA, USA. [6]Department of Pathology, The University of Texas MD Anderson Cancer Center, Houston, TX, USA. [7]Department of Surgery, Boston University School of Medicine, Boston, MA, USA.

References

1. Pohl H, Welch HG: The role of overdiagnosis and reclassification in the marked increase of esophageal adenocarcinoma incidence. *J Natl Cancer Inst* 2005, **97**(2):142–146.
2. Locke GR 3rd, Talley NJ, Fett SL, Zinsmeister AR, Melton LJ 3rd: Prevalence and clinical spectrum of gastroesophageal reflux: a population-based study in Olmsted County, Minnesota. *Gastroenterology* 1997, **112**(5):1448–1456.
3. Enzinger PC, Mayer RJ: Esophageal cancer. *N Engl J Med* 2003, **349**(23):2241–2252.
4. Siu KT, Rosner MR, Minella AC: An integrated view of cyclin E function and regulation. *Cell Cycle* 2012, **11**(1):57–64.
5. Stamatakos M, Palla V, Karaiskos I, Xiromeritis K, Alexiou I, Pateras I, Kontzoglou K: Cell cyclins: triggering elements of cancer or not? *World J Surg Oncol* 2010, **8**:111.
6. Galimberti F, Thompson SL, Liu X, Li H, Memoli V, Green SR, DiRenzo J, Greninger P, Sharma SV, Settleman J, Compton DA, Dmitrovsky E: Targeting the cyclin E-Cdk-2 complex represses lung cancer growth by triggering anaphase catastrophe. *Clin Cancer Res* 2010, **16**(1):109–120.
7. Liang Y, Gao H, Lin SY, Goss JA, Brunicardi FC, Li K: siRNA-based targeting of cyclin E overexpression inhibits breast cancer cell growth and suppresses tumor development in breast cancer mouse model. *PLoS One* 2010, **5**(9):e12860.
8. Keyomarsi K, Tucker SL, Buchholz TA, Callister M, Ding Y, Hortobagyi GN, Bedrosian I, Knickerbocker C, Toyofuku W, Lowe M, Herliczek TW, Bacus SS: Cyclin E and survival in patients with breast cancer. *N Engl J Med* 2002, **347**(20):1566–1575.
9. Kosacka M, Piesiak P, Porebska I, Korzeniewska A, Dyla T, Jankowska R: Cyclin A and Cyclin E expression in resected non-small cell lung cancer stage I-IIIA. *In Vivo* 2009, **23**(4):519–525.
10. Nakayama N, Nakayama K, Shamima Y, Ishikawa M, Katagiri A, Iida K, Miyazaki K: Gene amplification CCNE1 is related to poor survival and potential therapeutic target in ovarian cancer. *Cancer* 2010, **116**(11):2621–2634.
11. Jang SJ, Park YW, Park MH, Lee JD, Lee YY, Jung TJ, Kim IS, Choi IY, Ki M, Choi BY, Ahn MJ: Expression of cell-cycle regulators, cyclin E and p21WAF1/CIP1, potential prognostic markers for gastric cancer. *Eur J Surg Oncol* 1999, **25**(2):157–163.
12. Choi MG, Noh JH, An JY, Hong SK, Park SB, Baik YH, Kim KM, Sohn TS, Kim S: Expression levels of cyclin G2, but not cyclin E, correlate with gastric cancer progression. *J Surg Res* 2009, **157**(2):168–174.
13. Aamodt R, Jonsdottir K, Andersen SN, Bondi J, Bukholm G, Bukholm IR: Differences in protein expression and gene amplification of cyclins between colon and rectal adenocarcinomas. *Gastroenterol Res Pract* 2009, **2009**:285830.
14. Li JQ, Miki H, Ohmori M, Wu F, Funamoto Y: Expression of cyclin E and cyclin-dependent kinase 2 correlates with metastasis and prognosis in colorectal carcinoma. *Hum Pathol* 2001, **32**(9):945–953.
15. del Pizzo JJ, Borkowski A, Jacobs SC, Kyprianou N: Loss of cell cycle regulators p27(Kip1) and cyclin E in transitional cell carcinoma of the bladder correlates with tumor grade and patient survival. *Am J Pathol* 1999, **155**(4):1129–1136.
16. Cassia R, Moreno-Bueno G, Rodriguez-Perales S, Hardisson D, Cigudosa JC, Palacios J: Cyclin E gene (CCNE) amplification and hCDC4 mutations in endometrial carcinoma. *J Pathol* 2003, **201**(4):589–595.
17. Wang S, Wuu J, Savas L, Patwardhan N, Khan A: The role of cell cycle regulatory proteins, cyclin D1, cyclin E, and p27 in thyroid carcinogenesis. *Hum Pathol* 1998, **29**(11):1304–1309.
18. Sarbia M, Bektas N, Muller W, Heep H, Borchard F, Gabbert HE: Expression of cyclin E in dysplasia, carcinoma, and nonmalignant lesions of Barrett esophagus. *Cancer* 1999, **86**(12):2597–2601.
19. Lin L, Prescott MS, Zhu Z, Singh P, Chun SY, Kuick RD, Hanash SM, Orringer MB, Glover TW, Beer DG: Identification and characterization of a 19q12 amplicon in esophageal adenocarcinomas reveals cyclin E as the best candidate gene for this amplicon. *Cancer Res* 2000, **60**(24):7021–7027.
20. Miller CT, Moy JR, Lin L, Schipper M, Normolle D, Brenner DE, Iannettoni MD, Orringer MB, Beer DG: Gene amplification in esophageal adenocarcinomas and Barrett's with high-grade dysplasia. *Clinical Cancer Res* 2003, **9**(13):4819–4825.
21. Umansky M, Yasui W, Hallak A, Brill S, Shapira I, Halpern Z, Hibshoosh H, Rattan J, Meltzer S, Tahara E, Arber N: Proton pump inhibitors reduce cell cycle abnormalities in Barrett's esophagus. *Oncogene* 2001, **20**(55):7987–7991.
22. Sarbia M, Stahl M, Fink U, Heep H, Dutkowski P, Willers R, Seeber S, Gabbert HE: Prognostic significance of cyclin D1 in esophageal squamous cell carcinoma patients treated with surgery alone or combined therapy modalities. *Int J Cancer* 1999, **84**(1):86–91.
23. Dulak AM, Schumacher SE, Van Lieshout J, Imamura Y, Fox C, Shim B, Ramos AH, Saksena G, Baca SC, Baselga J, Tabernero J, Barretina J, Enzinger PC, Corso G, Roviello F, Lin L, Bandla S, Luketich JD, Pennathur A, Meyerson M, Ogino S, Shivdasani RA, Beer DG, Godfrey TE, Beroukhim R, Bass AJ: Gastrointestinal adenocarcinomas of the esophagus, stomach, and colon exhibit distinct patterns of genome instability and oncogenesis. *Cancer Res* 2012, **72**(17):4383–4393.
24. Yasui W, Kuniyasu H, Yokozaki H, Semba S, Shimamoto F, Tahara E: Expression of cyclin E in colorectal adenomas and adenocarcinomas: correlation with expression of Ki-67 antigen and p53 protein. *Virchows Arch* 1996, **429**(1):13–19.
25. Hur K, Kim JR, Yoon BI, Lee JK, Choi JH, Oh GT, Kim DY: Overexpression of cyclin D1 and cyclin E in 1,2-dimethylhydrazine dihydrochloride-induced rat colon carcinogenesis. *J Vet Sci* 2000, **1**(2):121–126.
26. Ma Y, Fiering S, Black C, Liu X, Yuan Z, Memoli VA, Robbins DJ, Bentley HA, Tsongalis GJ, Demidenko E, Freemantle SJ, Dmitrovsky E: Transgenic cyclin E triggers dysplasia and multiple pulmonary adenocarcinomas. *Proc Natl Acad Sci U S A* 2007, **104**(10):4089–4094.
27. Huang LN, Wang DS, Chen YQ, Li W, Hu FD, Gong BL, Zhao CL, Jia W: Meta-analysis for cyclin E in lung cancer survival. *Clin Chim Acta* 2012, **413**(7-8):663–668.
28. Corin I, Larsson L, Bergstrom J, Gustavsson B, Derwinger K: A study of the expression of Cyclin E and its isoforms in tumor and adjacent mucosa, correlated to patient outcome in early colon cancer. *Acta Oncol* 2010, **49**(1):63–69.
29. Bondi J, Husdal A, Bukholm G, Nesland JM, Bakka A, Bukholm IR: Expression and gene amplification of primary (A, B1, D1, D3, and E) and secondary (C and H) cyclins in colon adenocarcinomas and correlation with patient outcome. *J Clin Pathol* 2005, **58**(5):509–514.
30. Ioachim E: Expression patterns of cyclins D1, E and cyclin-dependent kinase inhibitors p21waf1/cip1, p27kip1 in colorectal carcinoma: correlation with other cell cycle regulators (pRb, p53 and Ki-67 and PCNA) and clinicopathological features. *Int J Clin Pract* 2008, **62**(11):1736–1743.
31. Bedrosian I, Lu KH, Verschraegen C, Keyomarsi K: Cyclin E deregulation alters the biologic properties of ovarian cancer cells. *Oncogene* 2004, **23**(15):2648–2657.
32. Hu Y, Bandla S, Godfrey TE, Tan D, Luketich JD, Pennathur A, Qiu X, Hicks DG, Peters JH, Zhou Z: HER2 amplification, overexpression and score criteria in esophageal adenocarcinoma. *Mod Pathol* 2011, **24**(7):899–907.
33. Yoon HH, Shi Q, Sukov WR, Wiktor AE, Khan M, Sattler CA, Grothey A, Wu TT, Diasio RB, Jenkins RB, Sinicrope FA: Association of HER2/ErbB2 expression and gene amplification with pathologic features and prognosis in esophageal adenocarcinomas. *Clin Cancer Res* 2012, **18**(2):546–554.

12

The prevalence of gastric heterotopia of the proximal esophagus is underestimated, but preneoplasia is rare - correlation with Barrett's esophagus

Ulrich Peitz[1,2]* , Michael Vieth[3], Matthias Evert[4], Jovana Arand[1], Albert Roessner[5] and Peter Malfertheiner[1]

Abstract

Background: The previously reported prevalence of gastric heterotopia in the cervical esophagus, also termed inlet patch (IP), varies substantially, ranging from 0.18 to 14%. Regarding cases with adenocarcinoma within IP, some experts recommend to routinely obtain biopsies from IP for histopathology. Another concern is the reported relation to Barrett's esophagus. The objectives of the study were to prospectively determine the prevalence of IP and of preneoplasia within IP, and to investigate the association between IP and Barrett's esophagus.

Methods: 372 consecutive patients undergoing esophagogastroduodenoscopy were carefully searched for the presence of IP. Biopsies for histopathology were targeted to the IP, columnar metaplasia of the lower esophagus, gastric corpus and antrum. Different definitions of Barrett's esophagus were tested for an association with IP.

Results: At least one IP was endoscopically identified in 53 patients (14.5%). Histopathology, performed in 46 patients, confirmed columnar epithelium in 87% of cases, which essentially presented corpus and/or cardia-type mucosa. Intestinal metaplasia was detected in two cases, but no neoplasia. A previously reported association of IP with Barrett's esophagus was weak, statistically significant only when short segments of cardia-type mucosa of the lower esophagus were included in the definition of Barrett's esophagus.

Conclusions: The prevalence of IP seems to be underestimated, but preneoplasia within IP is rare, which does not support the recommendation to regularly obtain biopsies for histopathology. Biopsies should be targeted to any irregularities within the heterotopic mucosa. The correlation of IP with Barrett's esophagus hints to a partly common pathogenesis.

Keywords: Gastric heterotopia, Inlet patch, Esophagus, Preneoplasia, Intestinal metaplasia, Barrett's esophagus

Background

Islands of gastric mucosa in the proximal esophagus are commonly designated as inlet patches (IP). They are considered to be heterotopic in nature in that they represent remnants of the columnar lining of the fetal esophagus. Discussed sequelae of clinical significance are laryngitis, esophagitis, esophageal web, stricture, ulcer, perforation, fistula or adenocarcinoma [1]. Severe sequelae are rare, reported only in individual case reports. More than fifty cases of adenocarcinoma arising from an IP have been reported between 1950 and 2016 (literature reviews [2, 3], recent case reports [2, 4–12]). Some experts recommend to take biopsies from IP in order to detect neoplastic or preneoplastic alterations [13–15], or advise follow-up examinations [15, 16]. Before such recommendations can be generalized, more data on the prevalence of preneoplastic alterations in IP are needed.

Data on the very prevalence of IP diverge a lot. Prospective studies have yielded higher prevalences, ranging from 1 to 14% [15, 17–33], than studies with retrospective design, 0.18 to 1.6% [13, 17, 34–41].

* Correspondence: u.peitz@raphaelsklinik.de
[1]Clinic of Gastroenterology, Hepatology, and Infectious Diseases, Otto-von-Guericke University, Leipziger Str. 44, D 30120 Magdeburg, Germany
[2]Clinic of Gastroenterology, Raphaelsklinik, Münster, Germany

Preneoplastic conditions or lesions of IP are not yet defined. IP may contain any type of mucosa of the normal stomach, i.e. antrum, corpus or cardia mucosa, but also intestinal metaplasia [15, 19, 21, 26, 27, 31, 35, 38, 39, 41, 42]. In the stomach, *Helicobacter pylori* infection, mucosal atrophy and intestinal metaplasia (Correa cascade) increase the risk of gastric adenocarcinoma [43, 44]. In the lower esophagus, Barrett's esophagus is an established preneoplasia. But there are differing definitions of Barrett's esophagus regarding the type of columnar metaplasia. The risk for esophageal adenocarcinoma is lower with pure gastric metaplasia than with intestinal metaplasia. Among others, American and German guidelines require the presence of intestinal metaplasia to define Barrett's esophagus [45–47]. Retrospective publications have indicated that there is an association between the presence of IP and that of Barrett's esophagus [25, 29, 35, 36, 38, 48] or even adenocarcinoma of the lower esophagus [38, 48].

The aims of the study were to determine the prevalence of IP in a prospective endoscopic study, to characterize the type of columnar epithelium within these IP, in particular with respect to preneoplastic conditions, and to investigate the association between IP and Barrett's esophagus.

Methods
Patients
The study was based on patients referred for esophagogastroduodenoscopy (EGD) to the endoscopy unit of the University Magdeburg. Prior to starting the prospective study, the prevalence of IP was determined retrospectively. By searching the electronic files from January 1996 through January 2002, fifty patients with endoscopic description of IP were retrieved out of 9928 EGD, corresponding to a frequency of 0.5%.

The prospective study lasted from February to June 2002. It was approved by the Ethics Committee of our university and conformed to the provisions of the Declaration of Helsinki. Patients gave written informed consent. During the five months period, the prevalence of IP was determined in consecutive patients endoscopically examined by one investigator (UP). Of the 444 EGDs he performed the following were excluded: emergency cases ($n = 31$), percutaneous endoscopic gastrostomy ($n = 5$), patients after esophagus resection ($n = 4$), malignant tumor ($n = 2$) or severe esophagitis ($n = 4$) in the proximal part of the esophagus, repetitive endoscopies during the study period ($n = 26$). All other patients with consent ($n = 372$) were included, irrespective of the indication. For statistical analysis, indications were dichotomized into dominant reflux symptoms ($n = 93$) versus the remainder ($n = 279$). Outpatients were 175, inpatients 197.

Endoscopy
EGD was performed using routine video-endoscopes (GIF Q 145, Olympus Optical, Hamburg, Germany). An endoscopic diagnosis of IP was made when an island of salmon red velvety mucosa was identified in the proximal esophagus. The number of IP and the maximum diameter of the largest IP were documented. An attempt was made to take biopsies from IP for histological evaluation in any patient concerned, but contraindications against biopsies or technical difficulties in taking biopsies were respected and documented. Biopsies from gastric antrum and corpus were obtained according to the updated Sydney protocol [49].

Any pathology revealed by EGD was documented, as was conscious sedation, mainly midazolam iv, partly in combination with pethidin iv. The quality of visualization of the esophageal mucosa was graded into a 3-point scale.

Any columnar epithelium extending more than 0.5 cm proximal to the esophago-gastric junction, be it in form of tongues, islands or circumferential areas, were documented as "columnar epithelium lined lower esophagus" (CLE) and, if not contraindicated, biopsied for histopathology according to guidelines on Barrett's esophagus [50, 51]. The length of CLE and the maximum diameter of IP were estimated using an open biopsy forceps, or, in cases with long segments, comparing the distance from the incisors.

Histopathology
Histological slides were stained with hematoxilin-eosin and a modified Giemsa stain (2%) to detect *Helicobacter pylori* bacteria. In cases with doubtful *Helicobacter pylori* status, Warthin-Starry stain was used in addition. Detection of goblet cells led to diagnosis of intestinal metaplasia.

Categories of Barrett's esophagus
Based on the endoscopically determined length of CLE and the histopathological detection of columnar epithelium with or without intestinal metaplasia, four categories with different definitions of Barrett's esophagus were tested as independent variables: (1) CLE of at least 0.5 cm length, any columnar epithelium; (2) CLE of at least 3 cm length, any columnar epithelium; (3) CLE of at least 0.5 cm length, columnar epithelium with intestinal metaplasia, (4) CLE of at least 3 cm length, columnar epithelium with intestinal metaplasia.

Statistics
The expected prevalence of IP was estimated at 6%, based on the average of previous data of prospective studies in the literature. To achieve a width of 5% for the 95%-confidence interval of the proportion of patients with IP (prevalence), a sample size of $n = 350$

was calculated. The differences between the proportions of cases with and without IP in relation to different independent variables were statistically analyzed using non-parametric tests. Two-sided P values of less than 0.05 were considered to be statistically significant. The statistical software used was IBM SPSS Statistics 24™.

Results

Out of the 372 patients included, at least one IP was identified endoscopically in 54 cases (14.5%, 95% confidence interval 10.9%–18.1%). Demographic data are shown in Table 1. More males than females had IPs detected (18 vs 11%), but the difference was not statistically significant. There was an insignificant trend for a higher prevalence of IP between 50 and 70 years of age compared to the prevalence in younger or older subjects (Fig. 1).

All IPs were located in the cervical part of the esophagus, mostly within 1 to 5 cm distal to the upper esophageal sphincter, but partly also at the level of the sphincter. Although the detection rate of IP increased with the grade of visualization, this correlation was not significant. There was no correlation with the use of conscious sedation.

A single IP was observed in 37 cases. In 17 patients there were multiple IPs; 2 of them in 9; 3 IPs in 5; and 5 to 7 IPs in 3 cases. The maximum diameter of the largest IP ranged from 0.2 to 4 cm (Fig. 2). A scatter diagram of the maximum diameter is shown in Fig. 3.

In 46 patients with visible IP, at least one biopsy could be targeted to the IP (1 biopsy in $n = 7$; 2 biopsies in $n = 24$; 3 in $n = 14$; and 5 in $n = 1$ patients). Reasons for not obtaining biopsies were uneasiness or retching in 6, and coagulation disorders in 2 patients. Columnar epithelium could be confirmed in $n = 40$ (87%) of these patients. Cardia- and corpus-type mucosa were found at an almost equal frequency (Table 2).

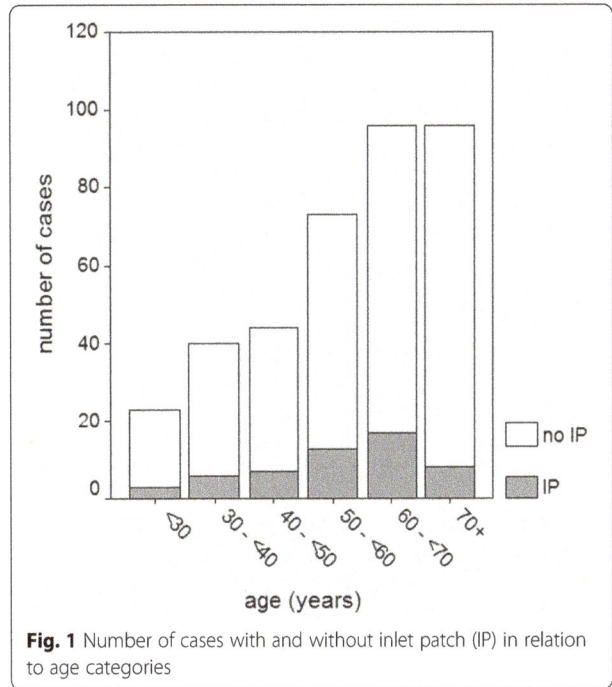

Fig. 1 Number of cases with and without inlet patch (IP) in relation to age categories

Biopsies from small IPs tended to contain more often cardia-type mucosa (Fig. 4), while those from larger IPs were more frequently composed of corpus mucosa. At the border between columnar and squamous cell epithelium, cardia-type mucosa was the predominant type of columnar mucosa (Fig. 5).

There were 277 patients with a complete set of biopsies from the gastric antrum and corpus, and, if endoscopically detected, from IP. The prevalence of IP in this subgroup was $n = 43$ (15.5%) by endoscopy, and $n = 36$ (12.9%) confirmed by histopathology. In gastric biopsies, *Helicobacter pylori* bacteria were detected in $n = 45$ (16%). Five of these

Table 1 Demographic data of patients with and without IP

	Patients with IP	Patients without IP	Level of statistical significance
Number	$n = 54$	$n = 318$	
Gender, number (percentage of columns)			Chi square test $p = 0.09$
Female	$n = 21$(39%)	$n = 163$ (49%)	
Male	$n = 33$ (61%)	$n = 155$ (51%)	
Age (years)			Mann-Whitney test $p = 0.44$
Minimum	19	18	
Median	57	60	
Maximum	89	93	

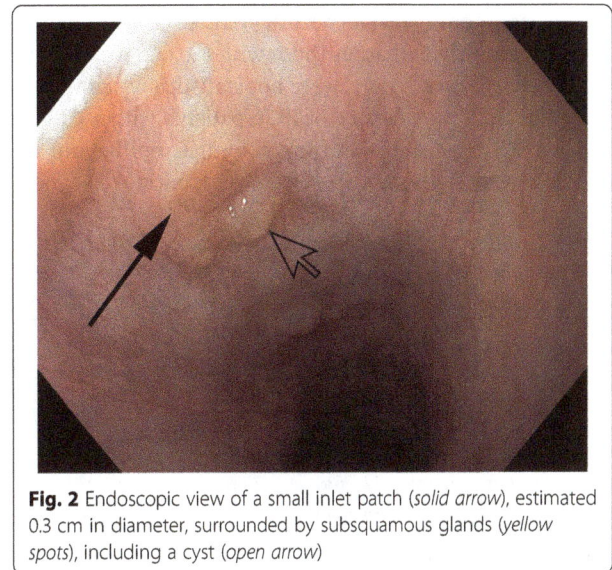

Fig. 2 Endoscopic view of a small inlet patch (*solid arrow*), estimated 0.3 cm in diameter, surrounded by subsquamous glands (*yellow spots*), including a cyst (*open arrow*)

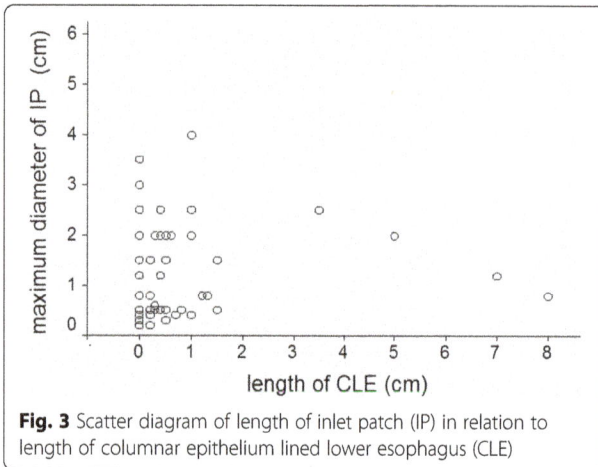

Fig. 3 Scatter diagram of length of inlet patch (IP) in relation to length of columnar epithelium lined lower esophagus (CLE)

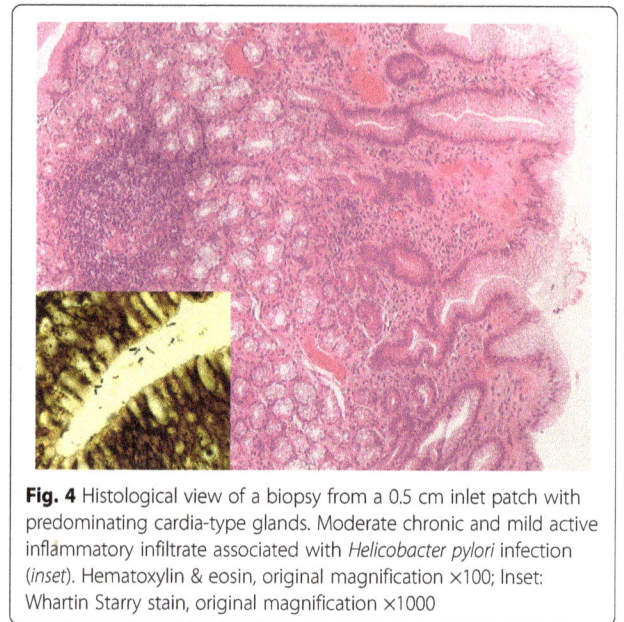

Fig. 4 Histological view of a biopsy from a 0.5 cm inlet patch with predominating cardia-type glands. Moderate chronic and mild active inflammatory infiltrate associated with *Helicobacter pylori* infection (*inset*). Hematoxylin & eosin, original magnification ×100; Inset: Whartin Starry stain, original magnification ×1000

were found with an IP, but only one had *Helicobacter pylori* detected also in his IP (Fig. 4). Overall, mild chronic inflammation of IP was present in 37, moderate in 4 cases (Figs. 4, 5 and 6). Active inflammatory infiltration of IP was always mild and occurred in 8 patients, including the one with *Helicobacter pylori*. The presence of chronic or active inflammation of IP was correlated neither with the presence of *Helicobacter pylori* infection of the stomach nor with any of the gastroesophageal reflux parameters mentioned below.

Within IP, we observed intestinal metaplasia in two cases (Fig. 6). One 59-year-old patient had a single IP of 0.5 cm diameter, the other, aged 65 years, a single IP of 2.5 cm. Both were males with reflux symptoms, but without CLE. In both cases intestinal metaplasia was focal. Only the latter patient exhibited focal intestinal metaplasia also in the corpus.

The relationship between IP and parameters of gastroesophageal reflux are shown in Table 3. Although the prevalence of IP was higher in patients with dominant reflux symptoms, hiatal hernia, reflux esophagitis, or Barrett's esophagus than in those without these respective conditions, these relations were not statistically significant. Only the higher prevalence of IP in patients with a CLE of at least 0.5 cm length and any columnar epithelium on histology was significant ($p = 0.02$, odds ratio 2.1). There

was no significant correlation between the grade of reflux esophagitis and the presence of IP, nor between the length of CLE and the presence of IP, and nor between the length of CLE and the maximum diameter of IP (Fig. 3).

In the total study sample, the following pathological findings were documented in addition to those of Table 3: esophageal thrush 3%, esophageal tumor 1%, esophageal varices 7%, esophageal peptic stenosis 1%, gastric ulcer 7%, gastric erosions 16%, gastric tumor 2%, previous distal gastric resection 2%, duodenal ulcer 2%, duodenal erosions 2%, duodenal stenosis 1%. None of these were significantly related to IP. A complete normal finding in

Table 2 Histology of IP in all patients with biopsy targeted to IP, and separately in two subgroups stratified according to maximum diameter of IP (percentages of columns)

	All patients with biopsy, n = 46	Maximum diameter of IP	
		<1 cm, n = 24	≥1 cm, n = 22
	Number (%)	Number (%)	Number (%)
Cardia mucosa	16 (35%)	10 (42%)	6 (27%)
Cardia plus corpus mucosa	12 (26%)	7 (29%)	5 (23%)
Corpus mucosa	12 (26%)	4 (17%)	8 (36%)
Only squamous epithelium	6 (13%)	3 (12%)	3 (14%)

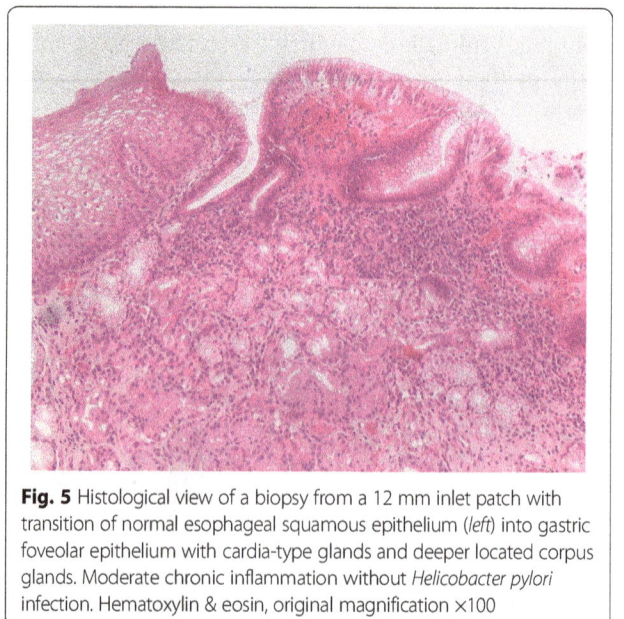

Fig. 5 Histological view of a biopsy from a 12 mm inlet patch with transition of normal esophageal squamous epithelium (*left*) into gastric foveolar epithelium with cardia-type glands and deeper located corpus glands. Moderate chronic inflammation without *Helicobacter pylori* infection. Hematoxylin & eosin, original magnification ×100

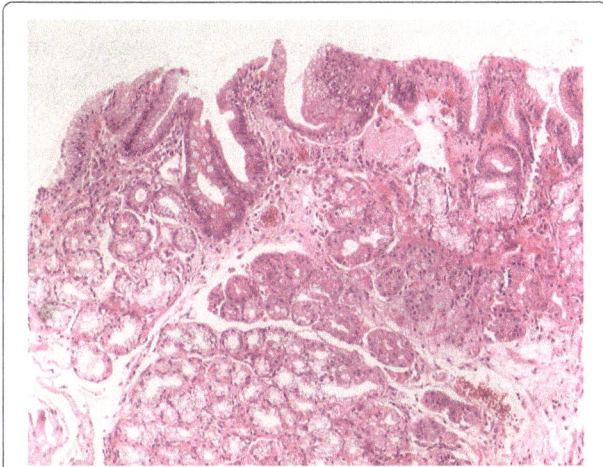

Fig. 6 Histological view of a biopsy from a 2.5 cm inlet patch with a combination of mucoid cardia-type and corpus-type glands and superficial focal intestinal metaplasia. Few subepithelial lymphocytes and plasma cells indicate a very mild chronic inflammatory reaction. Hematoxylin & eosin, original magnification ×100

the upper gastrointestinal tract was observed in 201 (54%) cases.

Discussion

The 14.5% prevalence of IPs revealed in this study is the highest ever reported as an English full text of a clinical study, to the best of our knowledge. But some studies report prevalences close to this, 10% by Borhan-Manesh et al. [18], 11% by Weickert et al. [27], 12% by Chung et al. [30] using narrow band imaging, 13% by Vesper et al. [33] and 14% by Kumagai et al. [23]. In an abstract, Ohara et al. [52] report even 21%, also using narrow band imaging. The same prevalence of 21% was yielded by an autopsy series of infants and children [53]. In contrast, in the retrospective part of our study, the prevalence was low (0.5%), within the range of previously reported

retrospective studies (0.18 to 1.6%) [13, 17, 34–41]. The discrepancy between retrospective and prospective studies is a clear indication that retrospective data comprise endoscopies in which IPs were often overlooked or neglected.

Nevertheless, IP should be looked for, and, if present, mentioned in examination reports. IP may give rise to benign or malignant sequelae, even though very rarely. Recent case reports on adenocarcinoma in IP include cases with small and flat lesions, fairly discernible from benign IP [6, 11]. Furthermore, IP should be distinguished from early esophageal squamous neoplasia, which also exhibits a flat red discoloration.

Like in the stomach and in Barrett's esophagus, intestinal metaplasia of IP may represent a preneoplastic condition. It has been described to occur in conjunction with an adenocarcinoma of IP [10, 54–56]. However, there are no long-term data on the risk of neoplasia emerging from intestinal metaplasia of IP. In those 40 cases with histologically confirmed IP of our study, the prevalence of intestinal metaplasia was $n = 2$ (5%), admittedly a number too small to representatively estimate the proportion. This proportion is of similar magnitude as in other studies reporting intestinal metaplasia in IP, ranging from 0 to 12% [15, 19, 21, 26, 27, 31, 35, 38, 39, 41, 42]. The two largest studies provided proportions of 1% [38] respectively 3% [39].

The high prevalence of IP in relation to the limited number of published cases with adenocarcinoma originating from IPs [2–12] challenges the recommendation given by some experts to obtain biopsies for histopathology from any IP [13–15]. Furthermore, taking biopsies in the proximal esophagus often provokes retching or coughing which makes it an uncomfortable or even risky approach. In our series, the low proportion of cases with intestinal metaplasia and the lack of any neoplasia within IP do not support such a recommendation.

Table 3 Relation of the prevalence of IP with gastroesophageal reflux parameters and with different categories of Barrett's esophagus

	Prevalence of IP in the condition	Prevalence of the condition in patients with IP	Prevalence of the condition in patients without IP	Level of statistical significance (Fisher's exact test, two-sided)
	Number (%)	Number (%)	Number (%)	
Dominant reflux symptoms	15/93 (16%)	15 (27%)	78 (24%)	$p = 0.61$
Hiatal hernia	13/83 (16%)	13 (24%)	70 (22%)	$p = 0.74$
Reflux esophagitis	14/75 (19)%	14 (26%)	61 (19%)	$p = 0.25$
CLE ≥ 0.5 cm	21/95 (22%)	21 (39%)	74 (23%)	$p = 0.02$
CLE ≥ 3 cm	4/18 (22)%	4 (7%)	14 (4%)	$p = 0.31$
CLE ≥ 0.5 cm with IM	7/30 (23%)	7 (13%)	23 (7%)	$p = 0.15$
CLE ≥ 3 cm with IM	3/14 (21%)	3 (6)%	11 (4%)	$p = 0.44$

CLE columnar epithelium lined lower esophagus (endoscopic diagnosis)
IM intestinal metaplasia (histopathologic diagnosis)

However, any irregularity of the mucosal surface of an IP identified on endoscopic examination should prompt taking targeted biopsies.

An high association of IP with Barrett's esophagus was reported in previous publications [25, 29, 35, 36, 38, 48], but not confirmed by other studies [13, 18, 57]. We tested four different definitions of Barrett's esophagus for an association with IP. The reason is that in different guidelines there are conflicting definitions with respect to the histopathological verification of Barrett's esophagus. Some guidelines consider the presence of intestinal metaplasia as mandatory [45–47], whereas others require only columnar epithelium [50, 58]. Cardia-type mucosa in the lower esophagus has consistently been shown to be an acquired type of mucosa [59–61], and is likely to be a precursor of intestinal metaplasia [62] and of adenocarcinoma as well [63]. Therefore, we took into account also cases with endoscopically detected columnar lining in the lower esophagus ("CLE") that exhibited only cardia-type mucosa on histological evaluation, but no intestinal metaplasia. Only for this category of CLE, there was a significant association with IP.

One limitation of the study is that patients from a tertiary referral center were examined rather than a sample from the general population. Certainly, such patients are not representative of the general population, but currently there are no data to give consistent evidence that IPs might be significantly correlated with any other pathology, except for the relation with Barrett's esophagus.

Another limitation is the delay between the study and its publication. Advanced endoscopic modalities like high density resolution, near focus and virtual chromoendoscopy were not yet applicable, but might ameliorate the detection rate of IP. However, Vesper et al. [33] found a high prevalence of IP (13.3%), which was comparable and not significantly different among standard definition videoendoscopy (12.7%), high definition endoscopy (14.4%), and narrow-band imaging (14.2%).

Endoscopic diagnosis of IP was confirmed by histopathology in 87%, which reduces the prevalence of IP to 12.6% as calculated for the whole study sample, or to 12.9% as counted in the subgroup of cases with a complete set of biopsies from stomach and esophagus. The most probable explanation for cases with endoscopic diagnosis of IP, but without histological confirmation, is unsuccessful targeting of the biopsy to a very small IP.

Half of our patients with IP had a maximum diameter of the largest IP of less than 1 cm (Table 2). The small IPs were mostly composed of cardia-type mucosa, whereas the larger ones were more likely to contain corpus mucosa centrally. In the vicinity of IPs within squamous epithelium, one frequently observes yellow spots (Fig. 2). These were not taken into account as IP in our study. They contain foci of subsquamous columnar epithelium, addressed by some pathologists as esophageal glands proper. Noteworthy, these yellow spots resemble those in squamous epithelium close to the squamocolumnar junction of the esophagogastric junction [64]. Esophageal submucosal glands are known to be clustered at either end of the esophagus [65]. A convincing though unproven concept is, that such foci represent a precursor of columnar metaplasia of the esophagus [66]. According to this concept, intraepithelial cysts erupt to the surface to build the columnar metaplasia. Our observation of very small IPs on the top of such yellow spots support the existence of such a dynamic process (Fig. 2).

Conclusions

The prevalence of IPs is often underestimated because IP may be overlooked or neglected. Regular biopsies for histopathology from any IP cannot be recommended because preneoplasia within IP is rare. Careful endoscopic inspection of IP, however, seems to be worthwhile in order to detect early malignancy and to differentiate IP from squamous cell neoplasia. The relation of IP with Barrett's esophagus, though clinically of minor relevance, may stimulate research on the common pathogenesis of IP and Barrett's esophagus.

Abbreviations
CLE: columnar epithelium lined lower esophagus; IM: intestinal metaplasia; IP: Inlet patch

Acknowledgements
We are grateful to all the patients who participated in this study. Special thanks go to the staff of the Endoscopy Unit of the Otto-von-Guericke University, Magdeburg, head Jutta Blumrich.

Funding
No funding was recieved.

Authors' contributions
UP designed the study, collected and analysed the data, performed the endoscopies and drafted the manuscript. MV, ME and AR were involved in designing the study, performed the histopathology and revised the manuscript critically for important intellectual content. JA was involved in designing the study, collecting and analyzing the data and drafting the manuscript. She revised the manuscript critically. PM was involved in designing the study, and revised the manuscript critically for important intellectual content. All authors read and approved the final manuscript.

Competing interests
The authors declare that they have no competing interests.

Author details
[1]Clinic of Gastroenterology, Hepatology, and Infectious Diseases, Otto-von-Guericke University, Leipziger Str. 44, D 30120 Magdeburg,

Germany. ²Clinic of Gastroenterology, Raphaelsklinik, Münster, Germany. ³Institute of Pathology, Klinikum Bayreuth, Bayreuth, Germany. ⁴Institute of Pathology, University Regensburg, Regensburg, Germany. ⁵Institute of Pathology, Otto-von-Guericke University, Magdeburg, Germany.

References

1. von Rahden BH, Stein HJ, Becker K, Liebermann-Meffert D, Siewert JR. Heterotopic gastric mucosa of the esophagus: literature-review and proposal of a clinicopathologic classification. Am J Gastroenterol. 2004;99(3):543–51.
2. Kitajima T, Kaida S, Lee S, Haruta S, Shinohara H, Ueno M, Suyama K, Oota Y, Fujii T, Udagawa H. Mixed adeno(neuro)endocrine carcinoma arising from the ectopic gastric mucosa of the upper thoracic esophagus. World J Surg Oncol. 2013;11:218.
3. Komori S, Osada S, Tanaka Y, Takahashi T, Nagao N, Yamaguchi K, Asano N, Yoshida K. A case of esophageal adenocarcinoma arising from the ectopic gastric mucosa in the thoracic esophagus. Rare Tumors. 2010;2(1):e5.
4. Kadota T, Fujii S, Oono Y, Imajoh M, Yano T, Kaneko K. Adenocarcinoma arising from heterotopic gastric mucosa in the cervical esophagus and upper thoracic esophagus: two case reports and literature review. Expert Rev Gastroenterol Hepatol. 2016;10(3):405–14.
5. Hudspeth VR, Smith DS, Pacicco T, Lewis JJ. Successful endoscopic resection of adenocarcinoma arising in an esophageal inlet patch. Dis Esophagus. 2016;29(7):880–2.
6. Probst A, Schaller T, Messmann H: Adenocarcinoma arising from ectopic gastric mucosa in an esophageal inlet patch: treatment by endoscopic submucosal dissection. Endoscopy 2015, 47 Suppl 1 UCTN:E337–338.
7. Nomura K, Iizuka T, Inoshita N, Kuribayashi Y, Toba T, Yamada A, Yamashita S, Furuhata T, Kikuchi D, Matsui A, et al. Adenocarcinoma of the cervical esophagus arising from ectopic gastric mucosa: report of two cases and review of the literature. Clin J Gastroenterol. 2015;8(6):367–76.
8. Ajmal S, Young JS, Ng T. Adenocarcinoma arising from cervical esophageal gastric inlet patch. J Thorac Cardiovasc Surg. 2015;149(6):1664–5.
9. Yasar B, Tarcin O, Benek D, Goksel S. Intramucosal adenocarcinoma arising from ectopic gastric mucosa in the upper esophagus treated successfully with endoscopic mucosal resection. J Gastrointest Cancer. 2014;45(Suppl 1):201–4.
10. Tanaka M, Ushiku T, Ikemura M, Shibahara J, Seto Y, Fukayama M. Esophageal adenocarcinoma arising in cervical inlet patch with synchronous Barrett's esophagus-related dysplasia. Pathol Int. 2014;64(8):397–401.
11. Möschler O, Vieth M, Müller MK: Endoscopic resection of an adenocarcinoma occurring in ectopic gastric mucosa within the proximal esophagus. Endoscopy 2014, 46 Suppl 1 UCTN:E24–25.
12. Verma YP, Chauhan AK, Sen R. Primary adenocarcinoma of the upper oesophagus. Ecancermedicalscience. 2013;7:314.
13. Akbayir N, Alkim C, Erdem L, Sokmen HM, Sungun A, Basak T, Turgut S, Mungan Z. Heterotopic gastric mucosa in the cervical esophagus (inlet patch): endoscopic prevalence, histological and clinical characteristics. J Gastroenterol Hepatol. 2004;19(8):891–6.
14. Klaase JM, Lemaire LC, Rauws EA, Offerhaus GJ, van Lanschot JJ. Heterotopic gastric mucosa of the cervical esophagus: a case of high-grade dysplasia treated with argon plasma coagulation and a case of adenocarcinoma. Gastrointest Endosc. 2001;53(1):101–4.
15. Poyrazoglu OK, Bahcecioglu IH, Dagli AF, Ataseven H, Celebi S, Yalniz M. Heterotopic gastric mucosa (inlet patch): endoscopic prevalence, histopathological, demographical and clinical characteristics. Int J Clin Pract. 2009;63(2):287–91.
16. Abe T, Hosokawa M, Kusumi T, Kusano M, Hokari K, Kagaya H, Watanabe A, Fujita M, Sasaki S. Adenocarcinoma arising from ectopic gastric mucosa in the cervical esophagus. Am J Clin Oncol. 2004;27(6):644–5.
17. Azar C, Jamali F, Tamim H, Abdul-Baki H, Soweid A. Prevalence of endoscopically identified heterotopic gastric mucosa in the proximal esophagus: endoscopist dependent? J Clin Gastroenterol. 2007;41(5):468–71.
18. Borhan-Manesh F, Farnum JB. Incidence of heterotopic gastric mucosa in the upper oesophagus. Gut. 1991;32(9):968–72.
19. Gutierrez O, Akamatsu T, Cardona H, Graham DY, El Zimaity HM. Helicobacter pylori and hetertopic gastric mucosa in the upper esophagus (the inlet patch). Am J Gastroenterol. 2003;98(6):1266–70.
20. Jabbari M, Goresky CA, Lough J, Yaffe C, Daly D, Cote C. The inlet patch: heterotopic gastric mucosa in the upper esophagus. Gastroenterology. 1985;89(2):352–6.
21. Jacobs E, Dehou MF. Heterotopic gastric mucosa in the upper esophagus: a prospective study of 33 cases and review of literature. Endoscopy. 1997;29(8):710–5.
22. Maconi G, Pace F, Vago L, Carsana L, Bargiggia S, Porro GB. Prevalence and clinical features of heterotopic gastric mucosa in the upper oesophagus (inlet patch). Eur J Gastroenterol Hepatol. 2000;12(7):745–9.
23. Kumagai Y. Incidence of heterotopic gastric mucosa in the upper esophagus (inlet patch). Progr Dig Endosc. 2005;66:19–21.
24. Korkut E, Bektas M, Savas B, Memmedzade F, Oztas E, Ustun Y, Idilman R, Ozdena A. Awareness of the endoscopist affects detection rate of heterotopic gastric mucosa in esophagus. Indian J Gastroenterol. 2009;28(2):75–6.
25. Yuksel I, Uskudar O, Koklu S, Basar O, Gultuna S, Unverdi S, Ozturk ZA, Sengul D, Arikok AT, Yuksel O, et al. Inlet patch: associations with endoscopic findings in the upper gastrointestinal system. Scand J Gastroenterol. 2008;43(8):910–4.
26. Alagozlu H, Simsek Z, Unal S, Cindoruk M, Dumlu S, Dursun A. Is there an association between helicobacter pylori in the inlet patch and globus sensation? World J Gastroenterol. 2010;16(1):42–7.
27. Weickert U, Wolf A, Schroder C, Autschbach F, Vollmer H. Frequency, histopathological findings, and clinical significance of cervical heterotopic gastric mucosa (gastric inlet patch): a prospective study in 300 patients. Dis Esophagus. 2011;24(2):63–8.
28. Cheng CL, Lin CH, Liu NJ, Tang JH, Kuo YL, Tsui YN. Endoscopic diagnosis of cervical esophageal heterotopic gastric mucosa with conventional and narrow-band images. World J Gastroenterol. 2014;20(1):242–9.
29. Al-Mammari S, Selvarajah U, East JE, Bailey AA, Braden B. Narrow band imaging facilitates detection of inlet patches in the cervical oesophagus. Dig Liver Dis. 2014;46(8):716–9.
30. Chung CS, Lin CK, Liang CC, Hsu WF, Lee TH. Intentional examination of esophagus by narrow-band imaging endoscopy increases detection rate of cervical inlet patch. Dis Esophagus. 2015;28(7):666–72.
31. Sahin G, Adas G, Koc B, Akcakaya A, Dogan Y, Goksel S, Yalcin O. Is cervical inlet patch important clinical problem? Int J Biomed Sci. 2014;10(2):129–35.
32. Govani SM, Metko V, Rubenstein JH. Prevalence and risk factors for heterotopic gastric mucosa of the upper esophagus among men undergoing routine screening colonoscopy. Dis Esophagus. 2015;28(5):442–7.
33. Vesper I, Schmiegel W, Brechmann T. Equal detection rate of cervical heterotopic gastric mucosa in standard white light, high definition and narrow band imaging endoscopy. Z Gastroenterol. 2015;53(11):1247–54.
34. Feurle GE, Helmstaedter V, Buehring A, Bettendorf U, Eckardt VF. Distinct immunohistochemical findings in columnar epithelium of esophageal inlet patch and of Barrett's esophagus. Dig Dis Sci. 1990;35(1):86–92.
35. Avidan B, Sonnenberg A, Chejfec G, Schnell TG, Sontag SJ. Is there a link between cervical inlet patch and Barrett's esophagus? Gastrointest Endosc. 2001;53(7):717–21.
36. Tang P, McKinley MJ, Sporrer M, Kahn E. Inlet patch: prevalence, histologic type, and association with esophagitis, Barrett esophagus, and antritis. Arch Pathol Lab Med. 2004;128(4):444–7.
37. Chen YR, Wu MM, Nan Q, Duan LP, Miao YL, Li XY. Heterotopic gastric mucosa in the upper and middle esophagus: 126 cases of gastroscope and clinical characteristics. Hepato-Gastroenterology. 2012;59(116):1123–5.
38. Neumann WL, Lujan GM, Genta RM. Gastric heterotopia in the proximal oesophagus ("inlet patch"): association with adenocarcinomas arising in Barrett mucosa. Dig Liver Dis. 2012;44(4):292–6.
39. Fang Y, Chen L, Chen DF, Ren WY, Shen CF, Xu Y, Xia YJ, Li JW, Wang P, Zhang AR, et al. Prevalence, histologic and clinical characteristics of heterotopic gastric mucosa in Chinese patients. World J Gastroenterol. 2014;20(46):17588–94.
40. Rodriguez-Martinez A, Salazar-Quero JC, Tutau-Gomez C, Espin-Jaime B, Rubio-Murillo M, Pizarro-Martin A. Heterotopic gastric mucosa of the proximal oesophagus (inlet patch): endoscopic prevalence, histological and clinical characteristics in paediatric patients. Eur J Gastroenterol Hepatol. 2014;26(10):1139–45.
41. Yu L, Yang Y, Cui L, Peng L, Sun G. Heterotopic gastric mucosa of the gastrointestinal tract: prevalence, histological features, and clinical characteristics. Scand J Gastroenterol. 2014;49(2):138–44.

42. Bogomoletz WV, Geboes K, Feydy P, Nasca S, Ectors N, Rigaud C. Mucin histochemistry of heterotopic gastric mucosa of the upper esophagus in adults: possible pathogenic implications. Hum Pathol. 1988;19(11):1301–6.

43. Meining A, Bayerdorffer E, Muller P, Miehlke S, Lehn N, Holzel D, Hatz R, Stolte M. Gastric carcinoma risk index in patients infected with helicobacter pylori. Virchows Arch. 1998;432(4):311–4.

44. Uemura N, Okamoto S, Yamamoto S, Matsumura N, Yamaguchi S, Yamakido M, Taniyama K, Sasaki N, Schlemper RJ. Helicobacter pylori infection and the development of gastric cancer. N Engl J Med. 2001;345(11):784–9.

45. Spechler SJ, Sharma P, Souza RF, Inadomi JM, Shaheen NJ. American Gastroenterological Association medical position statement on the management of Barrett's esophagus. Gastroenterology. 2011;140(3):1084–91.

46. Koop H, Fuchs KH, Labenz J, Lynen Jansen P, Messmann H, Miehlke S, Schepp W, Wenzl TG. S2k guideline: gastroesophageal reflux disease guided by the German Society of Gastroenterology: AWMF register no. 021–013. Z Gastroenterol. 2014;52(11):1299–346.

47. Shaheen NJ, Falk GW, Iyer PG, Gerson LB: ACG clinical guideline: diagnosis and Management of Barrett's esophagus. Am J Gastroenterol 2016, 111(1): 30–50; quiz 51.

48. Malhi-Chowla N, Ringley RK, Wolfsen HC. Gastric metaplasia of the proximal esophagus associated with esophageal adenocarcinoma and Barrett's esophagus: what is the connection? Inlet patch revisited. Dig Dis. 2000; 18(3):183–5.

49. Dixon MF, Genta RM, Yardley JH, Correa P. Classification and grading of gastritis. The updated Sydney system. International workshop on the histopathology of gastritis, Houston 1994. Am J Surg Pathol. 1996;20(10): 1161–81.

50. Boyer J, Robaszkiewicz M. Guidelines of the French Society of Digestive Endoscopy: monitoring of Barrett's esophagus. The Council of the French Society of digestive endoscopy. Endoscopy. 2000;32(6):498–9.

51. Sampliner RE. Updated guidelines for the diagnosis, surveillance, and therapy of Barrett's esophagus. Am J Gastroenterol. 2002;97(8):1888–95.

52. Ohara M. Incidence of heterotopic gastric mucosa in the upper esophagus in first time narrow banding image endoscopy of consecutive 900 patients. Gastrointest Endosc. 2010;71:AB316–7.

53. Variend S, Howat AJ. Upper oesophageal gastric heterotopia: a prospective necropsy study in children. J Clin Pathol. 1988;41(7):742–5.

54. Christensen WN, Sternberg SS. Adenocarcinoma of the upper esophagus arising in ectopic gastric mucosa. Two case reports and review of the literature. Am J Surg Pathol. 1987;11(5):397–402.

55. Lauwers GY, Scott GV, Vauthey JN. Adenocarcinoma of the upper esophagus arising in cervical ectopic gastric mucosa: rare evidence of malignant potential of so-called "inlet patch". Dig Dis Sci. 1998;43(4):901–7.

56. Chatelain D, Lajarte-Thirouard AS, Tiret E, Flejou JF. Adenocarcinoma of the upper esophagus arising in heterotopic gastric mucosa: common pathogenesis with Barrett's adenocarcinoma? Virchows Arch. 2002;441(4):406–11.

57. Van Asche C, Rahm AE Jr, Goldner F, Crumbaker D. Columnar mucosa in the proximal esophagus. Gastrointest Endosc. 1988;34(4):324–6.

58. Fitzgerald RC, di Pietro M, Ragunath K, Ang Y, Kang JY, Watson P, Trudgill N, Patel P, Kaye PV, Sanders S, et al. British Society of Gastroenterology guidelines on the diagnosis and management of Barrett's oesophagus. Gut. 2014;63(1):7–42.

59. Chandrasoma PT, Der R, Dalton P, Kobayashi G, Ma Y, Peters J, Demeester T. Distribution and significance of epithelial types in columnar-lined esophagus. Am J Surg Pathol. 2001;25(9):1188–93.

60. Chandrasoma PT, Der R, Ma Y, Peters J, Demeester T. Histologic classification of patients based on mapping biopsies of the gastroesophageal junction. Am J Surg Pathol. 2003;27(7):929–36.

61. Peitz U, Vieth M, Pross M, Leodolter A, Malfertheiner P. Cardia-type metaplasia arising in the remnant esophagus after cardia resection. Gastrointest Endosc. 2004;59(7):810–7.

62. Gatenby PA, Ramus JR, Caygill CP, Shepherd NA, Watson A. Relevance of the detection of intestinal metaplasia in non-dysplastic columnar-lined oesophagus. Scand J Gastroenterol. 2008;43(5):524–30.

63. Kelty CJ, Gough MD, Van Wyk Q, Stephenson TJ, Ackroyd R. Barrett's oesophagus: intestinal metaplasia is not essential for cancer risk. Scand J Gastroenterol. 2007;42(11):1271–4.

64. Paris Workshop on Columnar Metaplasia in the Esophagus and the Esophagogastric Junction, Paris, France, December 11–12 2004. Endoscopy 2005, 37(9):879–920.

65. Long JD, Orlando RC. Esophageal submucosal glands: structure and function. Am J Gastroenterol. 1999;94(10):2818–24.

66. Meining A, Bajbouj M. Erupted cysts in the cervical esophagus result in gastric inlet patches. Gastrointest Endosc. 2010;72(3):603–5.

13

Genetic polymorphisms of *NAMPT* related with susceptibility to esophageal Squamous cell carcinoma

Chuanzhen Zhang[1], Daojie Yan[2], Shanshan Wang[1], Changqing Xu[1], Wenjun Du[1], Tao Ning[3], Changhong Liu[1], Meijuan Zhang[1], Ruiping Hou[1] and Ziping Chen[1*]

Abstract

Background: Nicotinamide phosphoribosyl transferase (Nampt) plays a crucial role in tumorigenesis. The present study examines whether genetic polymorphisms of *NAMPT* are related to the risk of developing esophageal squamous cell carcinoma (ESCC).

Methods: A total of 810 subjects were enrolled in this study, including 405 ESCC patients and 405 healthy controls. Using polymerase chain reaction-restriction fragment length polymorphism (PCR-RFLP), genotypes at rs61330082, rs2505568 and rs9034 of *NAMPT* were identified. Haplotypes were constructed using PHASE software. Multivariate logistic regression models were used to evaluate the potentiating effects of the genotypes, alleles and haplotypes on the development of ESCC.

Results: The presence of genotypes CT and TT and allele T at rs61330082 was less frequent in ESCC cases than in controls (48.89% *vs.* 53.33%, $P < 0.01$, 95% CI: 0.33-0.68; 18.52% *vs.* 30.37%, $P < 0.01$, 95% CI: 0.22-0.50; 42.96% *vs.* 57.04%, $P < 0.01$, 95% CI: 0.38-0.61; respectively). No statistically significant differences existed in the distributions of genotypes or alleles at rs2505568 or rs9034 between ESCC cases and controls. Of five haplotypes constructed, haplotypes CTC, CTT and CAC were higher in ESCC cases ($P < 0.01$, OR = 1.57, 95% CI: 1.16-2.12; $P = 0.04$, OR = 1.72, 95% CI: 1.03-2.85; $P < 0.01$, OR = 3.39, 95% CI: 1.99-5.75; respectively) than in controls.

Conclusion: Genetic polymorphisms of *NAMPT*, specifically genotype CC and allele C at rs61330082 as well as haplotypes CTC, CTT and CAC, were significantly correlated with ESCC susceptibility.

Keywords: Nicotinamide phosphoribosyl transferase, Polymorphism, Haplotype, Esophageal squamous cell carcinoma, Susceptibility

Background

Esophageal cancer is relatively common throughout the world. In 2008, approximately 482,300 new esophageal cancer cases were diagnosed and 406,800 deaths occurred [1]. Notably, almost 90% of cancer cases in the so-called "Esophageal Cancer Belt," a region stretching from northern Iran through the Central Asian Republics to north-central China, are diagnosed as esophageal squamous cell carcinoma (ESCC). Common risk factors for ESCC include poor nutrition, a lack of adequate vitamin intake, tobacco smoking, excessive alcohol consumption, Barrett's Esophagus and mold pollution, among others [2]. In recent years, hereditary factors have also gained increasing attention for their role in the development of ESCC.

Nicotinamide phosphoribosyl transferase (Nampt) was first identified as pre-B-cell colony enhancing factor (PBEF). The *NAMPT* gene is located on chromosome7q22, spans 34.7 kb, has 11 exons and 10 introns, and produces cDNA of 2,357 kb translated into a 491-amino acid, 52-kDa protein that stimulates early B-cell formation [3]. Nampt was recently renamed "visfatin", as it is a visceral, fat-derived adipokine that might mimic insulin function [4], and it may exist both intracellularly (iNampt) and extracellularly (eNampt). Nampt is also known to act as a rate-limiting

* Correspondence: chenziping1966@163.com
[1]Digestive Department, Shandong Provincial Qianfoshan Hospital, Shandong University, Jingshi Road 16766#, Jinan 250014, China

enzyme in NAD biosynthesis, which is important because NAD availability is crucial for many vital cellular processes, including transcription regulation, DNA repair, cell cycle progression, apoptosis, calcium homeostasis, telomerase activity, antioxidation and oxidative stress, energy metabolism, circadian rhythm maintenance and chromatin dynamics regulation, and regulates factors of genomic stability and organismal metabolic homeostasis, including histone deacetylases (SirT1-T7), COOH-terminal binding proteins, CD38, poly(ADP-ribose) and polymerases [5,6]. Additionally, iNampt is involved in angiogenesis by activating the extracellular signal regulated kinase (ERK) 1/2 pathway and promoting the production of vascular endothelial growth factor (VEGF) and matrix metalloproteinase (MMP) 2/9 [7]. Independent of its enzymatic activity, eNampt plays a major role as a cytokine in the regulation of immune response [8]. Nampt is one of a few emerging adipokines (eg. leptin, adiponectin) whose expressions are correlated with the development of a variety of cancers [9]. Furthermore, a series of studies showed that Nampt might be a good biomarker of malignant potential and stage progression [8,10,11].

NAMPT shows a high degree of evolutionary conservation, suggesting that only tiny genetic changes can profoundly affect protein function and its dependent events. To date, the relationship between *NAMPT* genetic polymorphisms and disease has only been examined in bladder cancer, obesity and acute lung injury [12-14]. The aim of this study was to be the first to explore the relationship between *NAMPT* genetic polymorphisms and susceptibility to ESCC. Therefore, this case–control study was conducted using subjects recruited in Anyang, China, an area of high ESCC incidence. Three SNPs of *NAMPT*, including rs61330082 in the promoter region and rs2505568 and rs9034 in the 3'untranslated region (3' UTR), were selected for this study because of their potential effects on the influence of Nampt expression.

Methods

Study subjects

A total of 405 ESCC patients were recruited from Anyang Tumor Hospital in Henan Province from February 2005 to July 2011. These subjects were diagnosed as having ESCC by qualified pathologists using endoscopic biopsies or surgical specimens, had no history of any other cancer and had not previously received chemotherapy or radiotherapy. The control group consisted of 405 gender- and age-matched (±1 year), healthy and genetically unrelated individuals recruited during the same time period from the same region. Each subject was required to sign an informed consent and complete a personal questionnaire, which included fields for demographic data and the related risk factors age, gender, tobacco smoking and alcohol consumption, prior to being included in this study. The ethic

approval was provided by the ethic committee of Shandong Provincial Qianfoshan Hospital, Shandong University.

DNA extraction

A 5-ml blood sample was collected from each subject, then genomic DNA was extracted using the Qiagen DNA Isolation Kit (Qiagen, Dusseldorf, Germany).

Genotyping

Genotypes at rs61330082, rs2505568 and rs9034 of *NAMPT* were identified by polymerase chain reaction-restriction fragment length polymorphism (PCR-RFLP). Sequencing primers for rs61330082 and rs2505568 were used as previously described [12], and primers for rs9034 were designed using PRIMER 5.0 software (Canada). Information on primer sequences, the sizes of PCR products, restriction enzymes, enzyme digestion temperatures and restriction products is shown in Additional file 1: Table S1. PCR amplification was performed in a 20-μl reaction mixture containing 50–100 ng genomic DNA, 0.4 μl dNTPs (10 mM, Promega, USA), 0.8 μl each primer (10 mM, SinoGenoMax Co., Ltd.), 0.5 U Hotstart Taq DNA polymerase (5 U/μL, Qiagen, Dusseldorf, Germany) and 2 μl 10× PCR buffer. The PCR mixture was incubated for 2 min initial denaturation at 94.0°C followed by 36 cycles of 30 s denaturation at 94.0°C, 50 s annealing at the respective annealing temperatures (61°C, 52°C and 61°C, respectively) and 1 min extension at 72.0°C. The final extension was carried out for 10 min at 72.0°C. The PCR products were digested overnight by restriction enzymes at 37.0°C, then the digested products were analyzed following electrophoresis on a 3% agarose gel and photographing under UV light. To confirm the existence of polymorphisms, 10% of PCR products were directly sequenced. The representative pictures about the PCR-RFLP results and sequencing analysis were added in Additional file 2: Figure S1.

Statistical analysis

Distribution of age between the cases and controls was compared using the Mann–Whitney U test, differences between the other demographic variables were compared using the McNemar test, and the observed genotype frequencies were tested for Hardy-Weinberg equilibrium using the chi-square test. PHASE 2.1 software (University of Chicago, USA) was used to construct haplotypes on the basis of the known genotypes and estimate haplotype frequencies. The possible effects of the genotypes, alleles and haplotypes on ESCC susceptibility were analyzed by odds ratio (OR) and 95% confidence interval (95% CI) using multivariate logistic regression models adjusted for age, gender, tobacco smoking and alcohol consumption. All tests were two-sided, and P values of < 0.05 were considered statistically significant. All statistical analyses were

Zconducted using Stata 11.2 software (StataCorp., College Station, TX, USA).

Results

Demographic information of the subjects

The potential influence of age, gender, tobacco smoking and alcohol consumption on ESCC susceptibility was considered. As summarized in Table 1, the results showed that there were no significant differences in age or gender between groups or in the distributions of gender, tobacco smoking and alcohol consumption.

Correlation of NAMPT genotypes and alleles with ESCC susceptibility

All genotypes at the three NAMPT SNPs of the cases and controls were identified, and their distributions were found to be in Hardy-Weinberg equilibrium ($P > 0.05$). Table 2 shows that a significantly smaller proportion of the cases possessed either genotype CT or TT at rs61330082 than the controls (48.89% vs. 53.33%, $P < 0.01$; 18.52% vs. 30.37%, $P < 0.01$; respectively). Analogously, the frequency of allele T at rs61330082 in the cases was significantly decreased compared with the controls (42.96% vs. 57.04%, $P < 0.01$). Thus, subjects with genotypes CT or TT or allele Tat rs61330082 were less susceptible to ESCC (OR = 0.47, 95% CI: 0.33-0.68; OR = 0.33, 95% CI: 0.22-0.50; OR = 0.48, 95% CI: 0.38-0.61; respectively). Notably, no subjects carried genotype AA at rs2505568 or genotype TT at rs9034. With respect to the distributions at the two sites, no significant differences were found between the cases and controls ($P > 0.05$).

Correlation of NAMPT haplotypes with ESCC susceptibility

Five haplotypes were constructed using PHASE software. As summarized in Table 3, the presence of haplotypes a (TTC) and b (TAC) was less frequent in the cases than

Table 1 Demographic information of the subjects

Characteristics	Cases (n = 405)		Controls (n = 405)		P
	n	%	n	%	
Age (year; mean ± SD)	60.89 ± 7.83		60.93 ± 7.91		0.87[a]
Gender					
Male	240	59.26	240	59.26	-
Female	165	40.74	165	40.74	
Tobacco smoking					
Ever	183	45.19	171	42.22	0.43[b]
Never	222	54.81	234	57.78	
Alcohol consumption					
Ever	117	28.89	96	23.70	0.11[b]
Never	288	71.11	309	76.30	

[a]Mann–Whitney U test.
[b]McNemar test.

Table 2 Correlation of NAMPT genotypes and alleles with ESCC susceptibility

Genotype	Cases (n = 405)		Controls (n = 405)		P[a]	OR[a] (95% CI)
	n	%	n	%		
rs61330082						
CC	132	32.59	66	16.30	1.00	1.00
CT	198	48.89	216	53.33	<0.01	0.47 (0.33-0.68)
TT	75	18.52	123	30.37	<0.01	0.33 (0.22-0.50)
C Allele	462	57.04	348	42.96	1.00	1.00
T Allele	348	42.96	462	57.04	<0.01	0.48 (0.38-0.61)
rs2505568						
TT	168	41.48	171	42.22	1.00	1.00
AT	237	58.82	234	57.78	0.91	1.02 (0.77-1.34)
AA	0	0.00	0	0.00	-	-
T Allele	573	70.74	576	71.11	1.00	1.00
A Allele	237	29.26	234	28.89	0.92	1.02 (0.77-1.34)
rs9034						
TT	0	0.00	0	0.00	-	-
CT	51	12.59	36	8.89	1.00	1.00
CC	354	87.41	369	91.11	0.09	0.64 (0.38-1.07)
T Allele	51	6.30	36	4.44	1.00	1.00
C Allele	759	93.70	774	95.56	0.13	0.70 (0.45-1.10)

[a]Conditional logistic regression adjusted for risk factors (tobacco smoking, alcohol consumption).

in the controls (29.39% vs. 36.26%; 13.21% vs. 19.47%; respectively). Conversely, the presence of haplotypes CTC, CTT and CAC was more frequent in the cases than in the controls (36.17% vs. 30.91%; 4.81% vs. 2.94%; 14.92% vs. 8.92%; respectively). Each haplotype was then assessed for its ability to estimate susceptibility to ESCC (Table 4). Carriers with haplotypes TTC (–/a + a/a) or TAC (–/b + b/b) were less susceptible to ESCC ($P < 0.01$, OR = 0.61, 95% CI: 0.46-0.79; $P < 0.01$, OR = 0.69, 95% CI: 0.52-0.90; respectively) than those without these haplotypes (–/–). Conversely, individuals with haplotypes CTC, CTT or CAC (–/c + c/c, –/d + d/d or -e/e + e/e) were more

Table 3 Distributions of the estimated haplotype frequencies

Haplotypes	SNP positions			Cases (n = 405)		Controls (n = 405)	
	rs6133082	rs2505568	rs9034	n	%[a]	n	%[a]
a	T	T	C	238	29.39	294	36.26
b	T	A	C	107	13.21	158	19.47
c	C	T	C	293	36.17	250	30.91
d	C	T	T	39	4.81	24	2.94
e	C	A	C	121	14.92	72	8.92

[a]Conditional calculated by PHASE software.

Table 4 Correlation of *NAMPT* haplotypes with ESCC susceptibility

Haplotype	Cases (n = 405)		Controls (n = 405)		P^a	OR^a (95% CI)
	n	%	n	%		
a = TTC						
−/−[b]	258	63.70	204	50.37	1.00	1.00
−/a + a/a	147	36.30	201	49.63	<0.01	0.61 (0.46-0.79)
b = TAC						
−/−	237	58.52	195	48.15	1.00	1.00
−/b + b/b	168	41.48	210	51.85	<0.01	0.69 (0.52-0.90)
c = CTC						
−/−	111	27.41	147	36.30	1.00	1.00
−/c + c/c	294	72.59	258	63.70	<0.01	1.57 (1.16-2.12)
d = CTT						
−/−	354	87.41	372	91.85	1.00	1.00
−/d + d/d	51	12.59	33	8.15	0.04	1.72 (1.03-2.85)
e = CAC						
−/−	336	82.96	381	94.07	1.00	1.00
−/e + e/e	69	17.04	24	5.93	<0.01	3.39 (1.99-5.75)

[a]Logistic regression model, adjusted for age, gender, tobacco smoking and alcohol consumption.
[b]The minus sign (−) denotes any haplotype. For example: −/a indicates the a haplotype in combination with any other haplotype.

susceptible to ESCC ($P < 0.01$, OR = 1.57, 95% CI:1.16-2.12; $P = 0.04$, OR = 1.72, 95% CI:1.03-2.85; $P < 0.01$, OR = 3.39, 95% CI:1.99-5.75; respectively) than those without these haplotypes (−/−).

Discussion

Esophageal cancer has a poor prognosis, and in 2009, its mortality ranked the fourth and its incidence fifth among all reported cancers in China [2]. While esophageal cancer has been studied in depth, the specific mechanism by which it develops is still unclear. Given the known influence of genetic polymorphisms on certain types of cancer, it was important for this group to analyze the as yet unknown association between genetic polymorphisms and ESCC susceptibility, particularly since we are located within a high-ESCC-incidence region of China. For this study, *NAMPT* was selected as a basis for analyzing this association.

The adipokine Nampt was first reported as a pleiotropic protein, and is widely known as a key regulator of NAD, which is intimately involved in proliferation, cytokine production, immunological regulation and angiogenesis. Nampt is overexpressed in a variety of cancers, including that of the stomach and colorectal cavity [15,16], and its inhibitor FK866 is a widely studied anticancer agent [17].

In this study, the results demonstrated that the presence of genotypes CT and TT and allele T at rs61330082 of *NAMPT* was significantly decreased in the cases compared with the controls. It was therefore suggested that these genotypes or this allele might reduce ESCC susceptibility. In other words, genotype CC or allele C at rs61330082 might increase carrier susceptibility to ESCC. Considering the rs61330082 loci in the promoter region, its genetic mutation might influence the structure or function of Nampt protein. This finding is therefore commensurate with the probable roles of *NAMPT* in tumorigenesis and its elevated expression in gastric and colorectal cancers [15,16]. Although its expression did not vary in ESCC [18] and its genetic polymorphisms were never studied in ESCC, this result was consistent with a similar bladder cancer study by Zhang et al. [12].

Genotype AA at rs2505568 and genotype TT at rs9034 could not be detected in this study, which was a similar finding to Zhang's previous study [12]. Whether the limited sample size in that study was responsible for the absence of these genotypes in bladder cancer deserves further research. In spite of the importance of the 3' UTR on the regulation of gene expression, polymorphisms at rs2505568 and rs9034 were found to be independent risk factors for the development of ESCC, also partially coinciding with Zhang's study [12], although pathogenesis between ESCC and bladder cancer is comparatively limited.

Haplotype analysis assessed disease susceptibility more powerfully by analyzing the combined action of multiple loci. From the selected genetic sites, five haplotypes were constructed. The presence of haplotypes CTC, CTT or CAC was positively correlated with the development of ESCC, while the presence of haplotypes TTC or TAC protected carriers from ESCC. The determinant impact of allele C at rs61330082 among the three SNPs is thus implied.

This study had certain limitations worth noting. Specifically, the findings need to be confirmed by a larger sample of the population from more high-ESCC-incidence regions, and there are many more convenient and effective methods of confirming genotypes than PCR-PFLP. Additionally, functional studies and gene-environment interaction studies are needed to offer more authentic and integrative proof about the influence of *NAMPT* on ESCC.

Conclusions

In summary, genetic polymorphisms of *NAMPT* were significantly correlated with ESCC susceptibility in the studied Chinese population. Genotype CC and allele C at rs61330082 as well as haplotypes CTC, CTT and CAC were each risk factors for ESCC. Thus, these findings might provide one or more novel diagnostic indicators for ESCC.

Abbreviations
ESCC: Esophageal squamous cell carcinoma; Nampt: Nicotinamide phosphoribosyl transferase; PBEF: Pre-B-cell colony enhancing factor; ERK: Extracellular signal regulated kinase; VEGF: Vascular endothelial growth factor; MMP: Matrix metalloproteinase; PCR-RFLP: Polymerase chain reaction-restriction fragment length polymorphism.

Competing interests
The authors declare that they have no competing interests.

Authors' contributions
CZ devised the study concept and design, interpreted the data and drafted the manuscript. DY participated in patient selection. SW took charge of acquisition of data and statistical analysis. CX contributed to the study design and sample preparation. WD made contributions to revising the manuscript critically for important intellectual content. TN carried out sample preparation and data collection. CL was involved in the collection of samples and acquisition of data. MZ carried out DNA isolation. RH contributed to genotyping. ZC participated in devising the study concept and design, selecting samples, drafting the manuscript and providing final approval. All authors read and approved of the final manuscript.

Acknowledgments
This paper was supported by the Program of Shandong Province's Pharmaceutical Health and Technology Development (No HZ068). We thank all individuals who participated in this study and acknowledge the staff of the Laboratory of Genetics, Peking University School of Oncology.

Author details
[1]Digestive Department, Shandong Provincial Qianfoshan Hospital, Shandong University, Jingshi Road 16766#, Jinan 250014, China. [2]Infectious Diseases Hospital, Laiwu Hospital, Taishan Medical College, Laiwu, China. [3]Key Laboratory of Carcinogenesis and Translational Research (Ministry of Education), Laboratory of Genetics, Peking University School of Oncology, Beijing Cancer Hospital & Institute, Beijing, China.

References
1. Bray F, Center MM, Ferlay J, Ward E, Forman D. Global cancer statistics. CA Cancer J Clin. 2011;61:69–90.
2. Chen W, He Y, Zheng R, Zhang S, Zeng H, Zou HJ X. Esophageal cancer incidence and mortality in China, 2009. J Thoracic Dis. 2013;5:19–26.
3. Samal B, Sun Y, Stearns G, Xie C, Suggs S, McNiece I. Cloning and characterization of the cDNA encoding a novel human pre-B-cell colony-enhancing factor. Mol Cell Biol. 1994;14:1431–7.
4. Fukuhara A, Matsuda M, Nishizawa M, Segawa K, Tanaka M, Kishimoto K, et al. Visfatin: a protein secreted by visceral fat that mimics the effects of insulin. Science. 2005;307:426–30.
5. Shackelford RE, Mayhall K, Maxwell NM, Kandil E, Coppola D. Nicotinamide phosphoribosyltransferase in malignancy: a review. Genes Cancer. 2013;4:447–56.
6. Ying W. NAD+/NADH and NADP+/NADPH in cellular functions and cell death: regulation and biological consequences. Antioxid Redox Signal. 2008;10:179–206.
7. Kim S, Bae S, Choi K, Park S, Jun HO, Lee J, et al. Visfatin promotes angiogenesis by activation of extracellular signal-regulated kinase 1/2. Biochem Biophys Res Commun. 2007;357:150–6.
8. Garten A, Petzold S, Körner A, Imai S, Kiess W. Nampt: linking NAD biology, metabolism and cancer. Trends Endocrinol Metab. 2009;20:130–8.
9. Housa D, Housová J, Vernerová Z, Haluzík M. Adipocytokines and cancer. Physiol Res. 2006;55:233–44.
10. Srivastava M, Khurana P, Sugadev R. Lung cancer signature biomarkers: tissue specific semantic similarity based clustering of digital differential display (DDD) data. BMC Res Notes. 2012;5:617.
11. Bi T, Che X. Nampt/PBEF/visfatin and cancer. Cancer Biol Ther. 2014;10:119–25.
12. Zhang K, Zhou B, Zhang P, Zhang Z, Chen P, Pu Y, et al. Genetic variants in NAMPT predict bladder cancer risk and prognosis in individuals from southwest Chinese Han group. Tumor Biol. 2014;35:4031–40.
13. Blakemore AIF, Meyre D, Delplanque J, Vatin V, Lecoeur C, Marre M, et al. A rare variant in the visfatin gene (NAMPT/PBEF1) is associated with protection from obesity. Obesity. 2009;17:1549–53.
14. O'Mahony DS, Glavan BJ, Holden TD, Fong C, Black RA, Rona G, et al. Inflammation and immune-related candidate gene associations with acute lung injury susceptibility and severity: a validation study. PLoS One. 2012;7, e51104.
15. Nakajima TE, Yamada Y, Hamano T, Furuta K, Oda I, Kato H, et al. Adipocytokines and squamous cell carcinoma of the esophagus. J Cancer Res Clin Oncol. 2010;136:261–6.
16. Ghaemmaghami S, Mohaddes SM, Hedayati M, Gorgian MM, Dehbashi G. Resistin and visfatin expression in HCT-116 colorectal cancer cell line. Int J Mol Cell Med. 2013;2:143–50.
17. Pogrebniak A, Schemainda I, Azzam K, Pelka-Fleischer R, Nüssler V, Hasmann M. Chemopotentiating effects of a novel NAD biosynthesis inhibitor, FK866, in combination with antineoplastic agents. Eur J Med Res. 2006;11:313–21.
18. Nakajima TE, Yamada Y, Hamano T, Furuta K, Oda I, Kato H, et al. Adipocytokines and squamous cell carcinoma of the esophagus. J Cancer Res Clin Oncol. 2010;136:261–6.

14

Endoscopic optical diagnosis provides high diagnostic accuracy of esophageal squamous cell carcinoma

Kengo Nagai[1], Ryu Ishihara[1*], Shingo Ishiguro[2], Takashi Ohta[3], Hiromitsu Kanzaki[4], Takeshi Yamashina[1], Kenji Aoi[1], Noriko Matsuura[1], Takashi Ito[1], Mototsugu Fujii[1], Sachiko Yamamoto[1], Noboru Hanaoka[1], Yoji Takeuchi[1], Koji Higashino[1], Noriya Uedo[1], Hiroyasu Iishi[1], Masaharu Tatsuta[1], Yasuhiko Tomita[5] and Takashi Matsunaga[6]

Abstract

Background: Recent technological advances have stimulated the development of endoscopic optical biopsy technologies. This study compared the accuracy of endoscopic diagnosis using magnifying narrow-band imaging (NBI) and histologic diagnosis of esophageal squamous lesions.

Methods: Patients at high risk for esophageal squamous cell carcinoma were examined with endoscopy and subsequent biopsy. The lesions diagnosed as cancer on NBI and the lesions diagnosed as cancer on biopsy were resected endoscopically or surgically. Histological diagnoses of resected specimens, the reference standards in this study, were made by a pathologist who was blind to both the endoscopic and biopsy diagnoses. The primary outcome was the accuracy of endoscopic and biopsy diagnosis. A noninferiority trial design with a noninferiority margin of −10% was chosen to investigate the accuracy of endoscopic diagnosis using magnifying NBI.

Results: Between November 2010 and October 2012, a total of 111 lesions in 85 patients were included in the analysis. The accuracy of endoscopic diagnosis and biopsy diagnosis for all lesions was 91.0% (101/111) and 85.6% (95/111), respectively. The difference in diagnostic accuracy was 5.4% (95% confidence interval: −2.9%–13.7%). The accuracy of endoscopic diagnosis and biopsy diagnosis of invasive cancers was 94.9% (74/78) and 84.6% (66/78), respectively. The difference was 10.3% (95% confidence interval: 1.6%–19.0%) for invasive cancers. The lower bound of the 95% confidence interval was above the prestated −10% in both cases.

Conclusion: Noninferiority of endoscopic diagnosis by magnifying NBI to histologic diagnosis by biopsy was established in this study (p = 0.0001).

Keywords: Esophageal neoplasms, Esophageal cancer, Optical biopsy, Narrow-band imaging, Endoscopic diagnosis

Background

Esophageal cancer is the sixth most common cause of cancer-related mortality worldwide [1]. The overall survival of patients with esophageal cancer, regardless of histological type, remains poor. However, a favorable prognosis can be expected if this cancer is detected at an early stage [2-5].

Diagnosis of early esophageal cancers is based on the detection of suspicious lesions and histological evaluation of specimens taken from these suspicious lesions.

Endoscopically or surgically resected specimens with total biopsy of the lesions would provide the most accurate histologic diagnosis and can serve as the reference standard of histologic diagnosis. There are reports of discrepancy between diagnosis based on biopsy specimens and diagnosis based on endoscopically resected specimens, suggesting limited accuracy of biopsy diagnosis [6,7]. A high false-negative rate of biopsy diagnosis of esophageal,

* Correspondence: isihara-ry@mc.pref.osaka.jp
[1]Departments of Gastrointestinal Oncology, Osaka Medical Center for Cancer and Cardiovascular Diseases, 3-3, Nakamichi 1-chome, Higashinari-ku, Osaka 537-8511, Japan

gastric, and colon cancers has also been reported [8,9]. Such limitations in the accuracy of biopsy diagnosis may be associated with the sampling process or diagnostic process for small specimens. Taking 3 to 10 biopsy specimens would improve the accuracy of this technique [10-13]. However, multiple biopsies can increase the risk and cost of the procedure and potentially make subsequent endoscopic resection difficult [14-16].

Recent technological advances have stimulated the development of numerous optical methods. These methods allow for accurate evaluation and diagnosis of cancers in vivo and are thus termed optical biopsy techniques. Endoscopic optical biopsy techniques offer noninvasive real-time diagnosis. Some techniques currently being evaluated include optical coherence tomography [17,18], endocytoscopy [19], and narrow-band imaging (NBI) [20]. NBI is an imaging technique that enhances the visualization of mucosal microstructures and microvessels. Previous studies involving NBI and magnification have shown high diagnostic accuracy for esophageal squamous cell carcinoma [21-24]. Although many endoscopic techniques have preliminarily shown high accuracy rates, these technologies are still evolving, and the accuracy of endoscopic diagnosis has not yet been fully investigated. Endoscopic diagnosis has the advantage of providing noninvasive and real-time diagnosis without the additional cost of biopsy. If the accuracy of endoscopic diagnosis is comparable to that of histologic diagnosis of biopsy specimens, endoscopic optical biopsy can be used in some situations. However, few studies have compared the accuracy of endoscopic optical diagnosis with that of histologic biopsy diagnosis.

This study compared the accuracy of endoscopic diagnosis using magnifying NBI versus histologic diagnosis of esophageal squamous lesions. The accuracy was evaluated using lesions diagnosed as cancer on biopsy and lesions endoscopically diagnosed as cancer. Histologic diagnosis of resected specimens served as the reference standard. A noninferiority trial design was adopted under the consideration that a similar or slightly reduced accuracy of endoscopic diagnosis might be accepted because it would be balanced by other benefits such as less invasiveness, less cost, and real-time results.

Methods

Patients

The study protocol was approved by the Ethics Committee of the Osaka Medical Center for Cancer and Cardiovascular Diseases. The study was registered in the University Hospital Medical Network Clinical Trials Registry (UMIN-CTR) as number UMIN 000004529. The patient inclusion criteria were the presence of esophageal neoplasia, a history of esophageal cancer treated by endoscopic resection, and current or past head and neck cancer.

Patients were excluded if they had undergone previous surgery, chemotherapy, or radiotherapy for esophageal cancer. Patients were also excluded if they had severe reflux esophagitis or an allergy to iodine.

Endoscopic examinations and biopsies

The endoscopic procedures were carried out using a high-resolution magnifying upper gastrointestinal endoscope (GIF-Q240Z or GIF-FQ260Z; Olympus, Tokyo, Japan) or a high-definition magnifying upper gastrointestinal endoscope (GIF-H260Z; Olympus). The structure-enhancement function of the video processor was set at a level of B8 (strongest enhancement level for microstructures) for NBI observation. A black soft hood (MB-162 for GIF-Q240Z and MB-46 for FQ260Z and GIF-H260Z; Olympus) was mounted on the tip of the endoscope to maintain an adequate distance between the tip of the endoscope zoom lens and the mucosal surface during magnifying observation. Initial routine inspection was carried out with white-light imaging. The surface vascular pattern of the lesion was then observed by magnifying NBI. These procedures were followed by chromoendoscopy with iodine solution.

Endoscopic diagnosis using magnifying NBI was made as follows. Cancer was diagnosed when well-demarcated brownish change of the epithelium and scattered brown dots or dilated, tortuous vessels of various sizes were identified (Figure 1) [24,25]. An undetermined status was assigned when an obscure brownish change or obscure scattered brown dots were present (Figure 2). The absence of cancer was diagnosed when no brownish change or scattered brown dots were present (Figure 3). Biopsy specimens were taken from iodine-unstained lesions or lesions that were diagnosed as cancer or undetermined on NBI.

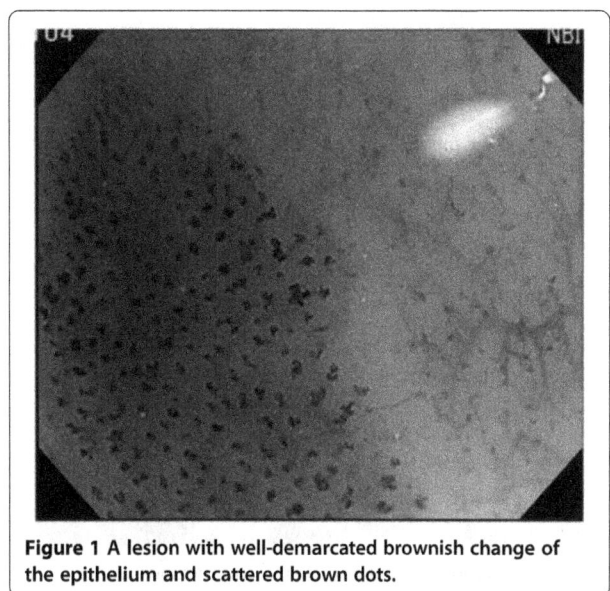

Figure 1 A lesion with well-demarcated brownish change of the epithelium and scattered brown dots.

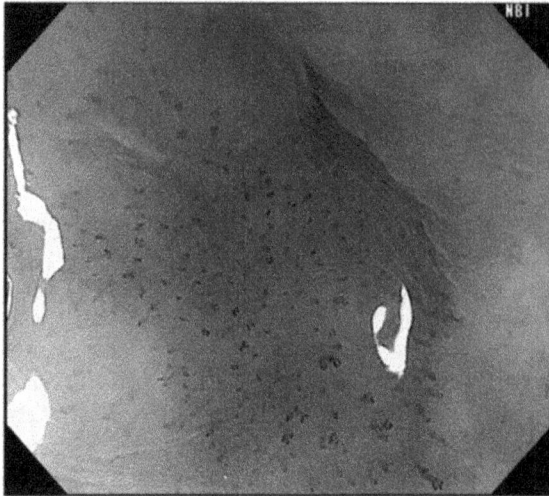

Figure 2 A lesion with obscure brownish change and obscure scattered brown dots.

Lesions in the cervical esophagus were excluded from the analysis because endoscopic observation and biopsy of these lesions are usually difficult. Lesions of ≤5 mm were also excluded from the analysis because most of them would likely be removed by biopsy. The endoscopic reports, which included lesion sizes but not endoscopic diagnoses, were sent to the pathologist. Biopsy specimens were embedded in paraffin and subjected to staining with hematoxylin and eosin. Pathologists with special qualifications made histological diagnoses of cancer based on structural and cytological abnormalities.

Endoscopic resection and histologic assessment

The lesions diagnosed as cancer on NBI and the lesions diagnosed as high-grade intraepithelial neoplasia or

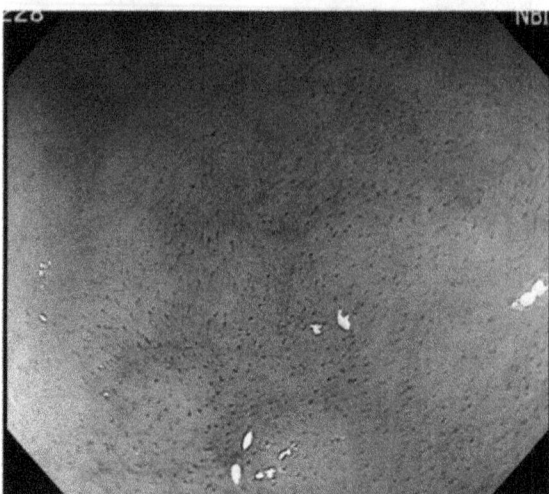

Figure 3 A lesion without any dilated and tortuous vessels.

cancer on biopsy were resected endoscopically or surgically. Lesions were also resected when they showed an obvious pink color change after iodine staining [26,27]. Resected specimens were embedded in paraffin and subjected to hematoxylin and eosin staining. Another pathologist with special qualifications (S.I.) who was blind to the endoscopic and biopsy diagnoses made the histological diagnoses according to the WHO criteria for the classification of early gastrointestinal neoplasia [28]. Lesions with structural and cytological abnormalities reaching the upper half of the squamous epithelium were diagnosed as cancer in situ, also termed high-grade intraepithelial neoplasia [28]. The lesions were also diagnosed as cancer based on obvious cytological abnormalities of the squamous epithelium, even when the abnormalities were confined to the lower half of the squamous epithelium [29]. The depth of cancer involvement was classified according to the Japanese Classification of Esophageal Carcinoma [29]. Written informed consent was obtained from all patients prior to enrollment.

Statistical analysis

The index lesion for the study was squamous cell carcinoma, including carcinoma in situ. For the statistical analysis, the histological results of resected specimen served as the reference standard. Evaluation was performed on a per-lesion basis, and the lesion was considered to be the unit of analysis. For patients with more than one lesion, each lesion was considered to be an independent observation for statistical purposes.

The primary outcome variable in this study was the accuracy of endoscopic diagnosis and biopsy diagnosis. The specificity, positive predictive value (PPV), negative predictive value (NPV), and accuracy were calculated as follows: Sensitivity = correctly diagnosed cancers/total cancers; Specificity = correctly diagnosed noncancers/total noncancers; PPV = total cancers/total lesions diagnosed as cancers; NPV = total noncancers/total lesions diagnosed as noncancers; and Accuracy = correctly diagnosed lesions/total lesions.

A noninferiority trial design was chosen to investigate the accuracy of endoscopic diagnosis using magnifying NBI. In a noninferiority trial, a slightly reduced diagnostic accuracy might be accepted if it is balanced by other secondary benefits; in the case of optical biopsy using magnifying NBI, these benefits include less invasiveness, less cost, and real-time results. Noninferiority of endoscopic diagnosis is established when the difference between endoscopic diagnosis and biopsy diagnosis is not smaller than the prespecified noninferiority margin. We chose a noninferiority margin (D) of −10% at the outset of this trial because we considered that this level would balance the clinical efficacy and secondary benefits. Previous studies have reported that the diagnostic accuracy of optical biopsy using magnifying NBI is approximately 90% [23]. Therefore, we hypothesized that optical biopsy diagnosis and histological diagnosis of biopsy specimens would achieve an accuracy of 90%. The study required at least 110 lesions for a 10% threshold of noninferiority and a statistical power of 80% with statistical significance set at $p < 0.05$. McNemar's test was used to compare the accuracy of endoscopic diagnosis and biopsy diagnosis. For all analyses, a p value of <0.05 was considered statistically significant.

Subgroup analysis was performed to compare the outcomes among subgroups divided according to lesion size and cancer invasion depth (cancer in situ or invasive cancer) to confirm the consistency of the results.

Results

Primary endpoint

Between November 2010 and October 2012, a total of 300 patients who fulfilled our criteria underwent endoscopic examination (Figure 4). A total of 193 lesions were detected in these patients, and 111 lesions in 85 patients were included in the analysis. Of the 111 lesions, 100 lesions were diagnosed as HGIN or cancer by magnifying

NBI. Eight lesions were diagnosed as undetermined by magnifying NBI but as cancer by histologic diagnosis of the biopsy specimens. Two lesions were diagnosed as no cancer by magnifying NBI but as cancer by histologic diagnosis of the biopsy specimens. One lesion was diagnosed as no cancer by magnifying NBI and histologic diagnosis of the biopsy specimens but as cancer by iodine staining.

A single biopsy specimen was taken from the lesion in 105 of the 111 lesions, and 2 biopsy specimens were taken from the other 6 lesions. Of the 111 lesions, 78 were invasive cancer, 32 were intraepithelial cancer, and 1 was low-grade intraepithelial neoplasia. The median (range) lesion size was 20 mm (6–100 mm). In total, 23 lesions were located in the upper esophagus, 63 were in the mid-esophagus, and 25 were in the lower esophagus. The accuracy, sensitivity, and specificity of endoscopic diagnosis by magnifying NBI were 91.0% (101/111) (95% CI: 84.1%–95.6%), 90.9% (100/110) (95% CI: 83.9%–95.6%), and 100% (1/1) (95% CI: 2.5%–100.0%), respectively (Table 1). The accuracy, sensitivity, and specificity of histologic diagnosis of biopsy specimens were 85.6% (95/111) (95% CI: 77.7%–91.5%), 86.4% (95/110) (95% CI: 78.5%–92.2%), and 0% (0/1) (95% CI: 0.0%–97.5%), respectively (Table 1). The difference in diagnostic accuracy was 5.4% (95% CI: −2.9%–13.7%). The lower bound of the 95% confidence interval was above the prestated −10%; thus, the primary endpoint was reached and the noninferiority of endoscopic diagnosis by

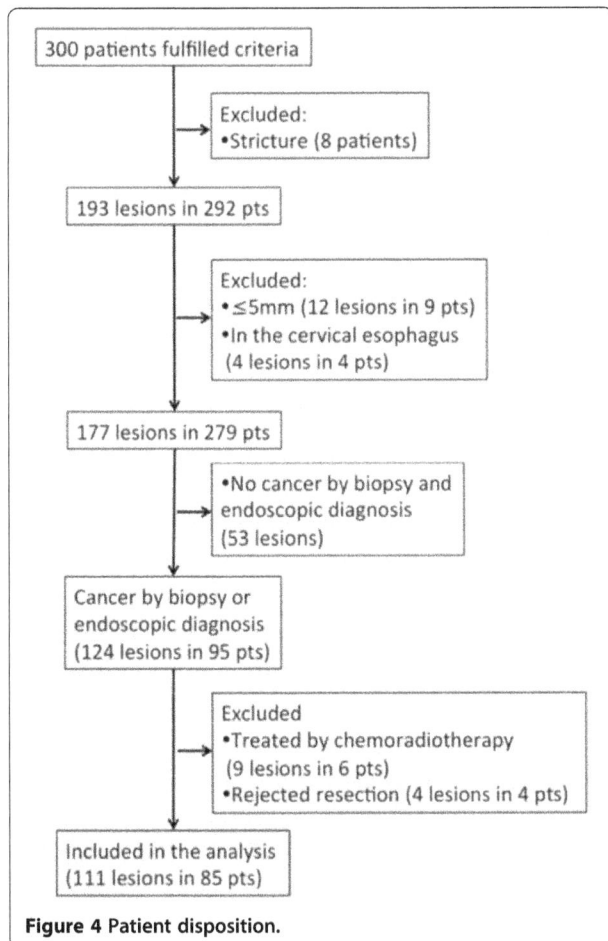

Figure 4 Patient disposition.

Table 1 Accuracy of endoscopic diagnosis and histologic diagnosis

	Endoscopic diagnosis	Histologic diagnosis
Sensitivity		
Value (95% CI[†])	90.9% (83.9–95.6%)	86.4% (78.5–92.2%)
No.lesions	100/110	95/110
Specificity		
Value (95% CI)	100% (2.5–100.0)	0% (0.0–97.5%)
No.lesions	1/1	0/1
Positive predictive value		
Value (95% CI)	100% (96.4–100.0%)	99.0% (94.3–100.0%)
No.lesions	100/100	95/96
Negative predictive value		
Value (95% CI)	9.1% (0.2–-41.3%)	0% (0–21.8%)
No.lesions	1/11	0/15
Accuracy		
Value (95% CI)	91.0% (84.1–95.6%)	85.6% (77.7–91.5%)
No.lesions	101/111	95/111

[†]CI: confidence interval.

magnifying NBI to histologic diagnosis by biopsy specimen was established (p = 0.0001) (Figure 5).

Subgroup analysis

The accuracy of endoscopic diagnosis in lesions ≤10 and >10 mm was 77.8% (21/27) (95% CI: 57.7%–91.4%) and 95.2% (80/84) (95% CI: 88.3%–98.7%), respectively. The accuracy of histologic diagnosis of biopsy specimens in lesions ≤10 and >10 mm was 74.1% (20/27) (95% CI: 53.7%–88.9%) and 89.3% (75/84) (95% CI: 80.6%–95.0%), respectively. The difference in the diagnostic accuracy was 3.7% (95% CI: –20.4%–27.8%, p = 0.13) in lesions ≤10 mm and 6.0% (95% CI: –1.7%–13.7%, p < 0.0001) in lesions >10 mm.

The accuracy of endoscopic diagnosis in epithelial lesions and invasive cancers was 81.8% (27/33) (95% CI: 64.5%–93.0%) and 94.9% (74/78) (95% CI: 87.4%–98.6%), respectively. The accuracy of histologic diagnosis of biopsy specimens in epithelial lesions and invasive cancers was 87.9% (29/33) (95% CI: 71.8%–96.6%) and 84.6% (66/78) (95% CI: 74.7%–91.8%), respectively. The difference in the diagnostic accuracy was –6.1% (95% CI: –24.8%–12.7%, p = 0.34) in epithelial lesions and 10.3% (95% CI: 1.6%–19.0%, p < 0.0001) in invasive cancers. With the exception of intraepithelial lesions, endoscopic diagnosis showed results preferable to those of histologic diagnosis of biopsy specimens, and the consistency of the results was confirmed in the subgroup analyses.

Retrospective analysis of misdiagnosis

Retrospective analysis of 15 cancers misdiagnosed as no cancer by biopsy was performed (Figure 6,7,8 and 9). Cytological abnormalities were confirmed in 13 of the 15 lesions. Of these 13 lesions with cytological abnormalities, 11 were misdiagnosed because the atypia was weak, and 2 were misdiagnosed because of concomitant inflammation.

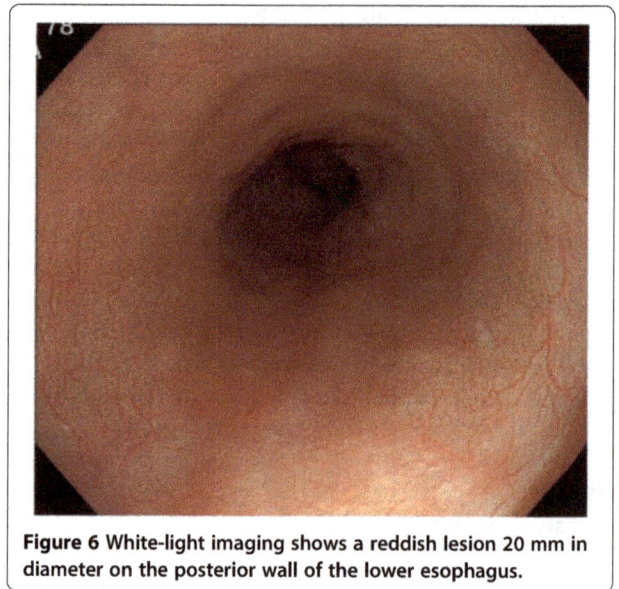

Figure 6 White-light imaging shows a reddish lesion 20 mm in diameter on the posterior wall of the lower esophagus.

Another two lesions were probably misdiagnosed due to sampling error because no cytological abnormalities were observed in the biopsy specimens.

Retrospective analysis of 10 cancers endoscopically misdiagnosed as undetermined or no cancer was performed. Of these 10 lesions, vascular change was not obvious in 4, brownish change of the epithelium was not obvious in 2, neither of these changes was obvious in 3, and the mucosal surface was not observed because of extensive keratosis in 1.

Discussion

The accuracy of endoscopic diagnosis and biopsy diagnosis was 91.0% (101/111) (95% CI: 84.1%–95.6%) and 85.6% (95/111) (95% CI: 77.7%–91.5%). The difference in diagnostic accuracy was 5.4% (95% CI: –3.9%–13.8%), and the noninferiority of endoscopic diagnosis by magnifying NBI to histologic diagnosis by biopsy was established (p < 0.001). Our study is unique because lesions diagnosed as cancer by endoscopic and biopsy examination were included in the study. This study is the first to show the accuracy of endoscopic diagnosis compared with biopsy diagnosis using a noninferiority trial design.

Diagnosis of gastrointestinal cancers is based on the detection of suspicious lesions and histological evaluation of biopsy specimens taken from these suspicious lesions. Although biopsy diagnosis serves as the gold standard pretreatment diagnosis, it is associated with high false-negative rates [8,9]. False-negative biopsy diagnosis may occur secondary to error in the specimen retrieval process. However, in this study, all biopsies were taken from the lesions, which was confirmed by recorded pictures. Focally distributed cancer can be missed by biopsy, even if the specimen is taken from the lesion.

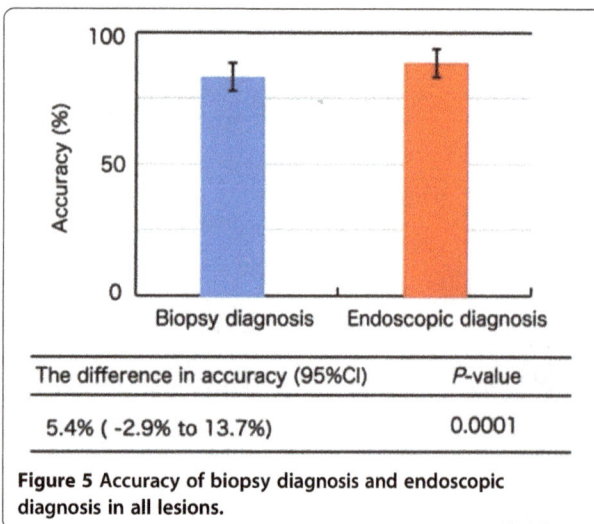

Figure 5 Accuracy of biopsy diagnosis and endoscopic diagnosis in all lesions.

The difference in accuracy (95%CI)	P-value
5.4% (-2.9% to 13.7%)	0.0001

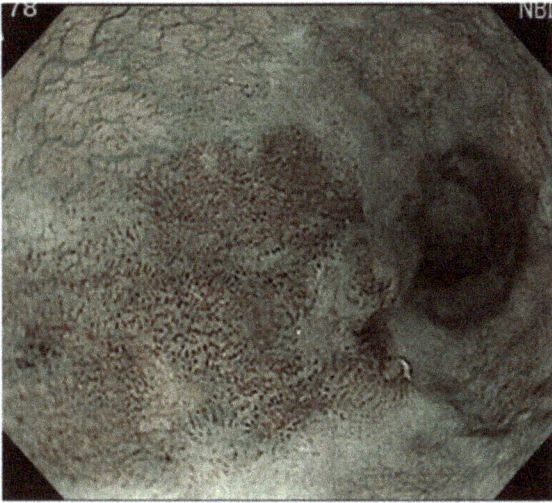

Figure 7 Narrow-band imaging shows well-demarcated brownish change of the epithelium and the presence of scattered brown dots.

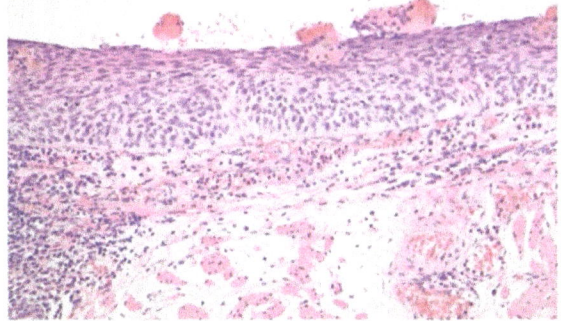

Figure 9 Histologic diagnosis of a resected specimen was cancer in situ.

Considering that only a small part can be examined by biopsy, this sampling error is a basic limitation of biopsy rather than technical error.

A single biopsy specimen was taken from the lesion in 105 of 111 lesions and from all 15 lesions with a false-negative biopsy diagnosis. Multiple biopsies may improve the accuracy of biopsy diagnosis. In previous reports, 3 to 4 biopsies [10], 4 to 6 biopsies [12], and 10 biopsies [13] are recommended to obtain high diagnostic accuracy. Multiple biopsies are acceptable for patients with advanced cancers that will be treated by surgical resection. However, multiple biopsies may cause problems for patients with early cancers because submucosal fibrosis caused by multiple biopsies sometimes interferes with the endoscopic resection process. Considering the potential disadvantage of

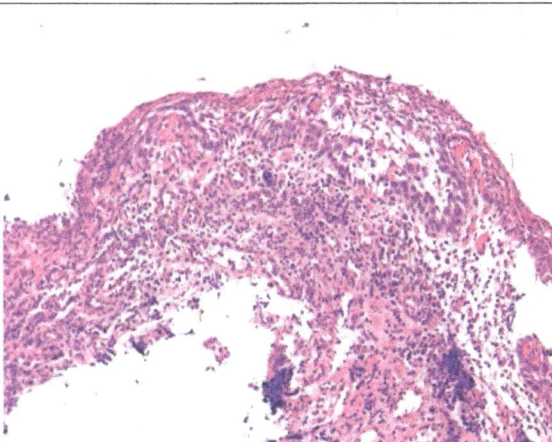

Figure 8 Biopsy diagnosis of cancer was not made because of inflammation.

multiple biopsies, the importance of endoscopic diagnosis rather than multiple biopsies for superficial lesions should be emphasized.

In recent years, several new endoscopic imaging techniques have been developed that may improve the detection and diagnosis of early esophageal cancer. NBI is a novel imaging technique that enhances the visualization of mucosal microstructures and microvessels. The addition of the magnification component has further allowed visualization of very minute mucosal details and hence histologic prediction in real time. Previous studies of NBI and magnification have shown a high diagnostic accuracy for esophageal squamous cell carcinoma, raising the expectation of optical biopsy in the clinical setting. However, the accuracy of endoscopic diagnosis has not been directly compared with that of other modalities. Before it can be regarded as a useful modality for diagnosis of cancer, it should be compared with the current standard modality of biopsy diagnosis. Therefore, we conducted the current study and showed the noninferiority of endoscopic diagnosis compared with the accuracy of biopsy diagnosis.

This study was conducted based on the assumption that biopsy diagnosis and endoscopic diagnosis are tested modalities and that only histologic diagnosis of resected specimens can be regarded as the reference standard. Based on these assumptions, unresected lesions were not included in the analysis because the reference standard of the resected specimens was not obtained in these lesions. However, even if those lesions were included as noncancer, the noninferiority of endoscopic diagnosis was established.

A noninferiority trial design was chosen to investigate the utility of endoscopic diagnosis compared with biopsy diagnosis. In a noninferiority trial, a slightly reduced clinical efficacy might be accepted if it is balanced by other secondary benefits; in the case of endoscopic diagnosis, these benefits include less invasiveness, lower cost, and real-time results. We chose a stringent and conservative noninferiority margin (Δ) of 10% [30] and showed the noninferiority of endoscopic diagnosis compared with biopsy diagnosis. In this study, lesions with obvious cytological abnormalities were diagnosed as cancer even when they were confined to the lower half of the squamous epithelium. There are some issues regarding the diagnosis of these lesions. In Western countries, these lesions are diagnosed as low-grade intraepithelial neoplasia and are not diagnosed as cancer. Therefore, we conducted subgroup analysis of invasive cancers. Noninferiority of the endoscopic diagnosis to biopsy diagnosis was also confirmed in this subgroup. Subgroup analyses were also performed among subgroups divided according to lesion size and intraepithelial lesions. The accuracy of endoscopic diagnosis was comparable with that of biopsy diagnosis in all subgroups, thus enhancing the reliability of the study conclusions.

This study is limited because all lesions were not confirmed by the reference standard of resected specimens. Considering the risk of endoscopic resection or surgical resection, resecting lesions diagnosed as noncancer by endoscopy or biopsy would not be acceptable.

Conclusions

This study showed that the accuracy of endoscopic diagnosis is comparable with that of biopsy diagnosis. This finding may facilitate the practical use of endoscopic optical diagnosis.

Competing interests
The authors declare that they have no competing interst.

Authors' contributions
RI, KN, NU, HK, TO, YTa, and SI planned the study. HK, RI, TO, YTo, and SI conducted the study. KN, HK, RI, TO, and TM collected the data. KN, HK, RI, TO, TY, KA, NM, TI, MF, SY, NH, KH, HI, MT and TM interpreted the data. KN and RI drafted the manuscript. All authors read and approved the final draft.

Author details
[1]Departments of Gastrointestinal Oncology, Osaka Medical Center for Cancer and Cardiovascular Diseases, 3-3, Nakamichi 1-chome, Higashinari-ku, Osaka 537-8511, Japan. [2]PCL Osaka Inc., Osaka, Japan. [3]Department of Gastroenterology, NTT West Osaka Hospital, Osaka, Japan. [4]Department of Gastroenterology and Hepatology, Okayama University Graduate School of Medicine, Okayama, Japan. [5]Departments of Pathology, Osaka Medical Center for Cancer and Cardiovascular Diseases, Osaka, Japan. [6]Departments of Medical Informatics, Osaka Medical Center for Cancer and Cardiovascular Diseases, Osaka, Japan.

References
1. Parkin DM, Bray F, Ferlay J, Pisani P: **Global cancer statistics, 2002.** *CA Cancer J Clin* 2005, **55**:74–108.
2. Yamashina T, Ishihara R, Nagai K, Matsuura N, Matsui F, Ito T, Fujii M, Yamamoto S, Hanaoka N, Takeuchi Y, Higashino K, Uedo N, Iishi H: **Long-term** outcome and metastatic risk after endoscopic resection of superficial esophageal squamous cell carcinoma. *Am J Gastroenterol* 2013, **108**:544–51.
3. Fujishiro M, Yahagi N, Kakushima N, Kodashima S, Muraki Y, Ono S, Yamamichi N, Tateishi A, Shimizu Y, Oka M, Ogura K, Kawabe T, Ichinose M, Omata M: **Endoscopic submucosal dissection of esophageal squamous cell neoplasms.** *Clin Gastroenterol Hepatol* 2006, **4**:688–94.
4. Igaki H, Kato H, Tachimori Y, Daiko H, Fukaya M, Yajima S, Nakanishi Y: **Clinicopathologic characteristics and survival of patients with clinical stage I squamous cell carcinomas of the thoracic esophagus treated with three-field lymph node dissection.** *Eur J Cardiothorac Surg* 2001, **20**:1089–94.
5. Yamamoto S, Ishihara R, Motoori M, Kawaguchi Y, Uedo N, Takeuchi Y, Higashino K, Yano M, Nakamura S, Iishi H: **Comparison between definitive chemoradiotherapy and esophagectomy in patients with clinical stage I esophageal squamous cell carcinoma.** *Am J Gastroenterol* 2011, **106**:1048–54.
6. Shimizu Y, Kato M, Yamamoto J, Ono Y, Katsurada T, Ono S, Mori Y, Nakagawa M, Nakagawa S, Itoh T, Asaka M: **Histologic results of EMR for esophageal lesions diagnosed as high-grade intraepithelial squamous neoplasia by endoscopic biopsy.** *Gastrointest Endosc* 2006, **63**:16–21.
7. Muehldorfer SM, Stolte M, Martus P, Hahn EG, Ell C: **Diagnostic accuracy of forceps biopsy versus polypectomy for gastric polyps: a prospective multicentre study.** *Gut* 2002, **50**:465–70.
8. Witzel L, Halter F, Grétillat PA, Scheurer U, Keller M: **Evaluation of specific value of endoscopic biopsies and brush cytology for malignancies of the oesophagus and stomach.** *Gut* 1976, **17**:375–7.
9. Szalóki T, Tóth V, Tiszlavicz L, Czakó L: **Flat gastric polyps: results of forceps biopsy, endoscopic mucosal resection, and long-term follow-up.** *Scand J Gastroenterol* 2006, **41**:1105–9.
10. Choi Y, Choi HS, Jeon WK, Kim BI, Park DI, Cho YK, Kim HJ, Park JH, Sohn CI: **Optimal number of endoscopic biopsies in diagnosis of advanced gastric and colorectal cancer.** *J Korean Med Sci* 2012, **27**:36–9.
11. Yalamarthi S, Witherspoon P, McCole D, Auld CD: **Missed diagnoses in patients with upper gastrointestinal cancers.** *Endoscopy* 2004, **36**:874–9.
12. Lal N, Bhasin DK, Malik AK, Gupta NM, Singh K, Mehta SK: **Optimal number of biopsy specimens in the diagnosis of carcinoma of the oesophagus.** *Gut* 1992, **33**:724–6.
13. Dekker W, Tytgat GN: **Diagnostic accuracy of fiberendoscopy in the detection of upper intestinal malignancy. A follow-up analysis.** *Gastroenterology* 1977, **73**:710–4.
14. Han KS, Sohn DK, Choi DH, Hong CW, Chang HJ, Lim SB, Choi HS, Jeong SY, Park JG: **Prolongation of the period between biopsy and EMR can influence the nonlifting sign in endoscopically resectable colorectal cancers.** *Gastrointest Endosc* 2008, **67**:97–102.
15. Ishiguro A, Uno Y, Ishiguro Y, Munakata A, Morita T: **Correlation of lifting versus non-lifting and microscopic depth of invasion in early colorectal cancer.** *Gastrointest Endosc* 1999, **50**:329–33.
16. Sweetser S, Baron TH: **Non-lifting sign from cold biopsy of sessile serrated polyp.** *Gastrointest Endosc* 2013, **78**:167–8.
17. Poneros JM, Brand S, Bouma BE, Tearney GJ, Compton CC, Nishioka NS: **Diagnosis of specialized intestinal metaplasia by optical coherence tomography.** *Gastroenterology* 2001, **120**:7–12.
18. Sivak MV Jr, Kobayashi K, Izatt JA, Rollins AM, Ung-Runyawee R, Chak A, Wong RC, Isenberg GA, Willis J: **High-resolution endoscopic imaging of the GI tract using optical coherence tomography.** *Gastrointest Endosc* 2000, **51**:474–9.
19. Kumagai Y, Kawada K, Yamazaki S, Iida M, Ochiai T, Momma K, Odajima H, Kawachi H, Nemoto T, Kawano T, Takubo K: **Endocytoscopic observation of esophageal squamous cell carcinoma.** *Dig Endosc* 2010, **22**:10–6.
20. Gono K, Obi T, Yamaguchi M, Ohyama N, Machida H, Sano Y, Yoshida S, Hamamoto Y, Endo T: **Appearance of enhanced tissue features in narrow-band endoscopic imaging.** *J Biomed Opt* 2004, **9**:568–77.
21. Yoshida T, Inoue H, Usui S, Satodate H, Fukami N, Kudo SE: **Narrow-band imaging system with magnifying endoscopy for superficial esophageal lesions.** *Gastrointest Endosc* 2004, **59**:288–95.
22. Muto M, Minashi K, Yano T, Saito Y, Oda I, Nonaka S, Omori T, Sugiura H, Goda K, Kaise M, Inoue H, Ishikawa H, Ochiai A, Shimoda T, Watanabe H, Tajiri H, Saito D: **Early detection of superficial squamous cell carcinoma in the head and neck region and esophagus by narrow band imaging: a multicenter randomized controlled trial.** *J Clin Oncol* 2010, **28**:1566–72.
23. Takenaka R, Kawahara Y, Okada H, Hori K, Inoue M, Kawano S, Tanioka D, Tsuzuki T, Uemura M, Ohara N, Tominaga S, Onoda T, Yamamoto K:

Narrow-band imaging provides reliable screening for esophageal malignancy in patients with head and neck cancers. *Am J Gastroenterol* 2009, **104**:2942–8.

24. Ishihara R, Inoue T, Uedo N, Yamamoto S, Kawada N, Tsujii Y, Kanzaki H, Hanafusa M, Hanaoka N, Takeuchi Y, Higashino K, Iishi H, Tatsuta M, Tomita Y, Ishiguro S: **Significance of each narrow-band imaging finding in diagnosing squamous mucosal high-grade neoplasia of the esophagus.** *J Gastroenterol Hepatol* 2010, **25**:1410–5.

25. Muto M, Nakane M, Katada C, Sano Y, Ohtsu A, Esumi H, Ebihara S, Yoshida S: **Squamous cell carcinoma in situ at oropharyngeal and hypopharyngeal mucosal sites.** *Cancer* 2004, **101**:1375–81.

26. Shimizu Y, Omori T, Yokoyama A, Yoshida T, Hirota J, Ono Y, Yamamoto J, Kato M, Asaka M: **Endoscopic diagnosis of early squamous neoplasia of the esophagus with iodine staining: high-grade intra-epithelial neoplasia turns pink within a few minutes.** *J Gastroenterol Hepatol* 2008, **23**:546–50.

27. Ishihara R, Yamada T, Iishi H, Kato M, Yamamoto S, Yamamoto S, Masuda E, Tatsumi K, Takeuchi Y, Higashino K, Uedo N, Tatsuta M, Ishiguro S: **Quantitative analysis of the color change after iodine staining for diagnosing esophageal high-grade intraepithelial neoplasia and invasive cancer.** *Gastrointest Endosc* 2009, **69**:213–8.

28. Gabbert HE, Shimoda T, Hainaut P, Nakamura Y, Field JK, Inoue H: **Squamous cell carcinoma of the esophagus.** In *Pathology and Genetics of the Digestive System: World Health Organization Classification.* Edited by Hamilton SR, Aaltonen LA. Lyon: IARC press; 2000:11–9.

29. Japan Esophageal Society: **Japanese Classification of Esophageal Cancer, tenth edition: part II and III.** *Esophagus* 2009, **6**:71–94.

30. Pint VF: **Non-inferiority clinical trials: concepts and issues.** *J Vasc Bras* 2010, **9**:145–51.

15

Leukotriene receptor expression in esophageal squamous cell cancer and non-transformed esophageal epithelium

M. Venerito[1†], C. Helmke[1†], D. Jechorek[2], T. Wex[1], R. Rosania[1], K. Antweiler[3], J. Weigt[1] and P. Malfertheiner[1*]

Abstract

Background: Leukotriene B4 (LTB4R and LTB4R2) and cysteinyl leukotriene receptors (CYSLTR1 and CYSLTR2) contribute to malignant cell transformation. We aimed to investigate the expression of LTB4R, LTB4R2, CYSLTR1 and CYSLTR2 in esophageal squamous cell carcinoma and adjacent non-transformed squamous epithelium of the esophagus, as well as in control biopsy samples from esophageal squamous epithelium of patients with functional dyspepsia.

Methods: Expression of LTB4R, LTB4R2, CYSLTR1 and CYSLTR2 was analyzed by immunohistochemistry (IHC) and quantitative reverse transcription-polymerase chain reaction (qRT-PCR) in biopsy samples of 19 patients with esophageal squamous cell cancer and 9 sex- and age-matched patients with functional dyspepsia.

Results: LTB4R, LTB4R2, CYSLTR1 and CYSLTR2 were expressed in all biopsy samples. Major findings were: 1) protein levels of all leukotriene receptors were significantly increased in esophageal squamous cell cancer compared to control mucosa ($p < 0.05$); 2) *CYSLTR1* and *CYSLTR2* gene expression was decreased in cancer tissue compared to control at 0.26–fold and 0.23–fold respectively; 3) an up-regulation of LTB4R (mRNA and protein expression) and a down-regulation of *CYSLTR2* (mRNA expression) in non-transformed epithelium of cancer patients compared to control ($p < 0.05$) was observed.

Conclusions: The expression of leukotriene receptors was deregulated in esophageal squamous cell cancer. Up-regulation of *LTB4R* and down-regulation of *CYSLTR2* gene expression may occur already in normal squamous esophageal epithelium of patients with esophageal cancer suggesting a potential role of these receptors in early steps of esophageal carcinogenesis. Larger studies are warranted to confirm these observations.

Keywords: Esophageal squamous cell cancer, Leukotriene receptors, Eicosanoids, Carcinogenesis

Background

The incidence of squamous cell carcinoma of the esophagus (ESCC) varies widely in the world, with age-adjusted incidence rates ranging from 5 to 100/100.000 inhabitants/year [1]. In Europe, the incidence of this subtype of esophageal cancer is of 5.4/100.000 for men and 1.1/100.000 for women, with highest rates in Scotland (13/100.000 for men and 4/100.000 for women) and lowest rates in Greece and Bulgaria (below 2/100.000 for men and 0.5/100.000 for women) [2]. In Germany the incidence is of 6–10/100.000, occurring four times more often in men than in women [3]. The prognosis is poor, with only 1 on 5 patients surviving 3 years or more after the initial diagnosis [4]. Many epidemiological studies have demonstrated that hazardous alcohol consumption and tobacco smoking increase the risk of ESCC [5–7].

Leukotrienes belong to the large group of eicosanoids that originate from the oxidative degradation of

* Correspondence: peter.malfertheiner@med.ovgu.de
†Equal contributors
[1]Department of Gastroenterology, Hepatology and Infectious Diseases, Otto-von-Guericke University Hospital, Leipziger Str. 44, 39120 Magdeburg, Germany

arachidonic acids [8]. Eicosanoids have pleiotropic effects on various cellular functions and numerous studies have shown their role in the pathogenesis of chronic inflammation and cancer [9, 10]. In particular, recent studies have shown an involvement of leukotriene receptors in the development of carcinomas of the pancreas, stomach, colon, urinary bladder and ovary [11–15].

We hypothesized that the expression of these receptors might be deregulated also in ESCC. Therefore, the expression pattern of the two leukotriene B4 receptors LTB4R and LTB4R2 and the two receptors for cysteinyl leukotrienes (CYSLTR1 and CYSLTR2) was studied by immunohistochemistry and quantitative reverse transcription-polymerase chain reaction (qRT-PCR) in a prospective study cohort of patients with esophageal squamous cell cancer. Tissue specimen from cancer and adjacent non-transformed squamous epithelium were analyzed. Gene expression may also be deregulated in adjacent non-transformed squamous epithelium of patients with esophageal squamous cell cancer [16]. Thus, a control group of patients with functional dyspepsia was recruited.

Methods
Study population
The study was conducted according to the declaration of Helsinki of 1975, as revised in 1983 and was approved by the Ethics Committee of the Otto-von-Guericke University Hospital of Magdeburg (No. 34/08). All subjects provided written informed consent before entering the study. Nineteen newly diagnosed patients with ESCC were prospectively enrolled from March 2009 to April 2010 at the Otto-von-Guericke University Hospital, Magdeburg, Germany. After overnight fasting all individuals underwent upper gastrointestinal endoscopy with videogastroscope (GIF Q145 or GIF Q180, Olympus Medical, Hamburg, Germany). The following exclusion criteria were applied: malignancies other than ESCC, lack of signed informed consent, clinically instable patient. None of the patients with ESCC had chemotherapy, radiotherapy or surgery prior to endoscopy. For each patient four biopsies each were collected from the tumor and from macroscopically non transformed mucosa. Two biopsies were sent to the pathologist for histology, one biopsy was immediately snap-frozen in liquid nitrogen and stored at -80 °C and one other was directly paraffin embedded. Narrow-band imaging was used to better demarcate neoplastic lesions from the surrounding normal non neoplastic mucosa. Lugol's chromoendoscopy was used to further investigate flat lesions suspicious of being cancerous.

Nine sex- and age-matched subjects (±4 years) undergoing upper GI endoscopy for dyspeptic symptoms were enrolled as control group. Exclusion criteria were: the presence of typical symptoms for gastro-esophageal reflux disease, the intake of proton pump inhibitors in the last 2 weeks, and/or the presence of esophageal erosions at endoscopy. Control biopsies were collected at least 2 cm cranial to the Z-line and subsequently snap frozen or directly paraffin embedded as mentioned above.

Structured questionnaire
Patients enrolled prospectively and controls were interviewed within 2 days before undergoing upper GI endoscopy using a structured questionnaire, providing information on demographics, medical history, smoking habits, alcohol intake and proton pump inhibitor (PPI) intake. The english version of the study questionnaire is shown in the Additional file 1. As there is no safe level of smoking [17], patients were classified into current smokers (within the past 12 months), former smokers and patients who never smoked. Alcohol consumption was consequently classified in 3 categories as most guidelines in different countries recommend that alcohol intake should not exceed 20g/day for men and 10g/day for women [18]: abstainers, low alcohol consumption (<20g/day for men, <10g/day for women) and hazardous alcohol consumption (≥20g/day for men, ≥10g/day women).

Extraction of total RNA, cDNA synthesis and quantitative RT-PCR
Biopsies were stored at -80 °C and subjected to a two-step RNA extraction protocol as described previously [19]. cDNA transcription was performed using 250 ng of total RNA amount. In a final volume of 40 µl, 20 units of AMV reverse transcriptase (Promega, Mannheim, Germany) in the buffer containing 1x reaction buffer, 0.5 mM dNTP (Roche, Mannheim, Germany), 10 mM random hexanucleotides and 50 units of placenta RNase inhibitor (all reagents from Promega) were utilized. After incubation at 42 °C for 1 h enzymes were inactivated at 95 °C for 10 min and the reaction mixture was kept frozen at -80 °C until enzymatic amplification. Quantitative RT-PCR was performed using an iCycler (BioRad, Munich, Germany). A typical 30 µl reaction mixture consisted of 15µl HotStarTaq™ Master Mix, 1.2 µl of the RT-reaction, 0.3 µl SYBR-Green I (1:10.000) (Molecular Probes, Eugene, USA), and 0.25 µM of the specific primers for the gene analyzed. Primary denaturation and activation of Taq-polymerase at 95 °C for 15 min was followed by 40 cycles with denaturation at 94 °C for 30 s, annealing at 60 °C for 30 s, and elongation at 72 °C for 30 s. The initial template mRNA amounts were calculated by determining the time point at which the linear increase of sample PCR product started, relative to the corresponding points of a standard curve; these are given as artificial units. All PCR products were cloned into the pDIRECT™ (Qiagen, Hilden, Germany) and used as internal standard for PCR. All PCR

standard curves had correlation coefficients >0.95. β-actin mRNA amounts were used to normalize the cDNA contents of the different samples. The following primers were used for the RT-PCR analysis: *β-actin* (fw: 5'-cat-gcc-atc-ctg-cgt-ctg.gac-c-3', rev: 5'-aca-tgg-tgg-tgc-cgc-cag-aca-g-3'), *LTB4R* (fw: 5'-tca-gca-cca-tca-ggg-cag-tga-c-3', rev: 5'-ctg-acc-ctg-gga-ttg-gca-tca-g-3'), *LTB4R2* (fw: 5'-ggg-tgt-aaa-ggg-acg-tgc-aca-g-3', rev: 5'-gct-tgt-gct-gtt-tcc-tgg-caa-g-3'), *CYSLTR1* (fw: 5'-caa-tag-tgt-cat-ggc-atg-tgg-c-3', rev: 5'-gct-tgc-ttc-tga-gaa-caa-acg-c-3'), *CYSLTR2* (fw: 5'-AGG-ATT-GAA-GCA-GGC-ATT-GG C-3', rev: 5'-aaa-gtg-gag-gtc-cca-gaa-tcg-g-3').

Immunohistochemical staining and cell count

Immunohistochemical analysis was performed using the avidin-biotin complex immunostaining method and the automated immunohistochemistry slide staining system by Ventana NexES (Ventana Medical System, Strasbourg, France). Tissue sections were deparafinized, dehydrated and underwent antigen retrieval using a Dako protocol. Slides were incubated with specific primary rabbit polyclonal antibodies for LTB4R, LTB4R2, CYSLTR1 or CYSLTR2 (Cayman chemicals, catalogue number 120114, dilution 1:100; Acris, catalogue number SP4368P, dilution 1:25; GeneTex Inc., catalogue number GTX70519, dilution 1:100; Lifespan Biosciences, catalogue number LS-A2255, dilution 1:100, respectively) either. All primary antibody incubations were followed by PBS-washing. Positive immunohistochemical reactions were revealed using the iVIEW[TM] DAB Detection Kit (Ventana, Germany). Specimens were counterstained with hematoxylin and mounted with DEPEX[TM]. Specificity of immunostaining was checked with non-immune serum. Samples were examined independently by CH and DJ. For LTB4R, LTB4R2, CYSLTR1 and CYSLTR2, the staining intensity (SI) and the percentage of positive cells (PP) were scored as followed: SI was classified in 0 (no staining), 1 (weak), 2 (moderate) and 3 (strong); PP: 0 (no positive cells), 1 (<10 %), 2 (10–50 %), 3 (51–80 %), 4 (>80 %). For each slide the immunoreactive score (IRS) was calculated as SI x PP with a possible maximum score of 12. The esophageal mucosa consists of different layers including (from the basal membrane to the lumen) basal stratum, spinosum stratum and superficial stratum. An example for an absent staining is shown in superficial cells of Fig. 1c (IRS = 0), whereas basal stratum shows a weak SI (SI score = 1) for 10–50 % of cells in the same picture (IRS = 2). A moderate staining is displayed in figure 1G (SI score = 2) for >80 % of cancer cells (IRS = 8). In 1H, superficial stratum shows a strong SI (SI score = 3) for >80 % cells (PP score = 4) resulting in an IRS of 12. For IRS assessment and statistical analysis we focused on the sole basal stratum where (cancer) stem cells are supposed to originate from [20].

Statistical analysis

All data were entered into a database and analyzed using the R - 2.15.0. statistic software (free download on http://www.r-project.org/). Wilcoxon signed-rank test and Mann-Whitney U test were used for comparisons of the groups where appropriate (2-sided). A statistical p-value <0.05 was considered as significant for all comparisons. In order to reduce the chances of obtaining false-positive results due to multiple comparisons ($k = 12$), Bonferroni correction was applied to the p-value of comparisons concerning immunohistochemistry of ESCC and basal stratum of non-transformed epithelium in cancer patients and control ($p < 0.05$).

Results

Overview on demographic population characteristics and tumor location, staging and grading

Baseline data of ESCC patients are presented in Table 1. The majority of subjects with ESCC and functional dyspepsia were male (14/19 and 5/9 respectively), and the mean age was 62 ± 11 years in cancer patients and 61.6 ± 12 years in controls. The most common symptoms reported at admission from patients with ESCC were loss of weight (60 %) and dysphagia (74.7 %), whereas only 28 % of patients reported heartburn and 25.3 % odynophagia.

For each patient the alcohol consumption was also recorded. In 94.7 % of cases (18 of 19) alcohol consume was accounted; 12/19 patients (63.2 %) were active alcohol consumer and 6/19 cases (31.6 %) were former drinker. 1 patient (5.3 %) never drank alcohol. According to the amount of alcohol, patients were considered low alcohol consumer (5/19, 41.7%) and high alcohol consumer (7/19, 58.3 %). Also smoking habits were recorded and 11/19 cases (57.9 %) were considered active smoker, whereas 8/19 patients (42.1 %) were former smoker in the last year. There was no never smoker in cancer patients.

Control group was composed by 9 sex-age matched patients with dyspeptic symptoms: 5 men (55.5 %) and 4 female (44.5 %). For 6/9 controls, smoking habits and alcohol intake were recorded: 3/ 6 controls had never smoked and further 3 controls were former smokers. Four out of 6 controls reported to consume alcohol currently whereas 2 controls were abstainers. In 3 cases questionnaires were not filled out before endoscopy. The use of sedation for endoscopy hampered to obtain missing information afterwards. Patients were not contacted again. No data on quantity of alcohol was available for controls.

In Fig. 2 an overview on tumor characteristics is presented. Tumor location was documented as distance from upper central incisor teeth. Distribution on upper (15 – 23 cm), mid-thoracic (23 – 32 cm) and lower

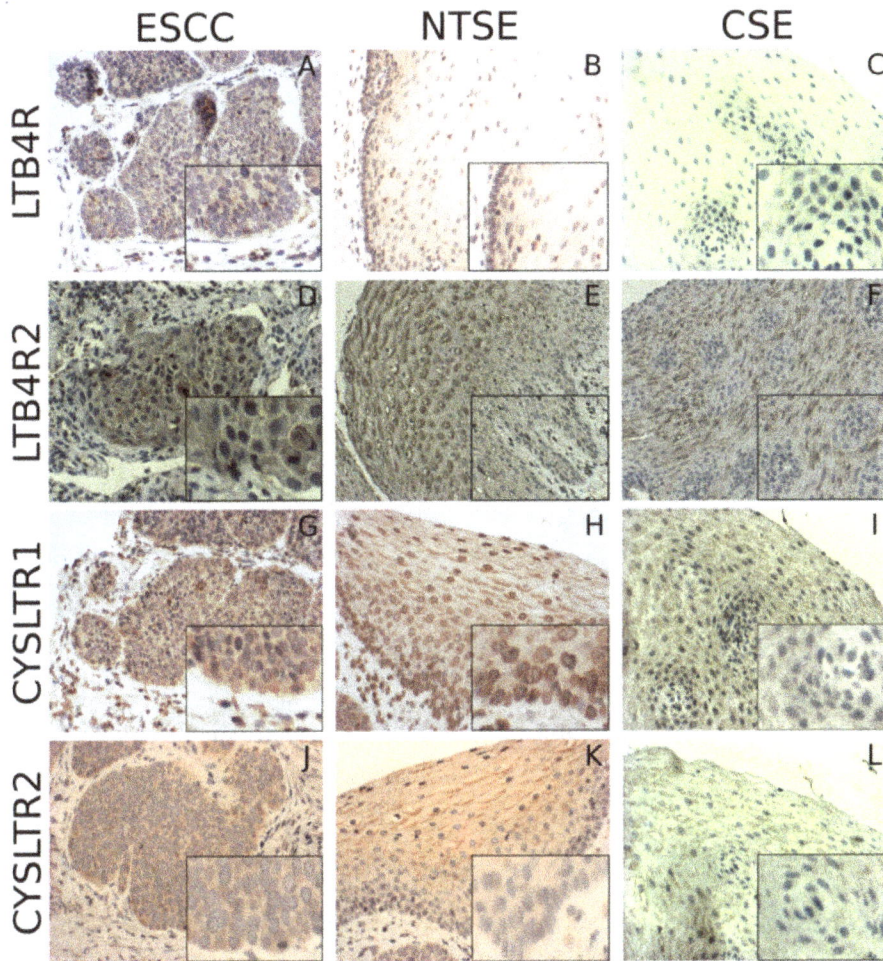

Fig. 1 Immunohistochemical localization of LTB4R/LTB4R2 and CYSLTR1/2. Leukotriene receptors are horizontally displayed from the top to the bottom. Vertical sections represent the distinct histological tissues examined. Images show sections with low (*large* picture) and higher (*right lower* corner) magnification example. In non-transformed mucosa of cancer patients and control mucosa, details display a representative section from basal stratum with adjacent submucosal tissue. Furthermore, control panels show a mucosal papilla with circularly oriented basal membrane. Positive receptor detection appears as brown staining (microscope: Nikon F200 camera 990). For LTB4R (**a-c**), the receptor is predominately located within the cytosol of cancer cells and normal esophageal epithelium. Within the non-transformed epithelia LTB4R reaches medium (**b**) to low (**c**) staining intensity in basal cells and a further reduction in luminal areas. The reactions for LTB4R2 also show a cytosolic receptor pattern (**d-f**). Non-cancerous tissues (E and F) present low LTB4R2 expression in basal strata. An up-regulation of LTB4R2 can be seen in superficial epithelial layers instead. CYSLTR1 results are demonstrated in the pictures below (**g-i**). Cancerous and non-cancerous epithelial esophageal cells present a cytosolic staining. As depicted, CYSLTR1 is also located within the nuclei of cancer cells and non-transformed mucosa of patients with cancer (**g** and **h**). A weak CYSLTR1 expression is present in basal stratum of the normal esophageal epithelium of cancer patients with up-regulation in superficial layers. CYSLTR1 staining remains low across all cellular layers of dyspeptic control. CYSLTR2 is also localized within the cytoplasm (**j-l**). Both groups with normal esophageal epithelium display a weak CYSLTR2 reactivity in basal compartments, whereas CYSLTR2 is up-regulated in luminal areas (**i** and **l**). ESCC = esophageal squamous cell cancer; NTSE = non-transformed squamous epithelium of cancer patients; CSE = control squamous epithelium

esophagus (32 – 40 cm) was 3 (15,8 %), 8 (42,1 %) and 8 (42,1 %).

With respect to the tumor grading, 0, 11/19 (57.9 %), 7/19 (36.8 %) and 1 (5.3 %) patients had G1, G2, G3 and G4, respectively.

According to the classification of the international Union Contre le Cancer [21] stage I, II, III and IV were present in 2/19 (10.5 %), 2/19 (10.5 %), 4/19 (21.1%) and 11/19 (57.9 %) patients, respectively. None of the patients in the control group had a malignancy of the upper GI tract.

Immunohistochemical expression of leukotriene receptors in ESCC, non-transformed epithelium of cancer patients and controls

Immunohistochemical staining was performed for all cancers (19/19) and control patients (9/9), as well as 15/19 normal esophageal epithelia of cancer patients. 4/19 biopsies from normal esophageal epithelia of cancer patients contained insufficient tissue for immunohistochemical evaluation. Raw data on immunohistochemical expression of leukotriene receptors are provided in the

Table 1 Baseline data of ESCC patients

	N = 19 (%)
Male/female	14/5 (73.6/26.4)
Mean age (years)	62 ± 11
Alcohol consumption	
Abstainer	1 (5.3)
Former drinking	6 (31.6)
Active drinking	12 (63.2)
Alcohol consumption (amount)	
Low[a]	5 (41.7)
High[b]	7 (58.3)
Smoking habits	
Never	0
Former smoker	8 (42.1)
Active smoker	11 (57.9)

Subjects were considered former drinkers of alcohol and former smokers when no consumption was declared within the past 12 month, respectively. The amount of male and female alcohol intake was differently classified into ([a]) low (<20g/day for men, <10g/day for women) and ([b]) high risk (≥20g/day for men, ≥10g/day women) intake. *ESCC* esophageal squamous cell cancer

Additional file 2. For each receptor staining, comparisons were performed between cancer tissue and basal strata of esophageal epithelium in cancer patients and control. An overview on LTB4R, LTB4R2, CYSLTR1 and CYSLTR2 receptors and their distinct expression profiles in cancers and non-malignant tissue is presented in Fig. 1. In cancerous and non-cancerous epithelial cells, leukotriene receptors were located within the cytoplasm. For CYSLTR1, nuclear receptor staining was also detected in 14/19 ESCC (74 %) as well as in 12/15 non-transformed mucosa specimen of patients with cancer (80 %) and 6/9 in control (66 %). In the present study we focused on the expression of leukotriene receptors in cancer tissue and basal epithelial cells of the esophageal mucosa. Statistical results regarding staining intensities of the different leukotriene receptors are shown in

Table 2. IRS of LTB4R was medium in cancer tissue and basal stratum of esophageal epithelium in cancer patients, whereas in control epithelium basal cells presented a weak reactivity. LTB4R protein expression was increased in cancer and non-transformed epithelium of cancer patients compared to control ($p < 0.05$), whereas no difference in LTB4R expression was observed between ESCC and adjacent non-transformed epithelium in cancer patients. IRS of LTB4R2, CYSLTR1 and CYSLTR2 receptors were medium in cancer tissue but low in normal epithelium of cancer patients and control basal stratum. Protein expression of LTB4R2 and CYSLTR2 was found to be significantly increased in cancer tissue compared to normal mucosa of cancer group and control ($p < 0.05$). With respect to CYSLTR1 expression, cancer tissue displayed a significant up-regulation compared to non-transformed squamous epithelium of cancer patients ($p < 0.05$) but not to control epithelium of dyspeptic patients. Protein expression of LTB4R2, CYSLTR1 and CYSLTR2 in basal stratum of non-transformed epithelium of cancer patients did not differ from the corresponding layer in control.

Immune cells infiltrating cancerous and non-cancerous tissue also presented a cytosolic and occasionally membranous leukotriene receptor expression for the various receptors.

Expression of *LTB4R/LTB4R2* and *CYSLTR1/CYSLTR2* mRNA in cancer tissue, non-transformed epithelium of cancer patients and control

Raw data on mRNA expression of leukotriene receptors are provided in the Additional file 2. Figure 3 shows the mRNA transcript level of *LTB4R/LTB4R2* and *CYSLTR1/CYSLTR2* in the 3 groups. The *LTB4R* mRNA showed an increase of the transcript in cancer tissue (1.69-fold) and non-transformed esophageal epithelium of cancer patients (2.24-fold) compared to control. The increase of

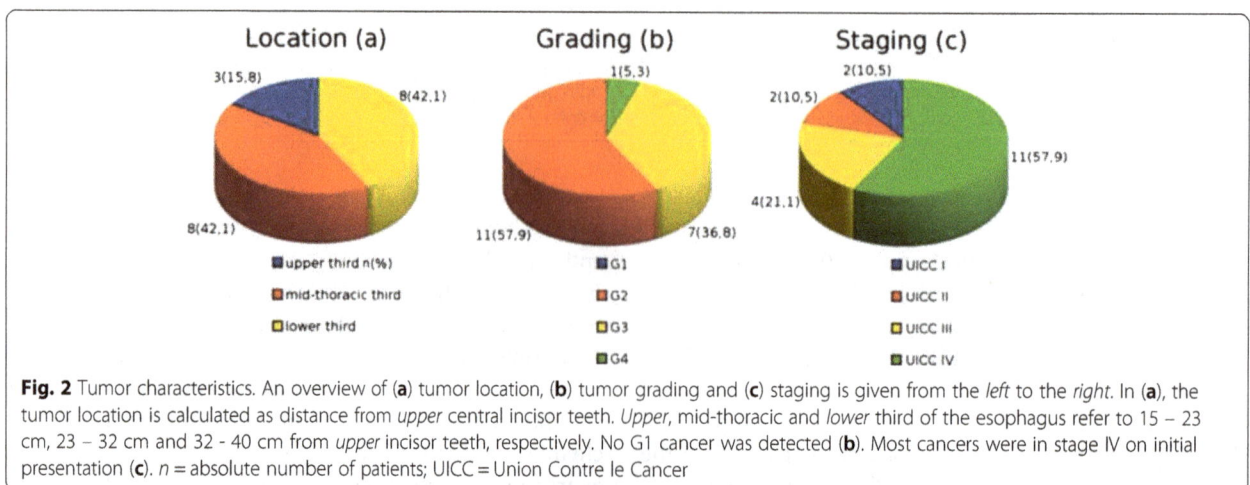

Fig. 2 Tumor characteristics. An overview of (**a**) tumor location, (**b**) tumor grading and (**c**) staging is given from the *left* to the *right*. In (**a**), the tumor location is calculated as distance from *upper* central incisor teeth. *Upper*, mid-thoracic and *lower* third of the esophagus refer to 15 – 23 cm, 23 – 32 cm and 32 - 40 cm from *upper* incisor teeth, respectively. No G1 cancer was detected (**b**). Most cancers were in stage IV on initial presentation (**c**). n = absolute number of patients; UICC = Union Contre le Cancer

Table 2 Immunohistochemical expression of leukotriene receptors

Immunoreactive score (IRS)

	LTB4R	LTB4R2	CYSLTR1	CYSLTR2
CSE median (range)	4 (0 - 8)	4 (4 - 6)	4 (4 - 8)	4 (-)
NTSE median (range)	8 (4 - 8)	4 (0 - 4)	4 (0 - 8)	4 (-)
ESCC median (range)	8 (4 - 12)	8 (4 - 12)	8 (4 - 12)	8 (4 - 12)
NTSE/CSE, p-value	**0.034**	0.588	1	1
ESCC/CSE, p-value	**0.0016**	**0.016**	0.252	**0.016**
ESCC/NTSE, p-value	1	**0.0059**	**0.047**	**0.0234**

IRS of all receptors are shown in the upper part of the table. Medians of IRS and corresponding range of staining intensities are shown for each group. In the lower part of the table comparisons between the different histological groups are shown. For statistical analysis, Wilcoxon signed-rank test was applied on groups of cancer patient whereas Mann-Whitney U test was used for inter-individual comparisons. All p-values were multiplied by k = 12 (Bonferroni correction) and considered significant when <0.05. Significant changes are displayed in bold letters. *ESCC* esophageal squamous cell cancer, *NTSE* non-transformed squamous epithelium of cancer patients, *CSE* control squamous epithelium; $p < 0.05$ (Wilcoxon signed-rank test, Mann-Whitney U test, Bonferroni correction k = 12)

LTB4R mRNA in normal mucosa of patients with cancer compared to control was statistically significant ($p < 0.05$). No significant differences were found between ESCC and non-transformed mucosa in cancer patients. The *LTB4R2* transcript showed no statistically significant

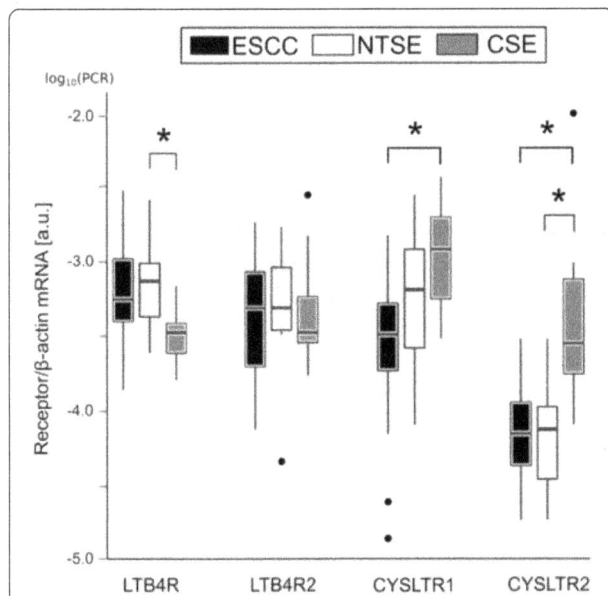

Fig. 3 mRNA expression of the leukotriene receptors in patients with esophageal squamous cell cancer (cancer and non-transformed mucosa) and in control. Logarithmic values were used to calculate the representation of each box plot. Median values (line within the box), and 25 % and 75 % quartiles (*upper* and *lower* box border) are shown. Brackets represent significant 2-group comparisons. Dots indicate values below or above the whiskers. a.u. = arbitrary units; ESCC = esophageal squamous cell cancer; NTSE = non-transformed squamous epithelium of cancer patients; CSE = control squamous epithelium; * = $p < 0.05$ (Wilcoxon-Test, Mann-Whitney U-Test)

difference between cancer tissue and the esophageal squamous epithelium (patients with ESCC and control). In cancer tissue, *CYSLTR1* showed a decrease to 0.26-fold in mRNA levels compared to control with statistical significance ($p < 0.05$). Between cancers and non-transformed mucosa of cancer patients, no differences were statistically detectable. The expression of *CYSLTR2* mRNA was reduced in cancer tissue to 0.23-fold and in normal epithelium of cancer patients to 0.25-fold compared to control. This reached statistical significance ($p < 0.05$).

Expression of leukotriene receptors and tumor stage

The clinical classification of tumor stages was performed according to UICC [21]. As the numbers of patients in stages I-III were small, stage I, II and III were grouped together and compared with stage IV. There was no observed difference in the expression of the receptors LTB4R, LTB4R2, CYSLTR1 and CYSLTR2 between the groups (Mann-Whitney U test).

Discussion

Herein we report for the first time the expression of leukotriene receptors in ESCC as well as in esophageal squamous epithelium of patients with and without esophageal neoplasia. The role of leukotriene receptors in immune cells is established [22], but their role in the esophageal mucosa has not been investigated so far, and thus future studies focusing on the physiological role of leukotriene receptors in the esophageal mucosa are warranted.

In the present study we report an up-regulation of LTB4R protein in ESCC compared to control. Similarly, a trend toward an up-regulation of *LTB4R* transcripts in ESCC compared to control was observed. An up-regulation of LTB4R protein has been reported in gastric and pancreatic cancer as well [15, 23]. However, combining the LTB4R antagonist LY293111 to gemcitabine did not add any benefit in terms of survival to chemotherapy-naïve patients with advanced pancreatic carcinoma [24]. Whether the use of a LTB4R antagonist might be an option for treating ESCC has not been studied yet. LTB4R expression was observed to be increased in the proliferative zone of gastric epithelium [25]. Moreover, in a placebo controlled trial on human volunteers, the oral LTB4-receptor antagonist VML295 diminished the proliferative epidermal activity after traumatically induced skin lesions [26]. LTB4R showed an up-regulation in proliferative areas of esophageal mucosa as well, suggesting a role of this receptor for the proliferation of esophageal squamous epithelium. Interestingly, an increased expression of LTB4R was observed also in non-transformed esophageal mucosa of cancer patients compared to control. This phenomenon suggests a potential role of LTB4R in early steps of esophageal carcinogenesis.

LTB4R2 protein expression is also up-regulated in ESCC whereas the specific transcripts did not show any difference between cancerous and non-cancerous epithelia. Previous studies have shown an increased LTB4R2 receptor expression in different epithelial cancers, suggesting a role of this receptor in cancer spread [27, 28]. In a recent study on an orthotopic breast cancer model, increasing the expression of the LTB4R2/LTB4/12(S)-HETE receptor system by lipopolysaccharide stimulation enhanced invasion of breast cancer cells, whereas its selective inhibition turned out in a reduced number of metastatic nodules [29]. Whether pharmacological inhibition of LTB4R2 might offer new options for treatment of ESCC has still to be determined.

LTB4R2 has not been described in normal esophageal mucosa before. The expression of LTB4R2 has been reported in different tissues and apart from its role in inflammatory cells LTB4R2 function needs to be clarified [30]. In a mice model, LTB4R2 was found to be expressed in colon cryptic cells and had a protective role against dextran sodium sulfate (DSS)-induced colitis, possibly by enhancing barrier function in epithelial cells of the colon [31]. A protective function of the LTB4R2 is to assume for the esophageal epithelium as well.

CYSLTR1 and CYSLTR2 proteins are up-regulated in ESCC, while the specific transcripts show a downregulation compared to the esophageal mucosa of dyspeptic patients. An increased expression of CYSLTR1 receptor protein was described in gastrointestinal and urological malignancies before [15, 32], whereas a loss of CYSLTR2 protein expression was shown in colon cancer cells compared to non-malignant intestinal cells [33]. According to functional studies, CYSLTR1 mediates preferentially pro-carcinogenic effects, whereas CYSLTR2 has been associated with anti-tumor mechanisms. In a recent study on colon cancer cells, CYSLTR1 signaling induced β-catenin translocation and the activation of β-catenin target genes, resulting in increased proliferation and migration of colon cancer cells [34]. Furthermore, CYSLTR1 expression was correlated with enhanced levels of anti-apoptotic proteins in colon cancer and CYSLTR1 transfection resulted in prolonged survival of Caco-2 cancer cells in vitro [35]. With respect to the CYSLTR2 function, a study on 329 colorectal cancers showed a more favorable prognosis for patients with high nuclear CYSLTR2 staining in combination with low nuclear CYSLTR1 receptor. Statistical analysis found high CYSLTR2 expression associated with a decreased risk of death [36]. In another study, aggressive CYSLTR2 negative breast cancer cells (MDA-MB-231) exhibited a decrease in migratory capacity after CYSLTR2 transfection which is associated with a reduction in metastatic potential [37]. Whether CYSLTR1 and CYSLTR2 might promote carcinogenesis and spread of ESCC needs to be addressed in future

studies. The observed discordance between CYSLTR1, CYSLTR2 protein expression and gene transcription can be explained by the presence of leukotriene receptor positive inflammatory cells infiltrating transformed and non-transformed tissue of cancer patients. An increase of β-actin in these leukocytes might have biased RT-PCR results in these patients mocking a total lower cysteinyl leukotriene receptor transcription. Furthermore, within the esophageal mucosa, spinosal and superficial cell layers constitute the main part of cellular mass. In the immunohistochemical analysis, the comparison was focused on the protein expression of cancer tissue and basal stratum only whereas in the RT-PCR all esophageal layers were analyzed. Thus, methodological aspects explain the differences between protein and mRNA expression pattern of the different leukotriene receptors.

The expression of CYSLTR1 and CYSLTR2 receptors was observed in non-transformed esophageal tissue as well. Similarly, non-transformed esophageal mucosa of cancer patients showed a significant reduction in CYSLTR2 mRNA transcription compared to the esophageal mucosa of dyspeptic control patients. Synthesis of cysteinyl leukotriene by the esophageal mucosa has been demonstrated, suggesting a physiological role of these receptors within the esophageal mucosa [38]. Further studies to define the role of cysteinyl leukotriene receptors in esophageal squamous epithelium are warranted.

The relatively small groups of patients and controls represent the major limitation of our study. This resulted in limited statistical power for some of the subgroups analysis and prevented stratified analysis by sex and some other risk modifiers. Moreover, the small number of recruited patients may be responsible for the lack of correlation between leukotriene receptor expression and ESCC stage (I-III versus IV). Larger studies may provide clearer results.

Furthermore, all inflammatory cells revealed a constant expression of leukotriene receptors. Cancerous and non-cancerous tissue of patients often showed a varying degree of inflammatory cell infiltration which may have influenced results of RT-PCR.

In addition, biopsies were not checked by microdissection for content of cancerous and non-cancerous tissue. Thus, the presence of non-transformed epithelium in cancer samples cannot be excluded and may have influenced results of mRNA analysis.

Another limitation is the observational character of this study. Although we explored leukotriene receptor expression in ESCC, the functional relevance of this finding remains to be determined. Functional research was not planned beforehand. Future in vitro analysis using siRNA knock-down techniques could clearly address this issue elucidating the role of leukotriene receptors in ESCC.

Conclusions

In the present study we report a deregulated expression of leukotriene receptors in esophageal squamous cell carcinoma. Furthermore, our results suggest a possible up-regulation of *LTB4R* and down-regulation of *CYSLTR2* gene expression also in the adjacent non-transformed squamous epithelium of the esophagus. Our data may implicate a potential role of these receptors in the early steps of esophageal carcinogenesis. Further studies with a larger number of patients and controls are warranted to validate our findings and to determine clinical implications for therapeutic and prevention purposes.

Abbreviations

cDNA, complementary desoxyribonucleic acid; CSE, control surface epithelium; CYSLTR1/2, cysteinyl leukotriene receptor 1/2; dNTP, desoxyribonucleic triphosphate; GI, gastrointestinal tract; IHC, immunohistochemistry; IRS, immunoreactive score; LTB4R, leukotriene B4 receptor 1; LTB4R2, leukotriene B4 receptor 2; mRNA, messenger ribonucleic acid; NTSE, non-transformed surface epithelium; PP, percentage of positive cells; PPI, proton pump inhibitor; qRT-PCR, quantitative reverse transcription-polymerase chain reaction; SI, staining intensity; UICC, Union Contre le Cancer

Acknowledgments

We thank Ingrid Bierwirth and Simone Phillipsen for technical assistance for PCR-analysis (Department of Gastroenterology). Our appreciation goes also to Claudia Miethke and Carola Kügler for their skillful help by performing immunohistochemistry (Institute of Pathology).

Funding

None.

Authors' contributions

MV, TW and PM designed this study. CH and MV enrolled patients and collected clinical data. MV and JW performed endoscopic procedures. CH and TW performed and evaluated quantitative reverse transcription-polymerase chain reactions. DJ and CH evaluated histopathologic sections. KA and CH conducted statistical analysis. The manuscript was drafted by CH, MV, RR and reviewed for content by TW, DJ and PM. All authors read and approved the final manuscript.

Competing interests

The authors declare that none of them has financial interests in context to this study.

Author details

[1]Department of Gastroenterology, Hepatology and Infectious Diseases, Otto-von-Guericke University Hospital, Leipziger Str. 44, 39120 Magdeburg, Germany. [2]Institute of Pathology, Otto-von-Guericke University Hospital, Leipziger Str. 44, 39120 Magdeburg, Germany. [3]Department of Biometrics and Medical Informatics, Otto-von-Guericke University Hospital, Leipziger Str. 44, 39120 Magdeburg, Germany.

References

1. Parkin DM, Bray FI, Devesa SS. Cancer burden in the year 2000. The global picture. Eur J Cancer. 2001;37:S4–S66.
2. Bosetti C, Levi F, Ferlay J, Garavello W, Lucchini F, Bertuccio P, Negri E, La Vecchia C. Trends in oesophageal cancer incidence and mortality in Europe. Int J Cancer. 2008;122:1118–29.
3. Muhr-Wilkenshoff F, Stahl M, Faiss S, Zeitz MSH. Current diagnosis and therapy of esophageal carcinoma. Z Gastroenterol. 2004;42:615–21.
4. Polednak AP. Trends in survival for both histological types of esophageal cancer in US surveillance, epidemiology and end results areas. Int J Cancer. 2003;105:98–100.
5. Zamboni P, Talamini R, La Vecchia C, Dal Maso L, Negri E, Tognazzo S, Simonato L, Franceschi S. Smoking, type of alcoholic beverage and squamous cell oesophageal cancer in northern Italy. Int J Cancer. 2000;86:144–9.
6. Freedman ND, Abnet CC, Leitzmann MF, Mouw T, Subar AF, Hollenbeck AR, Schatzkin A. A prospective study of tobacco, alcohol and the risk of esophageal and gastric cancer subtypes. Am J Epidemiol. 2007;165:1424–33.
7. Hashibe M, Boffetta P, Janout V, Zaridze D, Shangina O, Mates D, Szeszenia-Dabrowska N, Bencko V, Brennan P. Esophageal cancer in Central and Easrern Europe: tobacco and alcohol. Int J Cancer. 2007;120:1518–22.
8. Harizi H, Corcuff JB, Gualde N. Arachidonic-acid-derived eicosanoids: Roles in biology and immunopathology. Trends Mol Med. 2008;14:461–9.
9. Agarwal S, Reddy GV, Reddanna P. Eicosanoids in inflammation and cancer: The role of COX-2. Expert Rev Clin Immunol. 2009;5:145–65.
10. Singh RK, Gupta S, Dastidar S, Ray A. Cystenyl leukotrienes and their receptors: Molecular and functional characteristics. Pharmacology. 2010;85:336–49.
11. Seo JM, Cho KJ, Kim EY, Choi MH, Chung BC, Kim JH. Up-regulation of BLT2 is critical for the survival of bladder cancer cells. Exp Mol Ned. 2011;43:129–37.
12. Rocconi RP, Kirby TO, Seitz RS, Beck R, Straughn Jr JM, Alvarez RD, Huh WK. Lipoxygenase pathway receptor expression in ovarian cancer. Reprod Sci. 2008;15:321–6.
13. Nielsen CK, Campbell JI, Ohd JF, Mörgelin M, Riesbeck K, Landberg G, Sjölander A. A novel localization of the G-protein-coupled CysLT1 receptor in the nucleus of colorectal adenocarcinoma cells. Cancer Res. 2005;65:732–42.
14. Hennig R, Osman T, Esposito I, Giese N, Rao SM, Ding XZ, Tong WG, Büchler MW, Yokomizo T, Friess H, Adrian TE. BLT2 is expressed in PanINs, IPMNs, pancreatic cancer and stimulates tumour cell proliferation. Br J cancer. 2008; 99:1064–73.
15. Venerito M, Kuester D, Harms C, Schubert D, Wex T, Malfertheiner P. Up-regulation of Leukotriene receptor in gastric cancer. Cancer. 2011;3:3156–68.
16. Miyazaki M, Ohno S, Futatsugi M, Saeki H, Ohga T, Watanabe M. The relation of alcohol consumption and cigarette smoking to the multiple occurrence of esophageal dysplasia and squamous cell carcinoma. Surgery. 2002;131:S7–S13.
17. Bjartveit K, Tverdal A. Health consequences of smoking 1-4 cigarettes per day. Tob control. 2005;14:315–20.
18. Venerito M, Kohrs S, Wex T, Adolf D, Kuester D, Schubert D, Peitz U, Mönkemüller K, Malfertheiner P. Helicobacter pylori infection and fundic gastric atrophy are not associated with esophageal squamous cell carcinoma: a case-control study. Eur J Gastroenterol Hepatol. 2011;23:859–64.
19. Wex T, Treiber G, Lendeckel U, Malfertheiner P. A two-step method for the extraction of high-quality RNA from endoscopic biopsies. Clin Chem Lab Med. 2003;41:1033–7.
20. Rosekrans SL, Bart B, Vanesa M, van den Brink GR. Esophageal development and epithelial homeostasis. Am J Physiol Gastrointest Liver Physiol. 2015;309:G216–28.
21. Sobin LH, Gospodarowicz MK, Wittekind C. Digestive system tumours. TNM: Classification of malignant tumours. 7th ed. John Wiley & Sons; 2009. p. 66-72.
22. Nakamura M, Shimizu T. Leukotriene receptors. Chem Rev. 2011;111:6231–98.
23. Hennig R, Ding XZ, Tong WG, Schneider MB, Standop J, Friess H, Büchler MW, Pour PM, Adrian TE. 5-Lipoxygenase and leukotriene B(4) receptor are expressed in human pancreatic cancers but not in pancreatic ducts in normal tissue. Am J Pathol. 2002;161:421–8.
24. Saif MW, Oettle H, Vervenne WL, Thomas JP, Spitzer G, Visseren-Grul C, Enas N, Richards DA. Randomized double-blind phase II trial comparing gemcitabine plus LY293111 versus gemcitabine plus placebo in advanced adenocarcinoma of the pancreas. Cancer J. 2009;15:339–43.
25. Venerito M, Kuester D, Wex T, Roessner A, Malfertheiner P, Treiber G. The long-term effect of Helicobacter pylori eradication on COX-1/2, 5-LOX and leukotriene receptors in patients with a risk gastritis phenotype–a link to gastric carcinogenesis. Cancer Lett. 2008;270:218–28.

26. Seegers BA, Andriessen MP, van Hooijdonk CA, de Bakker ES, van Vlijmen-Willems IM, Parker GL, van Erp PE, van de Kerkhof PC. Pharmacological effects of a specific leukotriene B(4) receptor antagonist (VML 295) on blood leukocytes, cutaneous inflammation and epidermal proliferation. Skin Pharmacol Appl Skin Physiol. 2000;13:75–85.
27. Kim EY, Seo JM, Kim C, Lee JE, Lee KM, Kim JH. BLT2 promotes the invasion and metastasis of aggressive bladder cancer cells through a reactive oxygen species-linked pathway. Free Radic Biol Med. 2010;49:1072–81.
28. Seo JM, Park S, Kim JH. Leukotriene B4 receptor-2 promotes invasiveness and metastasis of ovarian cancer cells through signal transducer and activator of transcription 3(STAT3)-dependent up-regulation of matrix metalloproteinase 2. J Biol Chem. 2012;287:13840–9.
29. Park GS, Kim JH. Myeloid differentiation primary response gene 88-leukotriene B4 receptor 2 cascade mediates lipopolysaccharide-potentiated invasiveness of breast cancer cells. Oncotarget. 2015;6:5749–59.
30. Yokomizo T, Kato K, Terawaki K, Izumi T, Shimizu T. A second leukotriene B(4) receptor, BLT2. A new therapeutic target in inflammation and immunological disorders. J Exp Med. 2000;192:421–32.
31. Iizuka Y, Okuno T, Saeki K, Uozaki H, Okada S, Misaka T, Sato T, Toh H, Fukayama M, Takeda N, Kita Y, Shimizu T, Nakamura M, Yokomizo T. Protective role of the leukotriene B4 receptor BLT2 in murine inflammatory colitis. FASEB J. 2010;24:4678–90.
32. Matsuyama M, Yoshimura R. Cysteinyl-leukotriene1 receptor is a potent target for the prevention and treatment of human urological cancer. Mol Med Rep. 2010;3:245–51.
33. Magnusson C, Ehrnström R, Olsen J, Sjölander A. An increased expression of cysteinyl leukotriene 2 receptor in colorectal adenocarcinomas correlates with high differentiation. Cancer Res. 2007;67:9190–8.
34. Salim T, Sand-Demjek S, Sjölander A. The inflammatory mediator LTD4 induces subcellular β-catenin translocation and migration of colon cancer cells. Exp Cell Res. 2014;321:255–66.
35. Ohd JF, Nielsen CK, Campbell J, Landberg G, Löfberg H, Sjölander A. Expression of the leukotriene D4 receptor CysLT1, COX-2, and other cell survival factors in colorectal adenocarcinomas. Gastroenterology. 2003;124:57–70.
36. Magnusson C, Mezhybovska M, Lorinc E, Fernebro E, Nilbert M, Sjolander A. Low expression of CYsLT1R and high expression of CysLT2R mediate good prognosis in colorectal cancer. Eur J Cancer. 2010;46:826–35.
37. Magnusson C, Liu J, Ehrnstrom R, Manjer J, Jirstrom K, Andersson T, Sjolander A. Cysteinyl leukotriene receptor expression pattern affects migration of breast cancer cell s and survival of breast cancer patients. Int J Cancer. 2011;129:9–22.
38. Gupta SK, Peters-Golden M, Fitzgerald JF, Croffie JM, Pfefferkorn MD, Molleston JP, Corkins MR, Lim JR. Cysteinyl leukotriene levels in esophageal mucosal biopsies of children with eosinophilic inflammation: are they all the same? Am J Gastroenterol. 2006;101:1125–8.

Microcystic/reticular schwannoma of the esophagus: the first case report and a diagnostic pitfall

Mi Jin Gu* and Joon Hyuk Choi

Abstract

Background: Microcystic/reticular schwannoma is a recently described, rare, distinctive histological variant of schwannoma with a predilection for the gastrointestinal tract (GIT). The authors experienced the first case of a microcystic/reticular schwannoma occurring in the esophagus.

Case presentation: A 39-year-old male presented for an obstructive sensation during swallowing of several months duration. Endoscopy revealed a bulging mass with intact mucosa at 30 cm from incisors in the esophagus. The mass was excised and gross examination showed it was a well circumscribed, unencapsulated nodule, measuring 3.5×3.2×1.2 cm. On microscopic examination, the tumor showed a vague multinodular appearance with a pushing border and tumor cells arranged in a microcystic and reticular growth pattern with anastomosing and intersecting strands of spindle cells in a myxoid or collagenous/hyalinized stroma. Tumor cells showed diffuse nuclear and cytoplasmic positivity for S100.

Conclusions: The authors report the first case of microcystic/reticular schwannoma of the esophagus. Microcystic/reticular schwannoma is a distinctive histological variant of schwannoma with a benign clinical course. However, its histological findings are non-specific and may cause diagnostic difficulties. Awareness of this uncommon neoplasm with distinct histologic features is essential to prevent misdiagnosis.

Keywords: Schwannoma, Microcystic, Reticular, Esophagus

Background

Schwannomas are benign mesenchymal neoplasm and usually arise in the subcutaneous tissues of the distal extremities or in the head and neck region [1]. Gastrointestinal tract (GIT) schwannomas are rare and have histological and immunophenotypical features similar to those of non-GIT schwannomas. Several morphologic variants of schwannoma are recognized, that is, conventional, cellular, microcystic/reticular, plexiform, and melanotic schwannoma [1,2]. Microcystic/reticular schwannoma is a recently described, rare, distinctive histological variant of schwannoma with a predilection for the GIT. Twelve cases of microcystic/reticular schwannoma of the GIT have been reported in the English literature [1-4]. Herein, we report the first case of microcystic/reticular schwannoma of the esophagus and include a review of the literature.

Case presentation

A 39-year-old male presented for an obstructive sensation during swallowing of several months duration. During endoscopy, a bulging mass with intact mucosa was observed in the esophagus at 30 cm from incisors (Figure 1). Endoscopic ultrasonograpy revealed a homogeneously hypo- to iso-echoic mass measuring 2.3 cm in size in the submucosal layer. Mass excision via video-assisted thoracoscopic surgery (VATS) was performed. The resected mass was a well circumscribed, unencapsulated nodule, measuring 3.5×3.2×1.2 cm. Cut sections showed whitish yellow, homogeneously solid, rubbery tissue with a myxoid appearance (Figure 2). On microscopic examination, the tumor showed a vague multinodular appearance with a pushing border and was composed of elongate slender or plump spindle cells with oval nuclei and

* Correspondence: mjgu@yu.ac.kr
Department of Pathology, Yeungnam University College of Medicine, Daegu, Republic of Korea

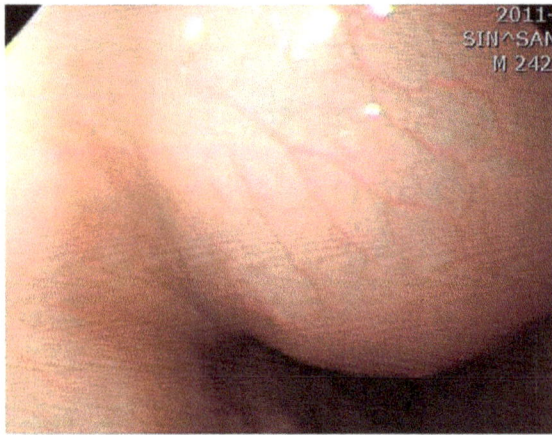

Figure 1 Endoscopic examination revealed a bulging mass with intact mucosa in the mid esophagus.

eosinophilic cytoplasm (Figure 3A). Its cells were arranged in a microcystic, reticular growth pattern with anastomosing and intersecting strands of spindle cells in a myxoid or collagenous/hyalinized stroma (Figure 3B,C). No cytologic atypia, necrosis, or mitosis was observed. In a collagenous/hyalinized area, hypocellular and hypercellular areas with vague nuclear palisading were observed, but no well-developed Verocay body was identified. Sparse perivascular lymphoplasma cell infiltrations were observed. However, prominent nodular lymphoplasmacytic infiltrates, thick and hyalinized vessels, hemorrhage with hemosiderin deposition, calcification, and cyst formation was absent, and the mitotic count did not exceed 1/50HPF. Tumor cells showed diffuse nuclear and cytoplasmic positivity for S100 (Figure 3D), but were negative for CD117, CD34, smooth muscle actin, synaptophysin, chromogranin, GFAP, and AE1/AE3. Throughout

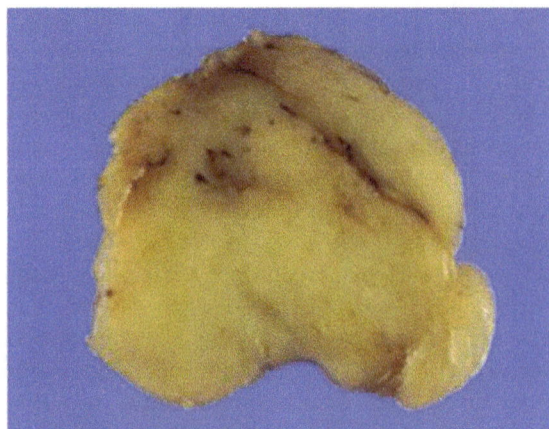

Figure 2 Gross findings. Cut surfaces showed whitish yellow, homogeneously solid, rubbery tissue with a myxoid appearance.

a follow-up of 27 months, the patient remained well without tumor recurrence or metastasis.

Discussion

Schwannomas account for 2 ~ 7% of mesenchymal GIT neoplasms and the stomach is the most common site [1]. In fact, More than 80% of benign esophageal tumors are leiomyomas [5]. Esophageal schwannomas are exceedingly rare, benign, and do not recur after complete excision [6]. Schwannoma has several morphologic variants, that is, conventional, cellular, microcystic/reticular, plexiform, and melanotic schwannoma. Schwannoma of the esophagus occur more frequently in women than in men and is usually encountered in the upper or mid esophagus. Recently, endoscopic ultrasonography-guided fine needle aspiration biopsy has been shown to be useful for preoperative diagnosis [5].

To the best of our knowledge, this is the first report of a microcystic/reticular schwannoma in the esophagus. However, 12 cases of reticular and microcystic schwannoma in the GIT have been reported [1-3] (Table 1); three in the stomach, two in each of the sigmoid colon, jejunum, and cecum, and one in each of the rectum, ascending colon, and small bowel. Nine of these 12 patients were female and three were male. Age at presentation ranged from 32 to 93 years (median 69 years), and tumors sizes ranged from 0.4 to 3.8 cm (mean 1.4 cm). Eleven of the 12 presented with a single mass and one with two masses. Neither recurrence nor metastasis was observed.

Our patient presented with a submucosal mass in the mid esophagus, which did not exhibit the conventional histological features of schwannoma, such as, nuclear palisading or Verocay body. Microscopically, the tumor showed a characteristic microcystic, reticular growth pattern with anastomosing and intersecting strands of spindle cells. Sparse perivascular lymphoplasma cell infiltrations were evident, but prominent nodular lymphoplasmacytic infiltrates were not observed. Liegl *et al.* also reported that lymphocytes cuffing with the germinal center were not observed in any of the case with a GIT location [1].

Therefore, variable entities should be considered to achieve a differential diagnosis, which includes gastrointestinal stromal tumor (GIST) with myxoid change, reticular variant of perineurioma, myoepithelial tumor, extraskeletal myxoid chondrosarcoma, low-grade fibromyxoid sarcoma (LGFMS), and ganglioneuroma with abundant myxoid stroma [1,2,7-10]. Gastrointestinal stromal tumors show a wide spectrum of histological features, but microcystic change is an unusual finding and immunoreactivity for CD117, CD34, and Dog-1 could aid the diagnosis of GIST. Histologically, reticular perineuriomas mimic microcystic/reticular schwannoma,

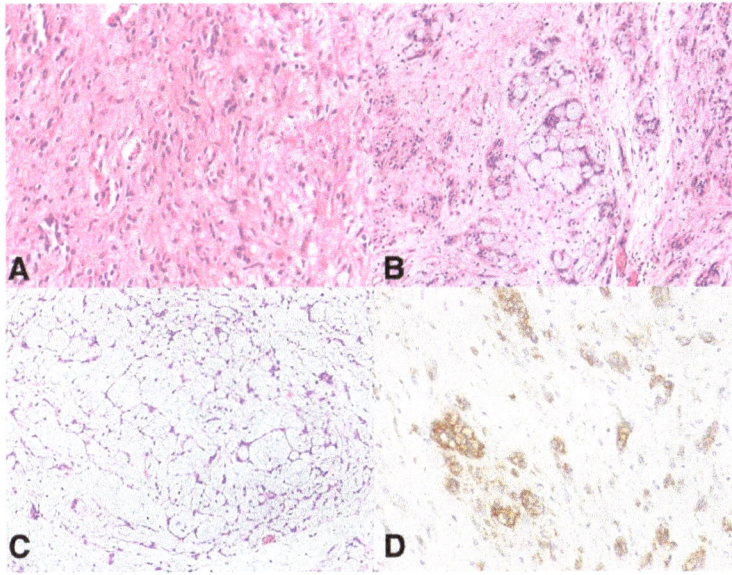

Figure 3 Microscopic findings. A) Elongate slender or plump spindle cells with oval nuclei and eosinophilic cytoplasm (original magnification 100×), **B-C)** Photograph showing a microcystic and reticular growth pattern with anastomosing and intersecting strands of spindle cells in myxoid or collagenous/hyalinized stroma (original magnification 100×). **D)** Immunohistochemistry showed strong positivity for S100 (original magnification 100×).

but they usually occur in superficial soft tissue of the hands and feet and exhibit a characteristic immunophenotype, that is, positivity for EMA and negativity for S100 and GFAP. Histological findings of myoepithelial tumors with a reticular growth pattern may overlap with those of microcystic/reticular schwannoma, although their immunoreactivities for epithelial and myoepithelial markers aid their differentiation from microcystic/reticular schwannoma. Extraskeletal myxoid chondrosarcoma may show features similar to those of microcystic/reticular schwannoma because the tumor is composed of branching and anastomosing cords in chondromyxoid stroma; however, a distinct microcystic change is an unusual finding. Molecular testing for *EWS* gene translocation and focal or scattered S100 staining can help exclude microcystic/reticular schwannoma. Low-grade fibromyxoid sarcoma is characterized by spindle cell tumor with bland histological findings, but has a fully aggressive behavior and a high rate of recurrence and metastasis. This tumor is composed of bland spindled to stellate cells in myxoid and fibrotic stroma. However, there are often prominent curvilinear and branching vessels in the myxoid area and the tumor

Table 1 Clinicopathological features of microcystic/reticular schwannoma of the GIT

Case	Sex	Age (y)	Site	Size (cm)	Status of last follow-up
1	F	73	Rectum	0.9	Died at 36 mo for colon cancer
2	F	72	Stomach	2.0	ANED 24 mo
3	M	68	Cecum	0.4	ANED 24 mo
4	F	93	Jejunum	1.6	ANED 7 mo
5	M	78	Small bowel	0.8	NA
6	F	63	Stomach	1.9	ANED 60 mo
7	F	70	Sigmoid colon	0.7	NA
8	F	32	Ascending colon	1.4	NA
9	F	67	Cecum	1.0	ANED 12 mo
10	F	67	Jejunum	2.2	ANED 12 mo
11	F	89	Stomach	3.8, 1.2	ANED 13 mo
12	M	61	Sigmoid colon	0.7	ANED 24 mo
Present case	M	39	Esophagus	3.5	ANED 27 mo

ANED, alive with no evidence of disease; NA, not available.

cells are negative for S-100 [8,9]. Ganglioneuroma usually presents as a large mass in the retroperitoneum or mediastinum that is composed of clusters of ganglion cells in a neuromatous stroma. Although ganglioneuroma with abundant myxoid stroma has been confused with microcystic/reticular schwannoma, tumor location and careful searching for ganglion cells can distinguish this entity from microcystic/reticular schwannoma [10].

Conclusions

We describe the first case of a microcystic/reticular schwannoma occurring in the esophagus. Microcystic/reticular schwannoma is a distinctive histological variant of schwannoma with a benign clinical course. However, many pathologists and gastroenterologist are unlikely to be familiar with this entity, which could cause diagnostic difficulties. Awareness of this uncommon neoplasm with a distinct histology is essential to prevent misdiagnosis.

Consents

A copy of the written informed consent provided by the patient prior to publication has been made available for review by the Editor-in-Chief of this journal.

Abbreviations
GIT: Gastrointestinal tract; GIST: Gastrointestinal stromal tumor.

Competing interest
None of the contributing authors have any conflict of interest, including specific financial interests or relationships and affiliations relevant to the subject matter or materials discussed in the manuscript.

Authors' contribution
GMJ and CJH collected references. GMJ analyzed pathological results and wrote the manuscript. Both authors read and approved the final manuscript.

Acknowledgments
The authors thank Professor Christopher Fletcher for reviewing the case and confirming the diagnosis.

References
1. Liegl B, Bennett MW, Fletcher CD: Microcystic/reticular schwannoma: A distinct variant with predilection for visceral locations. Am J Surg Pathol 2008, 32(7):1080–1087.
2. Chetty R: Reticular and microcystic schwannoma: A distinctive tumor of the gastrointestinal tract. Ann Diagn Pathol 2011, 15(3):198–201.
3. Trivedi A, Ligato S: Microcystic/reticular schwannoma of the proximal sigmoid colon: Case report with review of literature. Arch Pathol Lab Med 2013, 137(2):284–288.
4. Tozbikian G, Shen R, Suster S: Signet ring cell gastric schwannoma: Report of a new distinctive morphological variant. Ann Diagn Pathol 2008, 12(2):146–152.
5. Kitada M, Matsuda Y, Hayashi S, Ishibashi K, Oikawa K, Miyokawa N: Esophageal schwannoma: a case report. World J Oncol 2013, 11(2):253.
6. Kassis ES, Bansal S, Perrino C, Walker JP, Hitchicock C, Ross P, Daniel VC: Giant asymptomatic primary esophageal schwannoma. Ann Thorac Surg 2012, 93(4):e81–e83.
7. Lee SM, Goldblum J, Kim KM: Microcystic/reticular schwannoma in the colon. Pathology 2009, 41(6):595–596.
8. Evans HL: Low-grade fibromyxoid sarcoma: a clinicopathologic study of 33 cases with long-term follow-up. Am J Surg Pathol 2011, 35(10):1450–1462.
9. Billings SD, Giblen G, Fanburg-Smith JC: Superficial low-grade fibromyxoid sarcoma (Evans tumor): a clinicopathologic analysis of 19 cases with a unique observation in the pediatric population. Am J Surg Pathol 2005, 29(2):204–210.
10. Yokoi H, Arakawa A, Inoshita A, Ikeda K: Novel use of a Weerda laryngoscope for transoral excision of a cervical ganglioneuroma: a case report. J Med Case Rep 2012, 6:88.

17

A superficial esophageal cancer in an epiphrenic diverticulum treated by endoscopic submucosal dissection

Kuangi Fu[1,2*], Peng Jin[2], Yuqi He[2], Masanori Suzuki[1] and Jianqiu Sheng[2]

Abstract

Background: We report a unique case of a superficial esophageal cancer arising in a single diverticulum, diagnosed with magnifying image-enhanced endoscopy and then successfully treated by endoscopic submucosal dissection (ESD).

Case presentation: A 66-year-old man with alcohol-related liver injury visited our hospital for endoscopy for investigation of varix. Esophagogastroduodenoscopy showed no varix but a large epiphrenic diverticulum with an area of fainted redness just above the esophagogastric junction. Narrow band imaging revealed a sharply demarcated brownish dotted area, and dilated intra-epithelial papillary capillary loops (IPCL) were subsequently seen after magnification. Chromoendoscopy with 1% Lugol's iodine solution demonstrated a well-demarcated unstained area, approximately 20 mm in diameter. Endoscopic biopsy revealed a squamous cell carcinoma (SCC).

Conclusion: The tumor was completely resected by ESD without perforation. Histologically, it was an intraepithelial SCC without lympho-vascular invasion of cancer cells. No local recurrence or metastasis was detected at the last follow-up of 42 months.

Keywords: Epiphrenic diverticulum, Superficial esophageal cancer, Magnifying endoscopy, Narrow band imaging, Endoscopic submucosal dissection

Background

Cancer can arise from the normal mucosa near or within an esophageal diverticulum. However, cancer located within a diverticulum is a very rare phenomenon; only sporadic cases have been reported to date. The incidence has been reported to be between 0.3 and 3% [1]. Almost all cases were diagnosed at an advanced stage, treated by surgery or radiation, and with overall poor prognosis. Rarely cases are detected in early stage and surgical resection is favored as diverticula have a characteristically thin wall and endoscopic resection carries a real risk of perforation [2]. Herein, we describe a case of a superficial esophageal cancer developed in an epiphrenic esophageal diverticulum, diagnosed with magnifying image-enhanced endoscopy and subsequently treated by endoscopic submucosal dissection (ESD).

* Correspondence: fukuangi@hotmail.com
[1]Department of Gastroenterology, Kanma Memorial Hospital, 2-5, Nasushiobara city, Tochigi 325-0046, Japan
[2]Department of Gastroenterology, PLA Army General Hospital, Beijing 100700, China

Case presentation

A 66-year-old man with alcohol-related liver injury visited our hospital for endoscopy for investigation of varix. Esophagogastroduodenoscopy (Olympus; Japan) showed no varix but a large epiphrenic diverticulum just above the esophagogastric junction (Fig. 1a). An area of fainted redness was detected with white light endoscopy at the base of the diverticulum (Fig. 1b). Narrow band imaging (NBI) endoscopy (GIF-H260Z, Olympus) revealed a demarcated brownish dotted area (Fig. 2a). Dilated intra-epithelial papillary capillary loops (IPCL) classified as B1 according to Japan Esophageal Society classification were subsequently seen on magnification (Fig. 2b) [3, 4]. Chromoendoscopy with 1% Lugol's iodine solution demonstrated a well-demarcated unstained area, approximately 20 mm in diameter, corresponding to the reddish area (Fig. 3). Pink color sign was also seen in the unstained area about 2 min after iodine staining [5]. Endoscopic biopsy revealed a squamous cell carcinoma (SCC). The depth of invasion of the detected

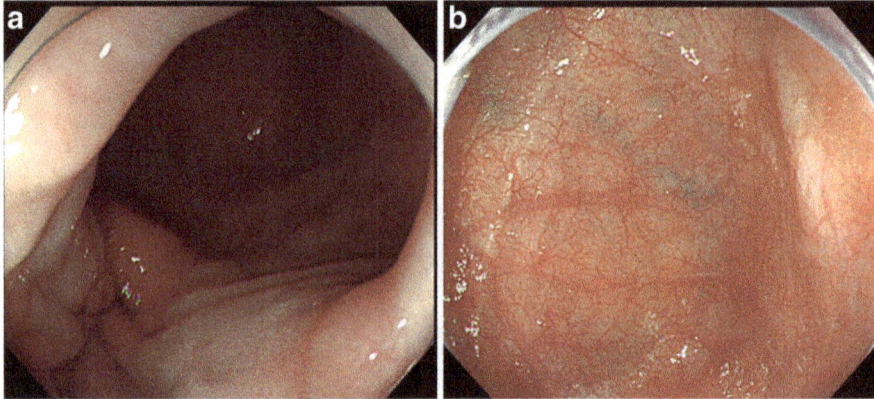

Fig. 1 a A large epiphrenic diverticulum just *above* the esophagogastric junction was seen during esophagogastroduodenoscopy. **b** An area of fainted redness was detected with white light endoscopy at the bottom of the diverticulum

tumor was estimated to remain within the mucosal epithelium (m1) or the lamina propria (m2), which carries almost no potential for nodal involvement. Therefore, ESD was proposed as an alternative to radical surgery and patient consent was obtained. Endoscopic submucosal dissection was conducted with the patient under general anesthesia. CO_2 was used for insufflation to decrease the risk of mediastinal emphysema or pneumothorax in the event of perforation. The lesion was well-lifted after submucosal injection of hyaluronic acid diluted with 10% glycerol at the ratio of 50%. The tumor was completely resected en bloc without complication (Fig. 4). Histologically, the resected specimen was a superficial cancer limited within the lamina propria (m2) without lympho-vascular invasion or marginal involvement of cancer cells. The patient had an uneventful hospital course and was discharged 1 week after ESD. No local recurrence or metastasis was detected at the last follow-up of 42 months (Fig. 5).

Discussion and conclusions

Cancers arising within esophageal diverticulum may be diagnosed at advanced stage despite their small size. As the muscular coat of a diverticulum is extremely thin or none, cancer arising within an esophageal diverticulum can easily extend into the mediastinal space relative to those arising from the normal mucosa apart from the diverticulum. This case was easily detected with the help of magnifying image-enhanced endoscopy in its early stage [3]. Our case illustrates the importance of meticulous endoscopic evaluation of depth invasion of esophageal cancers before removal, as surgery may be avoided in some cases. The changes in the IPCL pattern observed by magnifying NBI were reported to be useful for the qualitative diagnosis of cancerous/non-cancerous lesions and endoscopic diagnosis of invasion depth of cancers [6, 7]. Here we performed endoscopic resection of the lesion, as magnifying image-enhanced endoscopy provided an endoscopic diagnosis of a superficial cancer limited within the lamina propria (m2). It is commonly

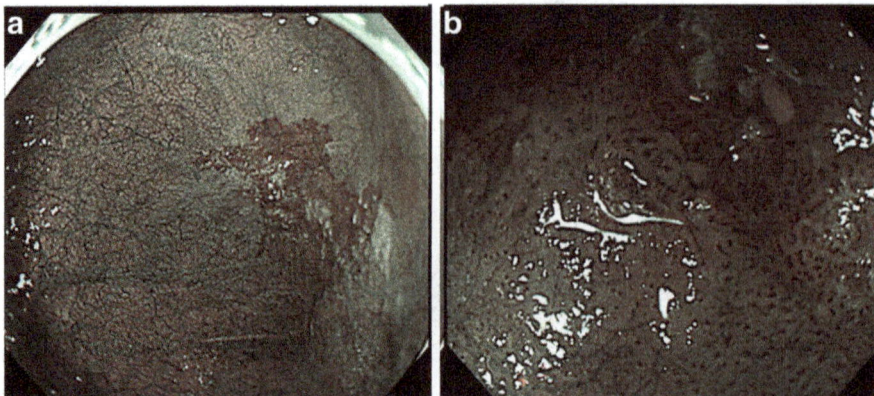

Fig. 2 a NBI revealed a demarcated *brownish dotted* area before magnification. **b** Dilated intra-epithelial papillary capillary loops (IPCL) were seen after magnifying NBI

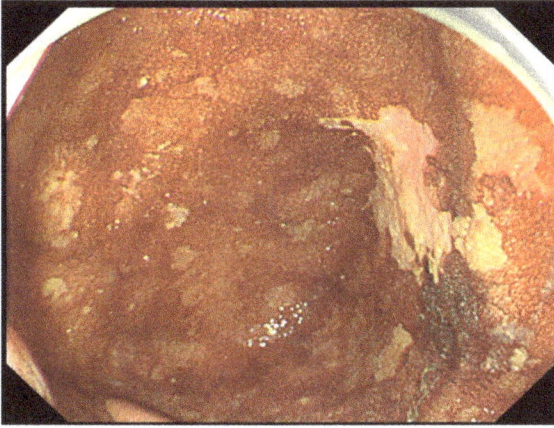

Fig. 3 At the *bottom* of the diverticulum, chromoendoscopy with 1% Lugol's iodine solution demonstrated a well-demarcated unstained area, approximately 20 mm in diameter

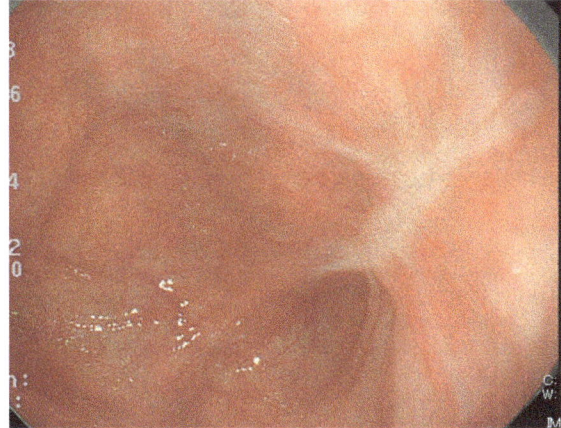

Fig. 5 *White light* endoscopy showed no local recurrence 42 months after ESD

accepted that esophageal cancers limited within m2 are extremely rarely associated with lymph node metastasis and therefore are good candidates for endoscopic resection [8].

Endoscopic ultrasonography (EUS) is commonly used for predicting the depth of tumor invasion in patients with superficial esophageal squamous cell carcinoma [9]. We did not utilize EUS in this case as part of the diagnostic workup, as it was difficult to appropriately approach the lesion located at the base of the diverticulum. Furthermore, diverticulum has a characteristically thin wall, which may be associated with higher risk of perforation during EUS [10].

Endoscopic mucosal resection (EMR) might be an alternative for local resection. There are three representative methods of EMR: endoscopic esophageal mucosal resection (EEMR)-tube method, EMR using a cap-fitted endoscope (EMRC) method and two-channel EMR

method. Generally, the incidence of perforation is lower than that of ESD. However, the lesion described here was not amenable to EMR as pulling the lesion back for resection would have resulted in frank perforation, likely 10 mm or larger in size, making endoscopic closure technically very difficult. Meanwhile, perforation during ESD is always smaller and linear, as the submucosal layer could be dissected under direct visualization [11]. To avoid undesirable perforation, we therefore planned to discontinue ESD if non-lifting sign positive was seen after appropriate submucosal injection. To achieve an appropriate submucosal dissection plane under the tumor for complete removal, mucosal incision and submucosal dissection were started from the oral side of the normal mucosa outside of the diverticulum as both of the submucosal and muscular layers of the diverticulum were expected to be much thinner than those of the normal esophagus histologically.

In conclusion, we report a case of a superficial esophageal cancer developing within an epiphrenic diverticulum. The lesion was correctly diagnosed with magnifying image-enhanced endoscopy and subsequently treated by ESD with long-term success.

Acknowledgements
We thank Dr. Dhavan Parikh (UC Davis Medical Center) for initial editing of this manuscript.

Funding
This work was supported by Capital city public health project (Grant No. Z141100002114007).

Authors' contributions
Concept of the manuscript- KF; lesion detection and ESD procedure- KF; literature review of the manuscript- MS; writing of the manuscript- KF, PJ, YH, JS; all authors have read and approved the final version of the manuscript.

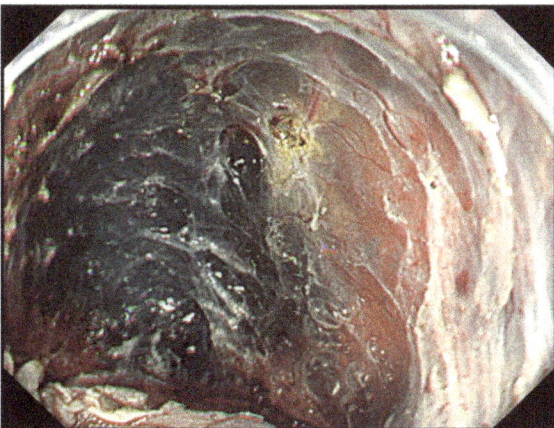

Fig. 4 Mucosal defect after ESD was shown and no definite perforation was seen endoscopically

Competing interests
The authors declare that they have no competing interests.

References
1. Benacci JC, Deschamps C, Trastek VF, Allen MS, Daly RC, Pairolero PC. Epiphrenic diverticulum: results of surgical treatment. Ann Thorac Surg. 1993;55:1109–13.
2. Honda H, Kume K, Tashiro M, Sugihara Y, Yamasaki T, Narita R, et al. Early stage esophageal carcinoma in an epiphrenic diverticulum. Gastrointest Endosc. 2003;57:980–2.
3. Muto M, Minashi K, Yano T, Saito Y, Oda I, Nonaka S, et al. Early detection of superficial squamous cell carcinoma in the head and neck region and esophagus by narrow band imaging: a multicenter randomized controlled trial. J Clin Oncol. 2010;28:1566–72.
4. Oyama T, Inoue H, Arima M, Momma K, Omori T, Ishihara R, et al. Prediction of the invasion depth of superficial squamous cell carcinoma based on microvessel morphology: magnifying endoscopic classification of the Japan esophageal society. Esophagus. 2017;14:105–12.
5. Shimizu Y, Omori T, Yokoyama A, Yoshida T, Hirota J, Ono Y, et al. Endoscopic diagnosis of early squamous neoplasia of the esophagus with iodine staining: high-grade intra-epithelial neoplasia turns pink within a few minutes. J Gastroenterol Hepatol. 2008;23:546–50.
6. Kumagai Y, Inoue H, Nagai K, Kawano T, Iwai T. Magnifying endoscopy, stereoscopic microscopy, and the microvascular architecture of superficial esophageal carcinoma. Endoscopy. 2002;34:369–75.
7. Sato H, Inoue H, Ikeda H, Sato C, Onimaru M, Hayee B, et al. Utility of intrapapillary capillary loops seen on magnifying narrow-band imaging in estimating invasive depth of esophageal squamous cell carcinoma. Endoscopy. 2015;47:122–8.
8. Takubo K, Aida J, Sawabe M, Kurosumi M, Arima M, Fujishiro M. Early squamous cell carcinoma of the oesophagus: the Japanese viewpoint. Histopathology. 2007;51:733–42.
9. Yoshinaga S, Oda I, Nonaka S, Kushima R, Saito Y. Endoscopic ultrasound using ultrasound probes for the diagnosis of early esophageal and gastric cancers. World J Gastrointest Endosc. 2012;4:218–26.
10. ASGE Standards of Practice Committee, Early DS, Acosta RD, Chandrasekhara V, Chathadi KV, Decker GA, Evans JA. Adverse events associated with EUS and EUS with FNA. Gastrointest Endosc. 2013;77:839–43.
11. Oyama T. Esophageal ESD: technique and prevention of complications. Gastrointest Endosc Clin N Am. 2014;24:201–12.

18

Endoscopic submucosal dissection under general anesthesia for superficial esophageal squamous cell carcinoma is associated with better clinical outcomes

Byeong Geun Song, Yang Won Min*, Ra Ri Cha, Hyuk Lee, Byung-Hoon Min, Jun Haeng Lee, Poong-Lyul Rhee and Jae J. Kim

Abstract

Background: Endoscopic submucosal dissection (ESD) has been widely accepted for treating superficial esophageal squamous cell carcinoma (SESCC). The aim of this study was to evaluate the efficacy and safety of ESD for SESCC and the effect of different sedation methods on their clinical outcomes.

Methods: We retrospectively analyzed a total of 169 patients (175 lesions) who underwent ESD for SESCC at Samsung Medical Center, Seoul, South Korea. Short-term and long-term clinical outcomes were evaluated and compared according to the sedation method (conscious sedation [CS] vs general anesthesia [GA]).

Results: En bloc resection, complete resection, and curative resection (CuR) were achieved in 93.7, 74.9, and 58.9% of cancers, respectively. Perforation and stricture occurred in 8.0 and 12.0% of lesions, respectively. During a mean follow-up period of 33.7 months for survival, 3 (3.0%) patients died without evidence of recurrence after achieving CuR. During a mean follow-up period of 32.5 months for recurrence, 1 (1.0%) patient experienced lymph node metastasis. Synchronous and metachronous cancer were found in 1.0% and in 3.0% of patients, respectively. Multivariate analysis revealed that GA was associated with a higher complete resection rate and a lower perforation rate as compared to CS (odds ratio 3.401, 95% confidence interval 1.317–8.785, $P = 0.011$ and odds ratio 0.067, 95% confidence interval 0.006–0.775, $P = 0.030$, respectively).

Conclusions: ESD is an oncologically effective treatment modality for SESCC, particularly when CuR is achieved. Applying GA for esophageal ESD could improve the clinical outcomes of ESD in patients with SESCC.

Keywords: Endoscopic submucosal dissection, Esophageal squamous cell carcinoma, General anesthesia, Sedation, Outcome

Background

Esophageal cancer was ranked the ninth for cancer incidence and the sixth for cancer death in 2013 [1]. Due to aging and growing population, esophageal cancer cases have increased compared to that in 1990. The majority of esophageal cancers are squamous cell carcinomas (SCCs) in the Middle East, Africa, Asia, and parts of Europe [2, 3]. Given the considerable morbidity and mortality of esophagectomy [4–6], endoscopic submucosal dissection (ESD)

has been used for superficial esophageal SCC (SESCC) without metastasis [7]. Furthermore, SESCC is frequently detected due to nationwide screening endoscopy for gastric cancer together with the development of advanced diagnostic techniques such as image-enhanced endoscopy in East Asia including Korea [8–11].

Safety and efficacy of ESD for early gastric cancer (EGC) have been sufficiently verified in many studies [12–14]. However, SESCC is different from EGC when considered for ESD. SESCC has a relatively higher risk of lymph node metastasis (LNM) even when it is confined to the mucosa [15, 16]. The risk of complications

* Correspondence: yangwonee@gmail.com
Department of Medicine, Samsung Medical Center, Sungkyunkwan University School of Medicine, 81 Irwon-ro, Gangnam-gu, Seoul 06351, South Korea

such as stricture and perforation is also higher in SESCC [17–19]. However, there is nonsurgical treatment option such as radiotherapy with or without chemotherapy after non-curative ESD for SESCC [20, 21]. Although several studies have reported the outcomes of ESD for SESCC, most of them were of small sample size and were performed in Japanese population [17, 18, 22–27]. Thus, there is still a need for further outcome data to be reported.

Given the relatively higher complication risk of esophageal ESD, ESD for SESCC is frequently performed under general anesthesia (GA). Indeed, a recent study reported that there was no perforation in 58 esophageal ESDs performed under GA [28]. However, till date, there has been no comparison between GA and conscious sedation (CS) in this aspect.

The aims of this study were (i) to evaluate the clinical outcomes of ESD for SESCC and (ii) to compare the short-term outcomes between ESD under CS and that under GA.

Methods
Patients
Patients who underwent ESD for SESCC at Samsung Medical Center, Seoul, South Korea, between March 2007 and June 2016 were eligible. Based on the final pathologic report, only SCC cases were included. All patients underwent endoscopic evaluation including chromoendoscopy with the Lugol's iodine dye-spraying method. Most of them also underwent endoscopic ultrasound (EUS) to confirm that the cancer was confined to the mucosa except those patients who had mucosal cancer confirmed by EUS which were performed prior to being referred to our institution. In addition, computed tomography (CT) scans of the chest and abdomen were performed in all patients prior to ESD to identify possible distant or local LNM. Finally, esophageal ESD was only performed for those SESCC that were confined to the mucosal layer without distant or local LNM excluding those with obvious SM invasion (Fig. 1). This study was conducted in accordance with the Declaration of Helsinki and approved by the Institutional Review Board at Samsung Medical Center (No. 2016–08-192).

Procedures and follow-ups
Six endoscopists performed esophageal ESD using standard technique as described elsewhere [29, 30]. At first, marking around the cancer is done 2–3 mm away from the edge which is well determined by Lugol's iodine chromoendoscopy. Then circumferential mucosal pre-cutting is performed after submucosal injection. After elevating the lesion by submucosal injection, submucosal layer under the lesion is dissected using various types of ESD knives (Fig. 2).

In the initial phase of the study period, esophageal ESD was mainly performed under CS. For sedation under CS, midazolam and pethidine were administered intravenously by the endoscopist. Since August 2012, selected cases were sedated using intravenous midazolam, propofol, and remifentanil by the anesthesiologist. Since March 2014, when anesthesia machine became available in the endoscopy room, almost all esophageal ESD were performed under GA with endotracheal intubation by the anesthesiologist. GA is induced with rocuronium, midazolam, and propofol and is maintained with propofol and remifentanil.

Six endoscopists performed esophageal ESD in the present study. Among them, three performed ESD under CS, and their mean experience of esophageal ESD was 23.7 cases. The other three performed ESD under CS or GA, and their mean experience was 34.7 cases.

Patients without any complications were discharged from the hospital at day 4 after ESD. To prevent post-ESD stricture, polyglycolic acid sheet application [31] or oral prednisolone administration [32, 33] was applied in patients with a large mucosal defect at the discretion of the endoscopist. Oral prednisolone administration was usually started at a dose of 30 or 40 mg/day, tapered gradually, and then discontinued after 8 weeks.

After curative ESD, upper endoscopy was performed at two months after ESD to exclude the presence of any residual tumor. Endoscopy and chest and abdomen CT scans were performed every 6 months for 3 years. From the 4th to the 5th year after ESD, endoscopy and CT scans were performed annually.

Data collection and definitions
Data in this study were obtained from a prospectively collected database of esophageal ESD. These data included demographics parameters (such as patient's age, gender, past medical history, and body mass index), tumor characteristics (such as the tumor location, endoscopic tumor morphology, gross and pathologic size of the tumor, pathology of the tumor, circumferential size of the tumor and post-ESD mucosal defect), and procedure-related factors (procedure time, method of sedation, and complications).

Tumor location was described according to the American Joint Committee on Cancer divisions of the esophagus [34]. Upper thoracic esophagus refers to the segment of esophagus at a distance of 20 cm to 25 cm from the incisor while middle thoracic esophagus, 25 cm to 30 cm and lower thoracic esophagus, 30 cm to typically, 40 cm. Esophagogastric junction refers to the region between the terminal end of the esophagus and beginning of the stomach at the cardiac orifice.

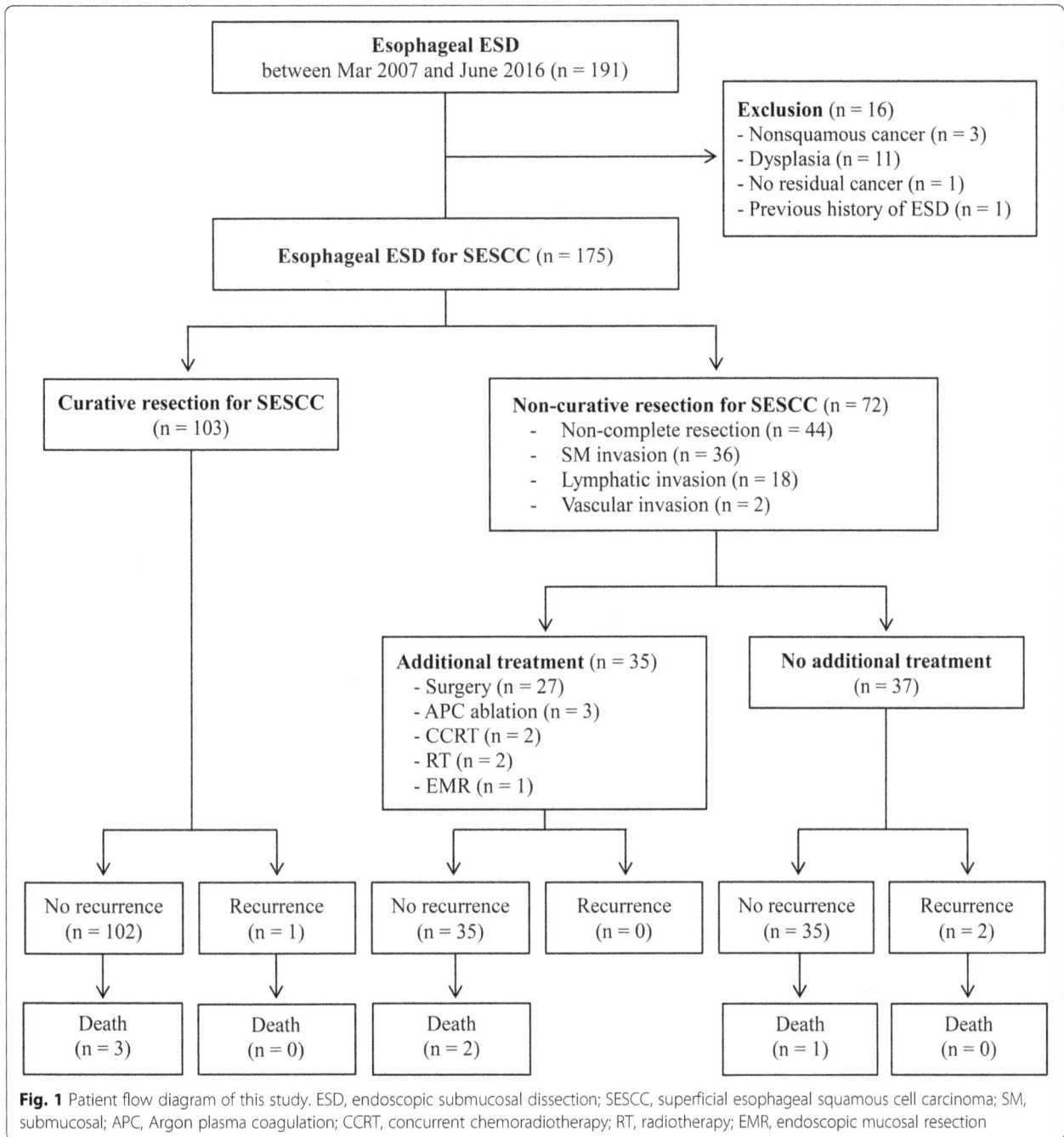

Fig. 1 Patient flow diagram of this study. ESD, endoscopic submucosal dissection; SESCC, superficial esophageal squamous cell carcinoma; SM, submucosal; APC, Argon plasma coagulation; CCRT, concurrent chemoradiotherapy; RT, radiotherapy; EMR, endoscopic mucosal resection

Assessments

Data were analyzed with respect to the en bloc resection (EnR) rate, complete resection (CR) rate, curative resection (CuR) rate, death rate, recurrence rate (local or distal recurrence), presence of synchronous and metachronous cancer, complications, procedure time, and length of hospital stay.

Resected specimens were fixed in formalin and serially sectioned perpendicularly at 2 mm intervals. Depth of invasion was classified into M1 (confined to the intraepithelium), M2 (confined to the lamina propria), M3 (confined to the muscularis mucosa), SM1 (submucosal invasion < 200 μm), and SM2&3 (submucosal invasion ≥200 μm) [35]. EnR was defined as resection of targeted lesions in one piece regardless of the depth of invasion or lymphovascular invasion (LVI). CR was defined as EnR with histologically confirmed tumor-negative margins. CuR was defined as CR without SM invasion, LVI, or poorly differentiated histology. Non-CuR was defined as tumors that did not fulfill the above criteria for CuR.

Local recurrence was defined as a histologically confirmed recurred SCC at the site of ESD after an initial

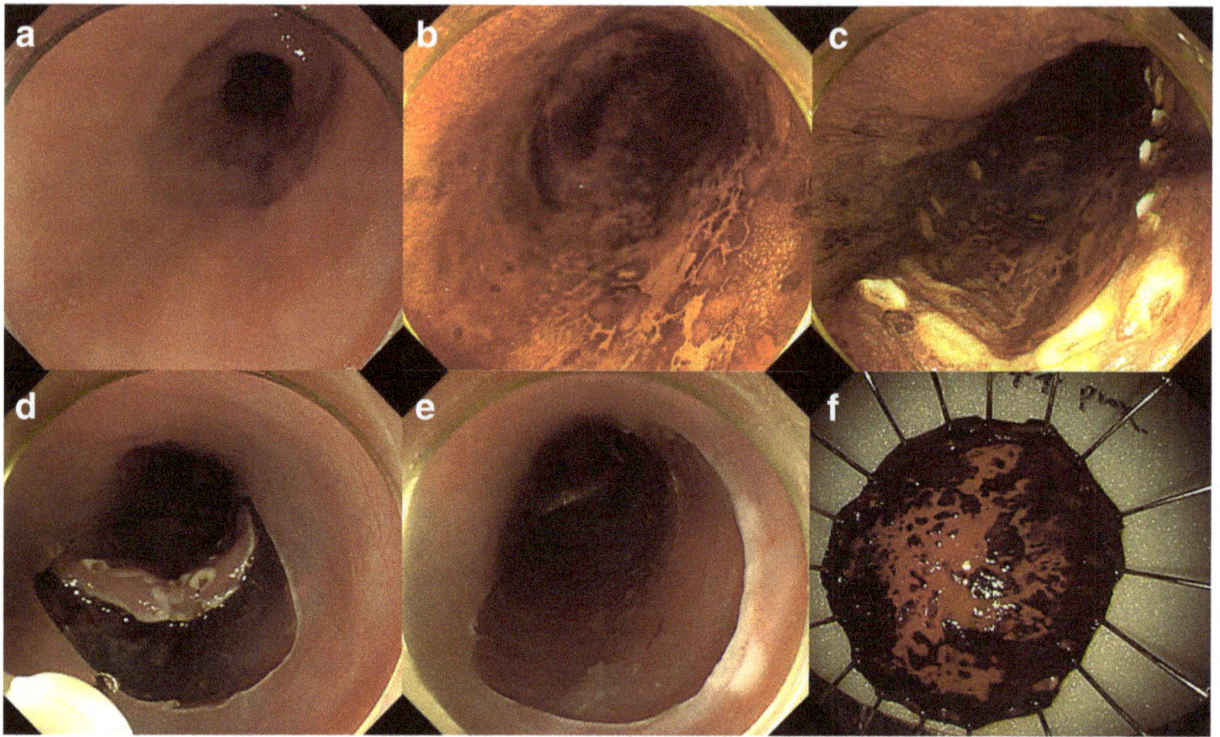

Fig. 2 Endoscopic submucosal dissection (ESD) procedure. **a** On the mid esophagus, a 2.6-cm-sized geographic mucosal hyperemia is noticed. **b** Lugol's solution is sprayed along the lesion to aid visualization. **c** Marking around the lesion is performed. **d** After submucosal injection, circumferential mucosal pre-cutting is performed. **e** After dissection of the submucosal layer, an artificial ulcer is seen. **f** Fixation of the resected specimen

CR. Distant recurrence was defined when a new malignant lesion was detected outside of the esophagus. Synchronous cancer was defined as a histologically confirmed recurred cancer at a different location from the ESD site within 1 year after ESD. Metachronous cancer was defined when recurred cancer was detected more than 1 year after ESD. Procedure time was defined as the interval of time between the first marking and the completion of submucosal dissection.

Complications

The incidence of ESD-related complications including perforation (micro-perforation and frank perforation), bleeding, and stricture were estimated per lesion. Micro-perforation was defined as radiographic evidence of free air or subcutaneous emphysema after ESD without gross perforation defects. Frank perforation was diagnosed when definite esophageal wall defect could be visualized during or after ESD. Bleeding related to ESD was defined as gastrointestinal bleeding that required further hemostatic treatment after the completion of ESD procedure and/or blood transfusion during or after the procedure. Stricture was defined as the presence of dysphagia requiring intervention.

Statistical analysis

Therapeutic efficacy (EnR, CR, and CuR rates) was assessed per lesion. Data were presented as means ± SD or number (%). Categorical variables were compared using Chi-square test or Fisher exact test while continuous variables were compared using Student's t test or Mann-Whitney rank sum test. Multivariate analysis was performed to evaluate whether GA was associated with better short-term outcomes. A p value of less than 5% was considered to be statistically significant. All statistical analyses were performed using SPSS version 23.0 (SPSS Inc., Chicago, IL, USA).

Results

Clinicopathologic characteristics

The clinicopathologic features of the 169 patients with 175 SESCC lesions were summarized in Table 1. The mean age was 64.5 ± 7.9 years. A total of 157 (92.9%) patients were men. Thirteen (7.4%), 46 (26.3%), 113 (64.6%), and 3 (1.7%) lesions were located in the upper-, middle-, lower-esophagus, and the gastroesophageal junction, respectively. Macroscopic type IIa, IIb, IIc, and mixed type were found in 26 (14.9%), 125 (71.4%), 21 (12.0%), and 3 (1.7%) tumors, respectively. The mean gross tumor size was 1.5 ± 0.9 cm and the mean

Table 1 Clinicopathologic characteristics of 169 patients with 175 superficial esophageal squamous cell carcinomas in this study

Variables	
Age (years)	64.5 ± 7.9
Gender, male	157 (92.9)
Body mass index (Kg/m^2)	23.6 ± 2.9
Smoking	
Current smoker	32 (18.9)
Ex-smoker	81 (47.9)
Never-smoker	56 (33.1)
Alcohol	
None	95 (56.2)
> 1 day/month	18 (10.7)
> 1 day/week	27 (16.0)
> 4 days/week	29 (17.2)
Diabetes mellitus (yes)	25 (14.8)
Hypertension (yes)	51 (30.2)
Tumor location	
Upper thoracic	13 (7.4)
Middle thoracic	46 (26.3)
Lower thoracic	113 (64.6)
Esophagogastric junction	3 (1.7)
Tumor morphology	
IIa	26 (14.9)
IIb	125 (71.4)
IIc	21 (12.0)
Mixed	3 (1.7)
Gross tumor size (cm)	1.5 ± 0.9
Pathologic tumor size (cm)	1.5 ± 0.8
Histologic differentiation	
Well differentiated	34 (19.4)
Moderately differentiated	140 (80.0)
Poorly differentiated	1 (0.6)
Circumferential size of the tumor (of lumen)	
< 1/4	50 (28.6)
≥ 1/4, < 1/2	109 (62.3)
≥ 1/2, < 3/4	16 (9.1)
≥ 3/4	0 (0)
Circumferential size of the post-ESD mucosal defect (of lumen)	
< 1/4	5 (2.9)
≥ 1/4, < 1/2	68 (38.9)
≥ 1/2, < 3/4	85 (48.6)
≥ 3/4	17 (9.7)
Depth of tumor invasion	
M1	26 (14.9)

Table 1 Clinicopathologic characteristics of 169 patients with 175 superficial esophageal squamous cell carcinomas in this study (Continued)

Variables	
M2	71 (40.6)
M3	42 (24.0)
SM1	10 (5.7)
SM2&3	26 (14.9)
Method of sedation	
Conscious sedation	93 (53.1)
General anesthesia	82 (46.9)

Data are presented as mean ± SD or number (%) of patients or lesions

pathologic tumor size of the resected specimen was 1.5 ± 0.8 cm. Thirty-four cancers (19.4%), 140 (80.0%), and 1 (0.6%) had well differentiated, moderately differentiated, and poorly differentiated histology, respectively. Most tumors (62.3%) had a circumferential size of < 1/2 but ≥1/4 of the lumen. Most post-ESD mucosal defect (48.6%) had a circumferential size < 3/4 but ≥1/2 of the lumen. Regarding the depth of tumor invasion, 26 (14.9%), 71 (40.6%), 42 (24.0%), 10 (5.7%), and 26 (14.9%) lesions were classified as M1, M2, M3, SM1, and SM2&3, respectively. Esophageal ESD was performed under CS for 93 (53.1%) lesions and under GA for 82 (46.9%) lesions.

Short-term outcomes and complications

Short-term outcomes were shown in Table 2. EnR was achieved for 164 (93.7%) lesions. CR was achieved for

Table 2 Short-term outcomes of endoscopic submucosal dissection for superficial esophageal squamous cell carcinoma

Variables	
En bloc resection (yes)	164 (93.7)
Complete resection (yes)	131 (74.9)
Non-complete resection	44 (25.1)
Piecemeal resection	10 (22.7)
Positive total margin	40 (90.9)
Positive lateral margin	30 (68.2)
Positive vertical margin	22 (50.0)
Curative resection (yes)	103 (58.9)
Non-curative resection	72 (41.1)
Non-complete resection	44 (61.1)
SM invasion	36 (50.0)
Positive lymphatic invasion	18 (25.0)
Positive vascular invasion	2 (2.8)
Procedure time (mins)	64.4 ± 46.2
Hospital stay (days)	6.7 ± 4.5

Data are presented as mean ± SD or number (%) of patients or lesions

131 (74.9%) lesions. Forty-four lesions with non-CR (25.1%) were due to piecemeal resection ($n = 10$) and positive resection margin ($n = 40$). CuR was achieved in 103 lesions (58.9%). Seventy-two lesions with non-CuR were due to non-CR ($n = 44$), SM invasion ($n = 36$), and LVI ($n = 20$). Among the 72 patients with non-CuR, 33 underwent additional treatment: 25 received surgery; 3 received argon plasma coagulation (APC) ablation; 2 received chemo-radiation therapy; 2 received radiation therapy; and 1 received further endoscopic mucosal resection (Fig. 1). The mean procedure time was 64.4 ± 46.2 mins and the mean duration of hospital stay was 6.7 ± 4.5 days.

Procedure-related perforation occurred in 14 (8.0%) lesions. Among 4 (2.3%) patients with frank perforation, 3 (1.7%) were controlled by immediate endoscopic clipping using Quickclips (Olympus, Tokyo, Japan) and 1 (0.6%) underwent operation. Among 10 (5.7%) patients with microperforation, 4 (2.3%) received endoscopic clipping and the remaining 6 (3.4%) had only conservative management including intravenous antibiotics and fasting. No patients with microperforation underwent operation. No patients experienced post-ESD bleeding that required blood transfusion or additional endoscopy for hemostasis.

Post-ESD stricture developed in 21 (12.0%) lesions which corresponded to 21 patients. The mean tumor size of these 21 lesions was 2.1 ± 0.8 cm. Of these 21 lesions, 10 lesions (47.6%) had a post-ESD mucosal defect size larger than 3/4 of the circumference of the lumen, 9 lesions (42.9%) were between 1/2 and 3/4 and the remaining 2 lesions (9.5%) were between 1/2 and 1/4. Twenty patients (11.4%) received balloon dilatation (median 2 sessions, range 1–11 sessions). Three (1.7%) received temporary fully covered esophageal metallic stent insertion, Bonastent (Standard Sci-Tech Inc., Seoul, South Korea), after balloon dilatations (4–10 sessions). One (0.6%) received temporary esophageal stent insertion without prior balloon dilatation. Preventive managements for post-ESD stricture were applied in 18 (10.3%) lesions with large mucosal defect. Among them, polyglycolic acid sheet, NEOVEIL (Gunze, Ayabe, Japan), were applied at the ESD-induced mucosal defect for 6 (3.4%) lesions and oral prednisolone was administered in 12 (6.9%). However, among these lesions that received preventive measures, post-ESD esophageal strictures occurred in 9 (50.0%) lesions (Table 3).

Long-term outcomes

The long-term outcomes of 99 patients achieving CuR were shown in Table 4 and Fig. 3. One-year, 3-year, and 5-year overall survival (OS) of these patients were 100, 97.3, and 93.8%, respectively. One-year, 3-year, and

Table 3 Complications of endoscopic submucosal dissection for superficial esophageal squamous cell carcinoma

Variables	
Perforation (yes)	14 (8.0)
Frank perforation	4 (2.3)
Clipping	3 (1.7)
Operation	1 (0.6)
Microperforation	10 (5.7)
Clipping	4 (2.3)
Conservative management	6 (3.4)
Bleeding (yes)	0 (0)
Stricture (yes)	21 (12.0)
Balloon dilatation	20 (11.4)
Balloon dilatation and temporary stent insertion	3 (1.7)
Temporary stent insertion	1 (0.6)
Preventive treatment for stricture (yes)	18 (10.3)
Polyglycolic acid sheet application	6 (33.3)
Stricture (yes)	4 (66.6)
Oral prednisolone	12 (66.6)
Stricture (yes)	5 (41.7)

Data are shown as number (%) of lesions

5-year recurrence-free survival (RFS) of them were 97.8, 91.5, and 91.5%, respectively. Specifically, during a mean follow-up period of 33.7 months (median 22.9 months, range 2.1–109.2 months) for OS, 3 patients died without esophageal cancer recurrence. During a mean follow-up period of 32.5 months (median 22.9 months, range 2.1–109.2 months) for recurrence, 1 (1.0%) patient experienced LNM and received concurrent chemo-radiation therapy. Esophageal cancer of this patient invaded lamina propria, but there was no LVI. Resection margin was

Table 4 Long–term outcome of 99 patients achieving curative resection

Variables	
Death (yes)	3 (3.0)
Esophageal cancer-related death (yes)	0 (0.0)
Distant recurrence (yes)	1 (1.0)
Lymph node metastasis	1 (1.0)
CCRT	1 (1.0)
Local recurrence (yes)	0 (0.0)
Synchronous cancer (yes)	1 (1.0)
APC ablation	1 (1.0)
Metachronous cancer (yes)	3 (3.0)
ESD	2 (2.0)
Ivor-Lewis operation	1 (1.0)

Data are presented as number (%) of patients
CCRT concurrent chemo-radiation therapy, *APC* argon plasma coagulation, *ESD* endoscopic submucosal dissection

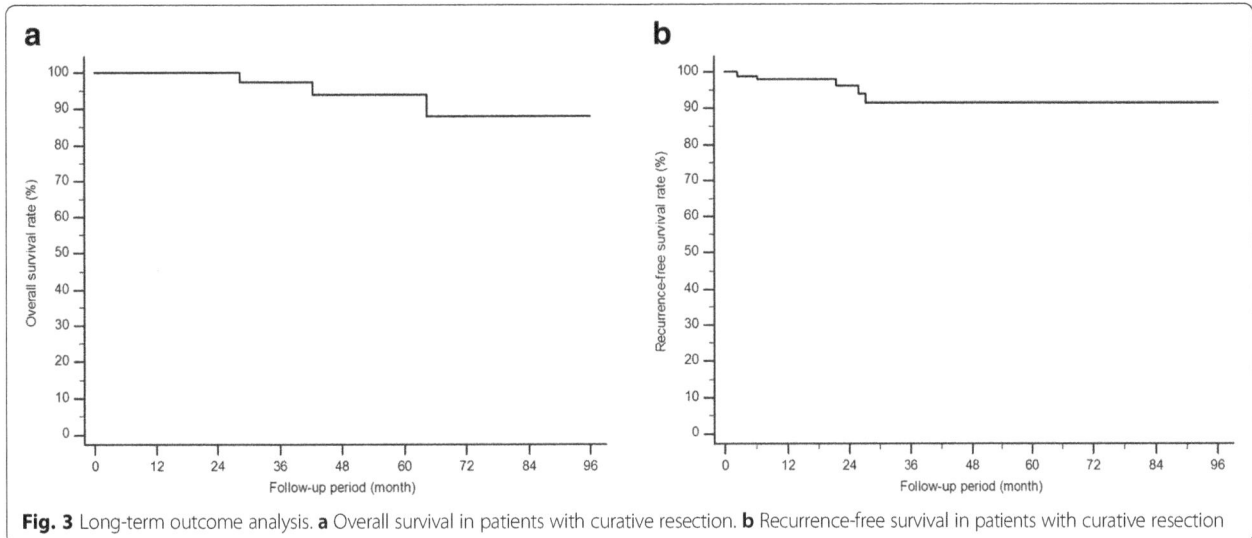

Fig. 3 Long-term outcome analysis. **a** Overall survival in patients with curative resection. **b** Recurrence-free survival in patients with curative resection

negative and the size was 1.2 ×1.3 cm. Two months after ESD, synchronous lesion close to the ESD scar was found. The patient received APC and was followed up without recurrence. However, after 18 months, CT showed a right supraclavicular lymph node enlargement and metastatic SCC was confirmed by histologic examination. Synchronous and metachronous cancers developed in 1 (1.0%) and 3 (3.0%) patients, respectively. The synchronous cancer located close to previous ESD-induced scar and was difficult to be removed by ESD. The patient denied surgery and the lesion was successfully treated with endoscopic ablation using APC. Of the 3 patients with metachronous cancers, 2 underwent repeat esophageal ESD and 1 received Ivor-Lewis operation.

Among the 70 patients with non-CuR, 3 died without esophageal cancer recurrence.

Clinicopathologic characteristics according to the sedation method

As shown in Table 5, there was no significant difference in terms of age, gender, and tumor location between patients/lesions receiving CS and those receiving GA. However, IIa tumor morphology (24.4% vs. 6.5%, $P <$ 0.001) was more frequent, gross tumor size (1.9 ± 1.0 vs. 1.2 ± 0.6 cm, $P <$ 0.001) and pathologic tumor size (1.8 ± 0.9 cm vs. 1.2 ± 0.6 cm, $P <$ 0.001) were larger in the GA group than those in the CS group. In addition, large circumferential size of tumor (≥ 1/2 of lumen) and post-ESD mucosal defect (≥ 3/4 of lumen) were more frequent in the GA group than those in the CS group (13.0% vs. 3.0%, $P =$ 0.005 and 17.1% vs. 3.2%, $P <$ 0.001, respectively). The first 10 ESDs were more frequent in the CS group than in the GA group (40.9% vs. 15.9%, $P <$ 0.001).

Short-term outcomes and perforation rate according to the sedation method

Short-term outcomes and complications according to the sedation method used for ESD were shown in Table 6. EnR rate was higher in the GA group than that in the CS group (100% vs. 88.2%, $P <$ 0.001). However, CR and CuR rates were not significantly different between the two groups. Procedure-related perforation occurred less in the GA group than that in the CS group (1.2% vs. 14.0%, $P =$ 0.002). Procedure time was longer in the GA group than that in the CS group (75.8 ± 47.1 min vs. 52.5 ± 42.4 min, $P =$ 0.001). Hospital stay was shorter in the GA group than that in the CS group (5.5 ± 1.1 days vs. 7.7 ± 5.9 days, $P <$ 0.001).

Multivariate analysis revealed that GA was associated with a higher CR rate and a lower perforation rate as compared to CS (odds ratio 3.401, 95% confidence interval 1.317–8.785, $P =$ 0.011 and odds ratio 0.067, 95% confidence interval 0.006–0.775, $P =$ 0.030, respectively, Table 7).

Discussion

Esophageal ESD has become widely accepted for the treatment of SESCC [17, 18, 23, 36, 37]. However, its indication and curative criteria have not been well established due to scanty outcome data. Thus, this study investigated the outcomes of ESD for SESCC based on a large Korean single center experience. To the best of our knowledge, this is the first study that demonstrates higher CR rate and less perforation rate in esophageal ESD under GA as compared to those under CS.

Our CuR rate (58.9%) was lower than that of the recent series [17, 18]. Park et al. [18] reported a higher CuR rate of 77.0% for esophageal ESD in treating superficial esophageal neoplasm ($n =$ 261). However, their

Table 5 Clinicopathologic features of patients and tumors according to the sedation method used for endoscopic submucosal dissection

Variables	Conscious sedation ($n = 93$)	General anesthesia ($n = 82$)	p-value
Age (years)	63.7 ± 8.0	65.3 ± 7.6	0.191
Gender, male	85 (91.4)	77 (93.9)	0.577
Tumor location			0.064
Upper thoracic	4 (4.3)	9 (11.0)	
Middle thoracic	21 (22.6)	25 (30.5)	
Lower thoracic	65 (69.9)	48 (58.5)	
Esophagogastric junction	3 (3.2)	0 (0.0)	
Tumor morphology			< 0.001
IIa	6 (6.5)	20 (24.4)	
IIb	77 (82.8)	48 (58.5)	
IIc	10 (10.8)	11 (13.4)	
Mixed	0 (0.0)	3 (3.7)	
Gross tumor size (cm)	1.2 ± 0.6	1.9 ± 1.0	< 0.001
Pathologic tumor size (cm)	1.2 ± 0.6	1.8 ± 0.9	< 0.001
Circumferential size of the tumor (of lumen)			0.005
< 1/4	24 (25.8)	26 (31.7)	
≥ 1/4, < 1/2	66 (71.0)	43 (52.4)	
≥ 1/2, < 3/4	3 (3.2)	13 (15.9)	
≥ 3/4	0 (0.0)	0 (0.0)	
Circumferential size of the post-ESD mucosal defect (of lumen)			< 0.001
< 1/4	4 (4.3)	1 (1.2)	
≥ 1/4, < 1/2	49 (52.7)	19 (23.2)	
≥ 1/2, < 3/4	37 (39.8)	48 (58.5)	
≥ 3/4	3 (3.2)	14 (17.1)	
Depth of tumor invasion			< 0.001
M1	20 (21.5)	6 (7.3)	
M2	38 (40.9)	33 (40.2)	
M3	22 (23.7)	20 (24.4)	
SM1	9 (9.7)	1 (1.2)	
SM2&3	4 (4.3)	22 (26.8)	
Experience of endoscopist, First 10 esophageal ESDs	38 (40.9)	13 (15.9)	< 0.001

Data are presented as mean ± SD or number (%) of patients or lesions

Table 6 Short-term outcomes and complications according to the sedation method used for endoscopic submucosal dissection

Variables	Conscious sedation ($n = 93$)	General anesthesia ($n = 82$)	p-value
En bloc resection (yes)	82 (88.2)	82 (100)	0.001
Complete resection (yes)	64 (68.8)	67 (81.7)	0.056
Curative resection (yes)	54 (58.1)	49 (59.8)	0.878
Perforation (yes)	13 (14.0)	1 (1.2)	0.002
Frank perforation	3 (3.2)	1 (1.2)	
Microperforation	10 (10.8)	0 (0.0)	
Procedure time (mins)	52.5 ± 42.4	75.8 ± 47.1	0.001
Hospital stay (days)	7.7 ± 5.9	5.5 ± 1.1	0.001

Data are presented as mean ± SD or number (%) of patients or lesions

Table 7 Multivariate analysis of factors associated with En bloc resection, complete resection, and procedure-related perforation

Variables	En bloc resection		Complete resection		Perforation	
	OR (95% CI)	p-value	OR (95% CI)	p-value	OR (95% CI)	p-value
Age	1.009 (0.921–1.105)	0.844	0.9991 (0.944–1.041)	0.713	1.029 (0.948–1.116)	0.494
Tumor location		0.950		0.376		0.647
Upper thoracic	1		1		1	
Middle thoracic	N/A	0.998	0.822 (0.171–3.959)	0.807	0.483 (0.034–6.948)	0.592
Lower thoracic	N/A	0.998	1.203 (0.276–5.240)	0.805	0.259 (0.020–3.309)	0.298
Esophagogastric Jx	N/A	1.000	0.140 (0.007–2.640)	0.189	N/A	0.999
Tumor morphology		0.734		0.955		0.933
IIa	1		1		1	
IIb	4.775 (0.318–71.736)	0.258	0.830 (0.253–2.728)	0.759	N/A	0.998
IIc	N/A	0.998	1.063 (0.225–5.030)	0.939	N/A	0.998
Mixed	N/A	1.000	0.511 (0.024–10.810)	0.666	N/A	1.000
Gross tumor size (cm)	0.294 (0.063–1.374)	0.120	1.320 (0.630–2.768)	0.462	0.907 (0.236–3.488)	0.888
Resected specimen size (cm)	1.147 (0319–4.126)	0.834	0.475 (0.228–0.989)	0.047	1.926 (0.580–6.397)	0.285
Depth of tumor invasion		0.744		0.228		0.924
Mucosal cancer	1		1		1	
SM invasion	1.467 (0.147–14.623)		0.567 (0.226–1.427)		0.916 (0.150–5.596)	
Experience of endoscopist		0.098		0.146		0.052
First 10 esophageal ESDs	1		1		1	
Further esophageal ESDs	0.226 (0.039–1.315)		0.513 (0.208–1.262)		0.289 (0.082–1.011)	
Method of sedation		0.996		0.011		0.030
Conscious sedation	1		1		1	
General anesthesia	N/A		3.401 (1.317–8.785)		0.067 (0.006–0.775)	

OR odds ratio, *CI* confidence interval, *ESD* endoscopic submucosal dissection

study population consisted of a significant number of dysplasia cases (70 cases, 26.8%) and less SESCCs with SM invasion cases (19 cases, 7.3%) as opposed to no dysplasia cases and higher SESCCs with SM invasion cases (36 cases, 20.6%) in our study. Similarly, in a Japanese multicenter study, CuR rate was reported to be higher at 76.2% (95% CI: 71.5–80.3%) for esophageal ESD in treating esophageal neoplasm (n = 368) [17]. They, too, included a significant number of dysplasia cases (111 cases, 30.2%). Furthermore, criteria for CuR was more inclusive as it was defined as a tumor within SM1 and thus, reducing the number of SESCC (23 cases, 6.3%) with SM invasion that meet the non-CuR criteria (SM2 or deeper invasion) [17].

Depth of tumor invasion is known to be associated with the risk of LNM [15, 38]. In a study assessing the accuracy of EUS for superficial esophageal cancers, the positive and negative predictive values of EUS for SM invasion were 67 and 86%, respectively [39]. According to a recent meta-analysis, the sensitivity and specificity of EUS for T1a staging (from T1b) was 0.85 (95% CI, 0.82–0.88) and 0.87 (95% CI, 0.84–0.90), respectively [40]. Although magnifying endoscopy with narrow-band

imaging has also been used for evaluating depth of tumor invasion, the additional benefit to white-light imaging is questionable [41, 42]. In addition to the depth of tumor invasion, LVI could be investigated for an accurate assessment of the risk of LNM. The risk of LNM is higher in M3 cancer with LVI than that in SM1 cancer without LVI [15, 38]. In this background, esophageal ESD could be applied as a reliable evaluation modality for LNM, although it is a therapeutic procedure for SESCC. Because we performed ESD for patients with SESCC even though minute SM invasion had already been suspected during EGD and EUS examinations, many SESCC cases with SM invasion ended up being included in the current study. This might have resulted in a lower CuR rate.

In this study, there was no death from esophageal cancer recurrence in patients who underwent CuR, and 3% of patients died from other causes. In a multicenter retrospective cohort study that investigated clinical outcomes of esophageal ESD for SESCC, 0.5% died from esophageal cancer, 5.6% died from other causes. Our study's result is comparable with this study [17]. EnR and CR rates were also similar to other study [24].

As the esophageal wall is thin and the lumen is narrow, a stable working field without rapid and/or unexpected movements rendered by GA could facilitate the performance of esophageal ESD with a decreased risk of complication. In this study, CR rate was higher and perforation rate was lower in ESD cases under GA compared to those under CS after adjusting several clinicopathologic factors including experience of endoscopist. Non-complete resection was the most common cause of non-CuR in this study. Thus, increasing CR rate by applying GA for esophageal ESD may improve oncologic outcomes in patients with SESCC. The increased cost of GA is only about US $30–40 in Korea as compared to conscious sedation. Although cost-effectiveness may be different among countries, this study could suggest that esophageal ESD under general anesthesia improves the clinical outcomes of ESD for esophageal cancer. However, although several clinicopathologic factors and experience of endoscopist were adjusted in the multivariate analysis, there is a significant time difference between ESD under CS and GA in this study with the time spent under GA being considerably longer than CS. There could be a risk of potential confounders like advancement of ESD techniques and learning curve effects which should act in favor of GA as GA was introduced in the latter part of the study. However, the ESD lesions resected under GA were considerably larger than the lesions under CS (1.9 ± 1.0 vs. 1.2 ± 0.6, $p < 0.001$). This is not surprising as endoscopist encountering large lesions would often seek GA as the preferred mode of sedation for a better working environment during ESD.

In this study, stricture was defined as the cases receiving intervention to relieve dysphagia. Although other studies also included cases where standard endoscope could not pass through the narrowed lumen, these cases usually undergo intervention. Thus, our stricture rate may not be underestimated. In this study, stricture rate was 12.0% despite the application of preventive managements for post-ESD stricture in cases with large post-ESD mucosal defect. Polyglycolic acid sheet and oral prednisolone could not reduce post-ESD stricture rate below 50% when applied to cases with a large mucosal defect. Stricture is the most common complication of esophageal ESD and its risk increases when the circumference of the mucosal defect is more than 75% of the luminal circumference [43]. Thus, development of effective strategy to reduce post-ESD stricture is imperative for a wider use of esophageal ESD. In this study, patients with stricture received median 2 sessions of balloon dilatation and/or temporary esophageal stent insertion. Considering the limited current treatment options for stricture, development of more effective prevention methods is required.

This study has some limitations. Firstly, it was a single center retrospective study. However, most data on characteristics of patients and tumors, procedure factors, and short-term ESD outcomes were obtained from a prospectively collected database which could minimize the risk of bias. Secondly, ESD under CS was performed in the earlier period of the present study while ESD under GA was in the latter. In addition to the effects of anesthesia per se, improvement of overall ESD technologies (knife, coagulator, etc.) and institutional experience, thus, might also affect the short-term outcomes of ESD with different anesthesia types. Thirdly, the follow-up period was short to demonstrate the definite long-term outcomes of ESD for SESCC. On the other hand, this study was a rather large case series. Lastly, poor outcomes of CS might contribute to statistically significant results. However, the major finding of this study is that CS is an independent risk factor for incomplete resection and perforation. Indeed, CR rate (81.7%) under GA is comparable to that (84.5%) of a recent Japanese multicenter study [17] and perforation rate (1.2%) under GA is even better than that (5.2%) of the study. Thus, GA appears to improve the outcomes of esophageal ESD.

Conclusion

Our results suggest that ESD is a safe and effective treatment for SESCC, particularly when CuR is achieved. Applying GA for esophageal ESD could improve the clinical outcomes of ESD in patients with SESCC.

Abbreviations

APC: Argon plasma coagulation; CR: Complete resection; CS: Conscious sedation; CT: Computed tomography; CuR: Curative resection; EGC: Early gastric cancer; EnR: En bloc reserction; ESD: Endoscopic submucosal dissection; EUS: Endoscopic ultrasound; GA: General anesthesia; LNM: Lymph node metastasis; LVI: Lymphovascular invasion; OS: Overall survival; RFS: Recurrence free survival; SCCs: Squamous cell carcinomas; SD: Standard deviation; SESCC: Superficial esophageal squamous cell carcinoma; SM: Submucosal

Funding

This paper was supported by the following grant (s): The National R & D Program for Cancer Control, Ministry of Health & Welfare, Korea (1720180).

Authors' contributions

SBG and MYW contributed to data acquisition, analysis, and interpretation and drafted the manuscript. CRR, LH, MBH, LJH, RPL contributed to the data interpretation and edited the manuscript. KJJ designed and coordinated the study, contributed to the data interpretation, and edited the manuscript. All the authors approved the final version of the manuscript.

Competing interests

The authors declare they have no competing interests.

References

1. Global Burden of Disease Cancer Collaboration, Fitzmaurice C, Dicker D, Pain A, Hamavid H, Moradi-Lakeh M, et al. the global burden of Cancer 2013. JAMA Oncol. 2015;1:505–27.
2. Ferlay J, Soerjomataram I, Dikshit R, Eser S, Mathers C, Rebelo M, et al. Cancer incidence and mortality worldwide: sources, methods and major patterns in GLOBOCAN 2012. Int J Cancer. 2015;136:E359–86.
3. Goda K, Singh R, Oda I, Omae M, Takahashi A, Koike T, et al. Current status of endoscopic diagnosis and treatment of superficial Barrett's adenocarcinoma in Asia-Pacific region. Dig Endosc. 2013;25(Suppl 2):146–50.
4. Ra J, Paulson EC, Kucharczuk J, Armstrong K, Wirtalla C, Rapaport-Kelz R, et al. Postoperative mortality after esophagectomy for cancer: development of a preoperative risk prediction model. Ann Surg Oncol. 2008;15:1577–84.
5. Chang AC, Ji H, Birkmeyer NJ, Orringer MB, Birkmeyer JD. Outcomes after transhiatal and transthoracic esophagectomy for cancer. Ann Thorac Surg. 2008;85:424–9.
6. Connors RC, Reuben BC, Neumayer LA, Bull DA. Comparing outcomes after transthoracic and transhiatal esophagectomy: a 5-year prospective cohort of 17,395 patients. J Am Coll Surg. 2007;205:735–40.
7. Takahashi H, Arimura Y, Masao H, Okahara S, Tanuma T, Kodaira J, et al. Endoscopic submucosal dissection is superior to conventional endoscopic resection as a curative treatment for early squamous cell carcinoma of the esophagus (with video). Gastrointest Endosc. 2010;72:255–64. 64.e1–2
8. Lee KS, Oh DK, Han MA, Lee HY, Jun JK, Choi KS, et al. Gastric cancer screening in Korea: report on the national cancer screening program in 2008. Cancer Res Treat. 2011;43:83–8.
9. Shimizu Y, Takahashi M, Yoshida T, Ono S, Mabe K, Kato M, et al. Endoscopic resection (endoscopic mucosal resection/ endoscopic submucosal dissection) for superficial esophageal squamous cell carcinoma: current status of various techniques. Dig Endosc. 2013;25(Suppl 1):13–9.
10. Kumagai Y, Monma K, Kawada K. Magnifying chromoendoscopy of the esophagus: in-vivo pathological diagnosis using an endocytoscopy system. Endoscopy. 2004;36:590–4.
11. Yoshida T, Inoue H, Usui S, Satodate H, Fukami N, Kudo SE. Narrow-band imaging system with magnifying endoscopy for superficial esophageal lesions. Gastrointest Endosc. 2004;59:288–95.
12. Choi LJ, Lee NR, Kim SG, Lee WS, Park SJ, Kim JJ, et al. Short-term outcomes of endoscopic submucosal dissection in patients with early Cancer: a prospective multicenter cohort study. Gut Liver. 2016;10:739–48.
13. Min BH, Kim ER, Kim KM, Park CK, Lee JH, Rhee PL, et al. Surveillance strategy based on the incidence and patterns of recurrence after curative endoscopic submucosal dissection for early gastric cancer. Endoscopy. 2015; 47:784–93.
14. Pyo JH, Lee H, Min BH, Lee JH, Choi MG, Lee JH, et al. Long-term outcome of endoscopic resection vs. surgery for early gastric Cancer: a non-inferiority-matched cohort study. Am J Gastroenterol. 2016;111:240–9.
15. Eguchi T, Nakanishi Y, Shimoda T, Iwasaki M, Igaki H, Tachimori Y, et al. Histopathological criteria for additional treatment after endoscopic mucosal resection for esophageal cancer: analysis of 464 surgically resected cases. Mod Pathol. 2006;19:475–80.
16. Soetikno R, Kaltenbach T, Yeh R, Gotoda T. Endoscopic mucosal resection for early cancers of the upper gastrointestinal tract. J Clin Oncol. 2005;23: 4490–8.
17. Tsujii Y, Nishida T, Nishiyama O, Yamamoto K, Kawai N, Yamaguchi S, et al. Clinical outcomes of endoscopic submucosal dissection for superficial esophageal neoplasms: a multicenter retrospective cohort study. Endoscopy. 2015;47:775–83.
18. Park HC, Kim DH, Gong EJ, Na HK, Ahn JY, Lee JH, et al. Ten-year experience of esophageal endoscopic submucosal dissection of superficial esophageal neoplasms in a single center. Korean J Intern Med. 2016;31:1064–72.
19. Kim GH, Jee SR, Jang JY, Shin SK, Choi KD, Lee JH, et al. Stricture occurring after endoscopic submucosal dissection for esophageal and gastric tumors. Clin Endosc. 2014;47:516 22.
20. Kawaguchi G, Sasamoto R, Abe E, Ohta A, Sato H, Tanaka K, et al. The effectiveness of endoscopic submucosal dissection followed by

21. Ikeda A, Hoshi N, Yoshizaki T, Fujishima Y, Ishida T, Morita Y, et al. Endoscopic submucosal dissection (ESD) with additional therapy for superficial esophageal Cancer with submucosal invasion. Intern Med. 2015; 54:2803–13.
22. Kim DH, Jung HY, Gong EJ, Choi JY, Ahn JY, Kim MY, et al. Endoscopic and oncologic outcomes of endoscopic resection for superficial esophageal neoplasm. Gut Liver. 2015;9:470–7.
23. Probst A, Aust D, Markl B, Anthuber M, Messmann H. Early esophageal cancer in Europe: endoscopic treatment by endoscopic submucosal dissection. Endoscopy. 2015;47:113–21.
24. Joo DC, Kim GH, Park DY, Jhi JH, Song GA. Long-term outcome after endoscopic submucosal dissection in patients with superficial esophageal squamous cell carcinoma: a single-center study. Gut Liver. 2014;8:612–8.
25. Park JS, Youn YH, Park JJ, Kim JH, Park H. Clinical outcomes of endoscopic submucosal dissection for superficial esophageal squamous neoplasms. Clin Endosc. 2016;49:168–75.
26. Yamashina T, Ishihara R, Nagai K, Matsuura N, Matsui F, Ito T, et al. Long-term outcome and metastatic risk after endoscopic resection of superficial esophageal squamous cell carcinoma. Am J Gastroenterol. 2013;108:544–51.
27. Ono S, Fujishiro M, Niimi K, Goto O, Kodashima S, Yamamichi N, et al. Long-term outcomes of endoscopic submucosal dissection for superficial esophageal squamous cell neoplasms. Gastrointest Endosc. 2009;70:860–6.
28. Yamashita K, Shiwaku H, Ohmiya T, Shimaoka H, Okada H, Nakashima R, et al. Efficacy and safety of endoscopic submucosal dissection under general anesthesia. World J Gastrointest Endosc. 2016;8:466–71.
29. Fujishiro M, Yahagi N, Kakushima N, Kodashima S, Muraki Y, Ono S, et al. Endoscopic submucosal dissection of esophageal squamous cell neoplasms. Clin Gastroenterol Hepatol. 2006;4:688–94.
30. Fujishiro M, Kodashima S, Goto O, Ono S, Niimi K, Yamamichi N, et al. Endoscopic submucosal dissection for esophageal squamous cell neoplasms. Dig Endosc. 2009;21:109–15.
31. Iizuka T, Kikuchi D, Yamada A, Hoteya S, Kajiyama Y, Kaise M. Polyglycolic acid sheet application to prevent esophageal stricture after endoscopic submucosal dissection for esophageal squamous cell carcinoma. Endoscopy. 2015;47:341–4.
32. Kataoka M, Anzai S, Shirasaki T, Ikemiyagi H, Fujii T, Mabuchi K, et al. Efficacy of short period, low dose oral prednisolone for the prevention of stricture after circumferential endoscopic submucosal dissection (ESD) for esophageal cancer. Endosc Int Open. 2015;3:E113–7.
33. Wang W, Ma Z. Steroid administration is effective to prevent strictures after endoscopic esophageal submucosal dissection: a network meta-analysis. Medicine (Baltimore). 2015;94:e1664.
34. Berry MF. Esophageal cancer: staging system and guidelines for staging and treatment. J Thorac Dis. 2014;6(Suppl 3):S289–97.
35. Japan Esophageal Society. Japanese classification of esophageal Cancer, 11th edition: part I. Esophagus. 2017;14:1–36.
36. Pimentel-Nunes P, Dinis-Ribeiro M, Ponchon T, Repici A, Vieth M, De Ceglie A, et al. Endoscopic submucosal dissection: European Society of Gastrointestinal Endoscopy (ESGE) guideline. Endoscopy. 2015;47:829–54.
37. Kuwano H, Nishimura Y, Oyama T, Kato H, Kitagawa Y, Kusano M, et al. Guidelines for diagnosis and treatment of carcinoma of the esophagus April 2012 edited by the Japan esophageal society. Esophagus 2015. 12:1–30.
38. Akutsu Y, Uesato M, Shuto K, Kono T, Hoshino I, Horibe D, et al. The overall prevalence of metastasis in T1 esophageal squamous cell carcinoma: a retrospective analysis of 295 patients. Ann Surg. 2013;257:1032–8.
39. Rampado S, Bocus P, Battaglia G, Ruol A, Portale G, Ancona E. Endoscopic ultrasound: accuracy in staging superficial carcinomas of the esophagus. Ann Thorac Surg. 2008;85:251–6.
40. Thosani N, Singh H, Kapadia A, Ochi N, Lee JH, Ajani J, et al. Diagnostic accuracy of EUS in differentiating mucosal versus submucosal invasion of superficial esophageal cancers: a systematic review and meta-analysis. Gastrointest Endosc. 2012;75:242–53.
41. Ebi M, Shimura T, Yamada T, Mizushima T, Itoh K, Tsukamoto H, et al. Multicenter, prospective trial of white-light imaging alone versus white-light

imaging followed by magnifying endoscopy with narrow-band imaging for the real-time imaging and diagnosis of invasion depth in superficial esophageal squamous cell carcinoma. Gastrointest Endosc 2015;81: 1355–61 e2.

42. Singh A, Konda VJ, Siddiqui U, Xiao SY, Waxman I. Use of narrow-band imaging with magnification to predict depth of invasion of early esophageal squamous cell cancer and to guide endoscopic therapy. Gastrointest Endosc. 2015;81:469–70. discussion 70

43. Jain D, Singhal S. Esophageal stricture prevention after endoscopic submucosal dissection. Clin Endosc. 2016;49:241–56.

19

Circular stripes were more common in Barrett's esophagus after acetic acid staining

Yating Sun[1], Shiyang Ma[1*], Li Fang[2], Jinhai Wang[1] and Lei Dong[1]

Abstract

Background: The diagnosis of Barrett's esophagus (BE) is disturbed by numerous factors, including correct gastroesophageal junction judgment, the initial location of the Z-line and the biopsy result above it. The acetic acid (AA) could help to diagnose BE better than high resolution imaging technology or magnifying endoscopy, by providing enhanced contrast of different epithelium. We have noticed AA could produce multiple white circular lines, forming circular stripes (CS), at lower esophagus, which hasn't been reported by others. This study aimed to investigate whether the CS is a special marker in BE patients.

Methods: A total of 47 BE patients and 63 healthy people were enrolled from March 2016 to October 2016, and 2% AA staining had been operated routinely at lower esophagus under high resolution gastroscopy. We observed whether there were CS after AA staining and the images were compared between the two groups.

Results: CS were confirmed in 42 patients (89.36%) in the BE group and 5 (7.94) in the control group (($\chi^2 = 72.931$, $P < 0.001$)). The average width of CS was 0.76 ± 0.25 cm in BE group, which was similar to that in the control group (0.88 ± 0.11 cm). Villous or punctate or reticular pattern usually existed above or below the CS.

Conclusions: CS could be found at lower esophagus in most BE patients with AA staining, and this special feature might be valuable in diagnosing, evaluating and following up of BE patients.

Keywords: Barrett's esophagus, Chromoendoscopy, Esophagogastric junction, Intestinal metaplasia

Background

Barrett's esophagus (BE) is defined as the replacement of squamous epithelium of the lower esophagus by single layer columnar epithelium [1–4], with or without the intestinal metaplasia (IM), which may be accompanied by risk of progression to carcinoma [4–6]. In recent years, the morbidity of esophageal squamous cell carcinoma and gastric carcinoma has been decreasing, while the incidence of esophageal adenocarcinoma is gradually increasing [5]. Therefore BE has attracted more attention as the most important precancerous lesion of esophageal adenocarcinoma.

The diagnosis of BE is disturbed by numerous factors clinically. Firstly, judgment for esophagogastric junction (EGJ) is subjective to some extent [7]. EGJ is usually defined by the top of the gastric folds, or the location of esophagus palisade blood vessel [8–13], both of which will be influenced by respiration, the volume of gas injected, the pressure of esophagus, even the relative position of diaphragmatic hiatus [9]. Secondly, the shape of the Z-line is another disturbing factor, and the biopsy result of columnar epithelium is meaningless if the initial or correct location of Z-line is wrong. Therefore, the accurate diagnosis of BE is based on correct EGJ judgment, the initial location of the Z-line, and the biopsy result above the Z-Line.

High resolution imaging technology and magnifying endoscopy have greatly improved the observation of mucosal micro-pattern. However, chromoendoscopy is irreplaceable. The acetic acid (AA) could provide better contrast of different epithelium. It is a kind of dye that can react specifically and reversibly with the columnar

* Correspondence: mashiyang123msy@163.com
[1]Department of Gastroenterology, the Second Affiliated Hospital of Xi'an Jiaotong University, No. 157 Xiwu Road, Xi'an, Shaanxi 710004, China

cells, however the exact mechanism is unclear yet. It is speculated that reversible degeneration of cellular proteins causes aceto-whitening reaction [14]. There are studies confirming that the AA used for BE epithelial staining could identify the mucosal microstructure especially highlight dysplasia and early cancer [15–18]. Meanwhile AA can increase the contrast between the squamous and columnar epithelium, producing white line at the junction which is coincident with Z-line in the healthy people. We have noticed that AA could produce multiple white circular lines, forming circular stripes (CS) at lower esophagus, and this feature was more common in BE patients. So a retrospective study was conducted to investigate whether the CS is a special marker for BE patients.

Methods

Patients

Both BE patients and control group participants were selected from Data of Endoscopy Center of The 2nd Affiliated Hospital of Xi'an Jiaotong University from March 2016 to October 2016.

Inclusion criteria: The BE patients should be diagnosed as full range or tongue type at least once before the research with pathological evidenc according to biopsy standard of ACG Clinical Guideline, 18 to 85 years old, male or female, outpatient or hospitalization. In this research, there are also some typical endoscope features can be seen to support BE diagnose, including columnar epithelium above esophagogastric junction (EGJ) where should be squamous epithelium normally, repositioned Z-line (upward the normal position > 0.5 cm) and the orange esophageal epithelium below the Z-line which is carnation in healthy people, and paliform vessel below the Z-line can be observed. If without the imaging evidence above, the patient will be removed out from the study.

In the control group, healthy physical examination participants with similar age and sex were selected. Esophageal AA staining was performed in both groups during the routine gastroscopy procedure and the images were fully integrated to identify the epithelial structure of lower esophagus near the Z-line.

Exclusion criteria: Patients with esophageal epithelial erosion which is always lead by gastroesphageal reflux disease (GERD) and will impact the mucosa observation after AA staining (Additional file 1), patients with esophageal or gastric cancer, patients with acute gastrointestinal bleeding, and patients with upper gastrointestinal surgery were excluded. Inappropriate patients, such as normal Z-line location in BE group, or BE in control group, were excluded either (Fig. 1).

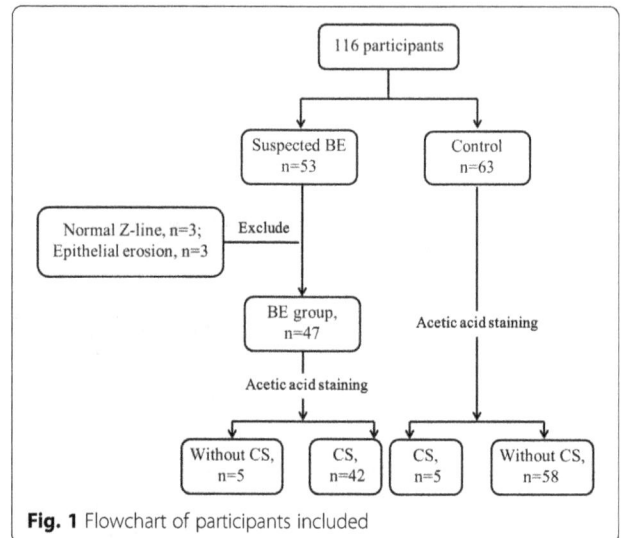

Fig. 1 Flowchart of participants included

Materials and equipments

AA was prepared as a 2% solution by diluting 5 mL of 6% acetic acid in (with) 10 mL of distilled water used for dyeing. High resolution gastroscopes (EG29-i10; PENTAX, Japan) were used for recording pictures and videos.

Protocol

The endoscope would be placed at the lower esophagus, or proximal end of the lesion if there was obvious metaplasia. The mucosa should be cleaned by injecting water before taking photos. Then 10 – 15 ml AA would be sprayed by spraying pipe onto cleaned mucosa, and further observation began after 30 s [19]. The biopsy were taken in and out of CS region with 1∼2 pieces separately. Patients were given spasmolytic (Anisodamine 10 mg im.) and sedation (Midazolam 5 mg im.) before the examination to reduce the discomfort.

Diagnostic criteria for CS

Made the Z-line and the submucosa of the esophageal folds evenly with moderate air under endoscope. The imaging features before AA staining were recorded. Thirty seconds after AA staining, the mucosa of lower esophagus and cardia turned white at the same time, which meaned the albino acetate reaction. Then, white linear stripes, so-called circular stripes, generally with a length of more than 0.5 cm, could be observed below the Z-line. These stripes had clear boundaries and distributed in circular or a certain quadrant. The images after AA staining were recorded. About 4–6 min later, the whitening area gradually returned to normal color and shape. This phenomenon is defined as CS positive in this study, which is approved and reviewed by two experienced endoscopic physicians.

All patients signed the informed consent of gastros-copy examination and AA staining. All aspects of the study were conducted using de-identified photographs and videos. Because all the photographs and videos existed before initiation of the study, this study was granted exempt status by the Xi'an Jiaotong University Human Research Committee.

Outcomes

The primary end point of the study was whether there were CS. The secondary outcome included the distribution and width of the CS, the length from the Z-line to the EGJ (presumed by CS) which was recorded using the Prague C&M criteria [20], the fine structure of the mucosa below the Z-line according to Guelrud M's study [21], and the clinical symptoms of patients in BE group.

Statistical methods

All analyses were performed with SPSS 18.0 software. χ^2 test or Fisher's exact test were used to compare the categorical variables. As the age for each group was normally distributed and had equal variance, t-test was conducted to test their mean difference. Statistical difference was considered to be significant at the level of 0.05.

Results

The general characteristics of the subject

A total of 110 people were enrolled in the study and there were 47 patients in the BE group. Consistent with our patient population, the majority of the patients were over-aged with a roughly equal distribution between males and females (Table 1). In the BE group, the main

clinical symptoms were not the same. 19 patients (40.42%) had acid reflux and heartburn, 12 (25.53%) had upper abdominal pain, 7 (14.89%) had abdominal distention, 5 (10.64%) had abdominal discomfort, and 4 (8.51%) had no typical symptom. In control group, there was no patient having symptom, consistent with the healthy screening population. There were not significant differences between two group of their taste preference (Table 1).

Outcomes

In the BE group, the average M length of BE epithelium was 1.35 ± 0.48 cm (Prague criteria), and the C length was 0.50 ± 0.32 cm (Table 2). There was no long segment BE patient, and there were 38 (80.85%) patients with 1 cm ≤ M < 3 cm and 9 (19.14%) patients with M < 1 cm respectively. After acetic acid staining, CS was showed in a total of 42 patients (89.36%) in the BE group, which was significantly higher than that in the control group (5/63, 7.94%). There was a significant difference between the two groups ($\chi^2 = 72.931$, $P < 0.001$). CS could be found in the control group, which indicating movement of Z-line in 5 cases. The average width of CS was 0.73 ± 0.25 cm in the BE group, which was similar with that in the control group (0.88 ± 0.11 cm, $t = -1.270$, $P = 0.211$).

In BE group, mucosa patterns were always abnormal above the CS, including 33.33% villous (Fig. 2a), 30.95% reticular and 33.33% punctate pattern. Blow the CS, the reticular (50.00%) and punctate patterns (45.24%) were observed after staining (Fig. 2b, c). There were some

Table 1 Baseline characteristics of the two groups

	BE group n = 47	Control group n = 63	χ^2	P value
Age, mean ± SD	53.68 ± 14.39	49.41 ± 11.51	1.728[a]	0.087
Female, n (%)	16 (34.0)	28 (44.4)	1.214	0.271
Fissure hernia, n (%)	6 (12.8)	4 (6.3)	1.341	0.320*
Taste preference				
Peppery	14 (29.79)	21 (33.33)	5.283	0.152
Sweet	11 (23.40)	18 (28.57)		
Sour	7 (14.89)	15 (22.22)		
Plain food	15 (31.91)	9 (14.29)		
Sympotoms (%)				
Acid reflux or heartburn	19 (40.42)	0		
Upper abdominal pain	12 (25.53)	0		
Abdominal distention	7 (14.89)	0		
Abdominal discomfort	5 (10.64)	0		
Asymptomatic	4 (8.51)	63 (100.00)		

*Fisher's exact test
[a]t value from t-test

Table 2 Results of gastroscopy and pathology in BE group vs control group

	BE group $n=47$	Control group $n=63$	χ^2 or t value	P value
M value(cm), mean ± SD	1.35 ± 0.48	–		
C value(cm), mean ± SD	0.50 ± 0.32	–		
CS below the Z-line, n(%)	42 (89.36)	5 (7.94)	72.931	< 0.001
Width of CS (cm), mean ± SD	0.73 ± 0.25	0.88 ± 0.11	-1.270[a]	0.211
Above the CS				
Punctate pattern, n (%)	14 (33.33)	1 (20.00)	–	*
Reticular pattern, n (%)	13 (30.95)	3 (60.00)	–	*
Villous pattern, n (%)	14 (33.33)	0 (0.00)	–	*
Below the CS				
Punctate pattern, n (%)	19 (45.24)	2 (40.00)	–	*
Reticular pattern, n (%)	21 (50.00)	2 (40.00)	–	*
Villous pattern, n (%)	0	0	–	*
Without the CS	5 (10.6)	58 (92.1)	72.931	< 0.001
Punctate pattern, n	2 (40.00)	1 (1.72)	–	*
Reticular pattern, n	2 (40.00)	0 (0.00)	–	*
Villous pattern, n	1 (20.00)	0 (0.00)	–	*
Pathology confirmed intestinal metaplasia (IM), n (%)	23 (48.94)	3 (4.76)	29.101	< 0.001
The region of CS, n (%)	8 (34.78)	2 (66.67)	–	*
Above the CS, n (%)	13 (56.52)	1 (33.33)	–	*
Below the CS, n (%)	2 (8.70)	0 (0.00)	–	*

*The sample size of the variable is too small to do the hypothesis testing
[a]t value from t-test

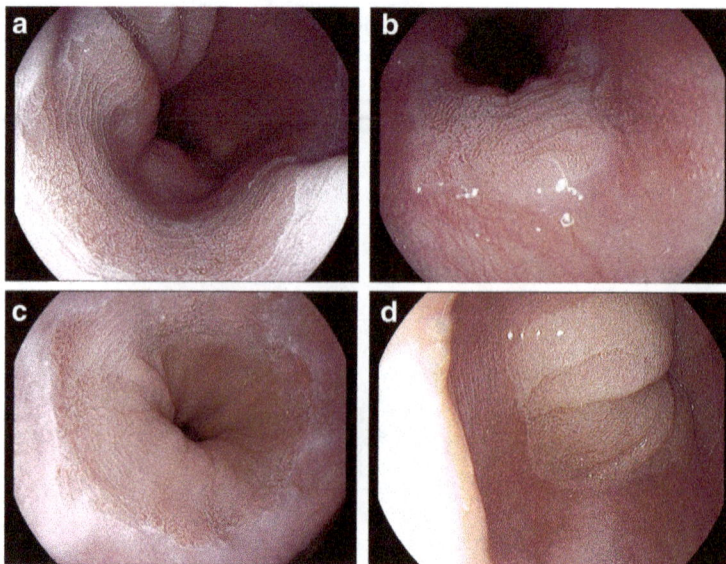

Fig. 2 Aceto-whitening reaction for the diagnosis of BE after instillation of 2% acetic acid. **a**, **b**, **c** After spraying acetic acid, the mucosal surface shows multiple CS near EGJ, with the surface pattern could be identified by either reticular or punctate or villous. **d** normal mucosa with punctate pattern without CS

abnormal mucosa patterns observed in control group (Table 2).

Without CS, the mucosa patterns were always normal, just 1 participant in control group without CS (1/58) was observed to have punctate pattern (Fig. 2d). But in BE group, although 5 patients didn't have CS, their mucosa patterns were all abnormal.

Pathological examination showed that 23 (48.94%) patients had intestinal metaplasia (IM), which was significant more than control group (3/63, 4.76%). The patients with IM all had CS meanwhile. In BE group, 34.78% IMs were detected in the region of CS, 56.52% were above the CS and just 8.70% were below the CS.

Discussion

Because the AA could give a good enhancement on the mucosa pattern at lower esophagus, we were using AA staining as a routine procedure for gastroscopy and the CS were unexpected discovery. In this study, CS were mostly observed in the BE group. There might be three potential mechanisms underneath this phenomenon.

Firstly, the CS might be caused by columnar epithelial metaplasia following squamous epithelium retraction. The AA might emphasize the gap between columnar epithelium in different periods. It could be found that the squamous epithelium was in circular pattern near the cardia in healthy people and the CS partially crossed from columnar epithelium to squamous epithelium (Fig. 3a, b), both supporting this explanation. However, the CS were only confined at the cardia within 2 cm. The emergence of new columnar epithelium in the

higher position no longer formed CS anymore and could be found in punctate, reticular or villous pattern while the previous two mainly. On the other hand, there could be absence of CS in 5 BE patients and villous or punctuate mucosa pattern were observed (Fig. 3c). Therefore, the generation of the CS cannot be fully explained only by the regression and metaplasia theory.

The second possible explanation was that the CS might be specifically performed at the EGJ region and its scope exactly represented the range of EGJ. The hypothesis, that EGJ was not a simple line, but a small portion of the lower esophagus to the cardia, was suggested by previous studies [22–24]. The dense squamous epithelium covering the EGJ might be the reason why we could less likely observe CS in the control group. When the squamous epithelium gradually became thinner or replaced by columnar epithelium, the CS would be revealed. However, more evidence needs to be found.

Thirdly, the CS might be the result of repeated hyperplasia and substitution of the cardiac epithelium. The columnar epithelium of the cardia in BE patients might be affected by inflammation [25] or mechanical motion, which led to the edema or protein change of epithelium cell. For example, some healthy people were observed with circular appearance of the cardia in the inferior position occasionally. However, there was difference between non-metaplastic CS and metaplastic CS, that stripes in the former were flatter, while the latter were often stacked (Fig. 3d).

Based on the above assumptions, CS might help to identify the EGJ, sometimes obscure in white light

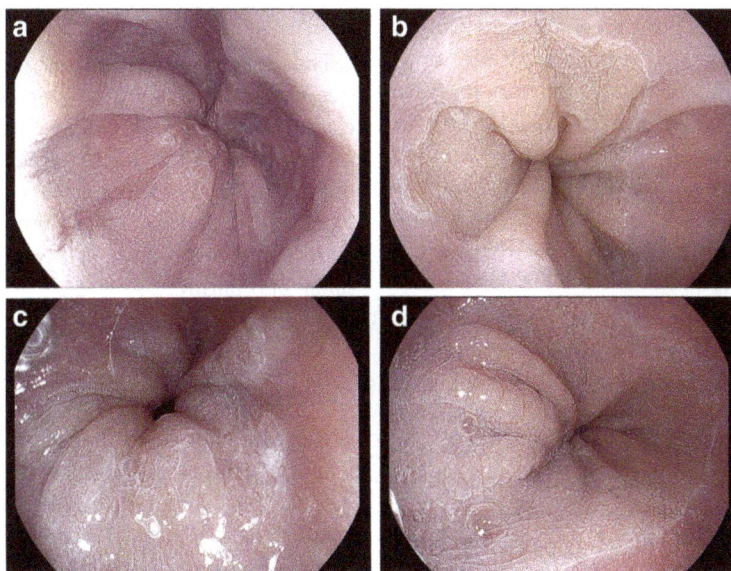

Fig. 3 Special features after instillation of the 2% acetic acid. **a** Squamous epithelium was in circular pattern near the cardia in healthy people, **b** CS partially crossed from columnar epithelium to squamous epithelium, **c** Absence of CS in 2 BE patients and only villous or punctuate mucosa pattern were observed, **d** Flat circular appearance was observed in healthy people

images, even in magnified or NBI images. EGJ is an important marker for endoscopists to get biopsy, which is necessary for the diagnosis of BE in some guidelines, such as British Society of Gastroenterology guidelines and American Gastroenterological Association on the diagnosis of BE [1, 9]. Most studies suggested that EGJ was a marker for pointing the initial position of squamous epithelium, and further evaluating distance between the EGJ and the ascending squamo-columnar junction (SCJ) precisely [1, 9–11, 26]. Paris Workshop showed that the EGJ was located in the abdomen, just below the diaphragmatic pinch with the upper margin of the longitudinal gastric folds coinciding with the SCJ in the normal situation. The length of the metaplastic columnar segment is the distance between the neo-formed SCJ and the anatomical EGJ [26], and the reliability of the evaluation depends on the precision of the determination of the EGJ under endoscopy [26]. Mistake in EGJ judgement has little influence on diagnosis of long-segment BE, however it would mislead the diagnosis of short or ultra-short segment BE, while the majority of the Asian BE patients are in short segment [11, 26–31]. Ishimura showed that the prevalence of long segment BE was extremely low in East Asia, while the prevalence of short segment BE was very high only in Japan [11], which was similar to Okita K and Amano Y [30, 31]. Chang CY showed that short segment BE (75.6%, $n = 31$) was more prevalent than long segment BE (24.4%, $n = 10$) in Chinese population [28, 29]. Therefore, more effective method is needed to determine EGJ. If the CS after AA staining are related to the newly hyperplastic columnar epithelium, the length of the BE epithelium can be evaluated from distal end of CS; if CS are limited to the EGJ region, then the proximal end can be borderline for hyperplastic epithelium. Multiple biopsies may prolong the time of procedure and increase patients' suffering, and cause too much bleeding to get the high-risk lesions [18, 32]. The CS helps to outline the target area and make emphasis on the microstructure of the surface. Meanwhile the fading effect after the AA staining can help to identify the abnormal mucosal lesions [14].

The research of the CS could also help to understand the origin and development of BE. Pathologists generally believe that the BE epithelium consists of three tissue types: [1] proximal end is intestinal epithelial cells including goblet cells, [2] in the middle, it is connection type epithelium that is cardiac mucosa without goblet cells, [3] the distal end is the basal epithelium contains both parietal cells and primary cells [33–36]. Our study indicates that CS may be a useful marker representing the connected epithelium perfectly and furthermore pathological evidences are required to support this theory.

It is generally believed that BE is closely associated with gastroesophageal reflux disease [1]. This study showed that BE patients mainly had gastroesophageal reflux symptoms, including acid reflux or heartburn, but 59.58% of patients had no symptoms of gastroesophageal reflux, which was similar to the literature reports 37–39]. These findings suggested that there may be other etiological factors, such as race, environment, diets, use of alcohol or smoking. Therefore, we should pay attention to the people without gastroesophageal reflux symptoms. Combined with magnifying endoscopy, Toyoda improved the mucosal microstructure classification through the study of patients with BE, including 3 types: normal pits, slit-reticular pattern, and gyrus-villous pattern. The sensitivity and specificity of gyrus-villous pattern for IM were 88.5% and 90.2%, and the overall accuracy was 90.0% [35]. In this study, we observed there was no IM in the punctate and the reticular area in the BE group, while the accuracy rate of IM was 100% in the villous area, which was consistent with Toyoda. This result suggested that AA staining combined with high resolution endoscopy could also improve the yielding of BE diagnosis without magnifying endoscopy, NBI or BLI, especially in screening.

The deficiency of this research was that the sample size was limited as a pilot study. In addition, we did not classify the different types of BE because of the small sample size. So further research is needed to explore the differences and the occurrence mechanism of different types of BE, and to explore the effectiveness of different endoscopic techniques in the diagnosis of BE epithelial range and nature.

Conclusion

This is the pilot study that mentions and describes CS as a special feature under high resolution endoscopy with AA staining, and CS may become an important reference in the diagnosis and treatment of BE.

Abbreviations
AA: Acetic acid; BE: Barrett's esophagus; CS: Circular stripes;
EGJ: Esophagogastric junction; IM: Intestinal metaplasia; SCJ: Squamo-columnar junction

Acknowledgments
We would like to thanks to the the cooperation of the nurses and Pathology department.

Authors' contributions
YS participated in the collection and analysis of data and writing of the manuscript. SM and LD participated in conception and oversight of the study, supervision, data analysis and manuscript editing. LF and JW participated in the data collection and analysis. All authors read and approved the final version of the manuscript.

Competing interests
The authors declare that they have no competing interests.

Author details
[1]Department of Gastroenterology, the Second Affiliated Hospital of Xi'an Jiaotong University, No. 157 Xiwu Road, Xi'an, Shaanxi 710004, China. [2]Endoscopy Center, Ankang People's Hospital, Ankang 401147, China.

References
1. Fitzgerald RC, di Pietro M, Ragunath K, et al. British Society of Gastroenterology guidelines on the diagnosis and management of Barrett's oesophagus. Gut. 2014;63:7–42.
2. Bennett C, Moayyedi P, Corley DA, et al. BOB CAT: a large-scale review and Delphi consensus for management of Barrett's esophagus with No Dysplasia, indefinite for, or low-grade Dysplasia. Am J Gastroenterol 2015; 110: 662–82 quiz 683.
3. Spechler SJ, Fitzgerald RC, Prasad GA, Wang KK. History, molecular mechanisms, and endoscopic treatment of Barrett's esophagus. Gastroenterology. 2010;138:854–69.
4. Pereira AD, Chaves P. Low risk of adenocarcinoma and high-grade dysplasia in patients with non-dysplastic Barrett's esophagus: results from a cohort from a country with low esophageal adenocarcinoma incidence. United European Gastroenterol J. 2016;4:343–52.
5. Hvid-Jensen F, Pedersen L, Drewes AM, Sørensen HT, Funch-Jensen P. Incidence of adenocarcinoma among patients with Barrett's esophagus. N Engl J Med. 2011;365:1375–83.
6. van der Burgh A, Dees J, Hop WC, van Blankenstein M. Oesophageal cancer is an uncommon cause of death in patients with Barrett's oesophagus. Gut. 1996;39:5–8.
7. Chandrasoma P, Makarewicz K, Wickramasinghe K, Ma Y, Demeester T. A proposal for a new validated histological definition of the gastroesophageal junction. Hum Pathol. 2006;37:40–7.
8. SA MC, Boyce HW Jr, Gottfried MR. Early diagnosis of columnar-lined esophagus: a new endoscopic criterion. Gastrointest Endosc. 1987;33:413–6.
9. Spechler SJ, Sharma P, Souza RF, Inadomi JM, Shaheen NJ. American Gastroenterological Association technical review on the management of Barrett's esophagus. Gastroenterology 2011;140:e18–e52; quiz e13.
10. Lee YC, Cook MB, Bhatia S, et al. Interobserver reliability in the endoscopic diagnosis and grading of Barrett's esophagus: an Asian multi-national study. Endoscopy. 2010;42:699–704.
11. Ishimura N, Amano Y, Sollano JD, et al. Questionnaire-based survey conducted in 2011 concerning endoscopic management of Barrett's esophagus in east Asian countries. Digestion. 2012;86:136–46.
12. Aida J, Vieth M, Ell C, et al. Palisade vessels as a new histologic marker of esophageal origin in ER specimens from columnar-lined esophagus. Am J Surg Pathol. 2011;35:1140–5.
13. Hoshihara Y. Complications of gastroesophageal reflux disease. 2. Endoscopic diagnosis of Barrett esophagus—can Barrett esophagus be diagnosed by endoscopic observation alone? Nihon Naika Gakkai Zasshi. 2000;89:85–90.
14. Chedgy FG, Subramaniam S, Kandiah K, Thayalasekaran S, Bhandari P. Acetic acid chromoendoscopy: improving neoplasia detection in Barrett's esophagus. World J Gastroenterol. 2016;22:5753–60.
15. Fortun PJ, Anagnostopoulos GK, Kaye P, et al. Acetic acid-enhanced magnification endoscopy in the diagnosis of specialized intestinal metaplasia, dysplasia and early cancer in Barrett's oesophagus. Aliment Pharmacol Ther. 2006;23:735–42.
16. Lambert R, Rey JF, Sankaranarayanan R. Magnification and chromoscopy with the acetic acid test. Endoscopy. 2003;35:437–45.
17. Longcroft-Wheaton G, Brown J, Basford P, Cowlishaw D, Higgins B, Bhandari P. Duration of acetowhitening as a novel objective tool for diagnosing high risk neoplasia in Barrett's esophagus: a prospective cohort trial. Endoscopy. 2013;45:426–32.
18. Tholoor S, Bhattacharyya R, Tsagkournis O, Longcroft-Wheaton G, Acetic BP. Acid chromoendoscopy in Barrett's esophagus surveillance is superior to the standardized random biopsy protocol: results from a large cohort study. Gastrointest Endosc. 2014;80:417–24.
19. Kaufman HB, Harper DM. Magnification and chromoscopy with the acetic acid test. Endoscopy. 2004;36:748–50.
20. Sharma P, Dent J, Armstrong D, et al. The development and validation of an endoscopic grading system for Barrett's esophagus: the Prague C & M criteria. Gastroenterology. 2006;131:1392–9.
21. Guelrud M, Herrera I, Essenfeld H, Castro J. Enhanced magnification endoscopy: a new technique to identify specialized intestinal metaplasia in Barrett's esophagus. Gastrointest Endosc. 2001;53:559–65.
22. Odze RD. Unraveling the mystery of the gastroesophageal junction: a pathologist's perspective. Am J Gastroenterol. 2005;100:1853–67.
23. Pathology ORD. Of the gastroesophageal junction. Semin Diagn Pathol. 2005;22:256–65.
24. Wallner B. Endoscopically defined gastroesophageal junction coincides with the anatomicalgastroesophageal junction. Surg Endosc. 2009;23:2155–8.
25. Savarino E, Marabotto E, Bodini G, et al. Epidemiology and natural history of gastro-esophageal reflux disease. Minerva Gastroenterol Dietol. 2017 Feb 17;
26. Paris workshop on columnar metaplasia in the esophagus and the esophagogastric junction, Paris, France, December 11–12, 2004. Endoscopy 2005;37:879–920.
27. Fock KM, Talley N, Goh KL, et al. Asia-Pacific consensus on the management of gastro-oesophageal reflux disease: an update focusing on refractory reflux disease and Barrett's oesophagus. Gut. 2016;65:1402–15.
28. Chang CY, Lee YC, Lee CT, et al. The application of Prague C and M criteria in the diagnosis of Barrett's esophagus in an ethnic Chinese population. Am J Gastroenterol. 2009;104:13–20.
29. Tseng PH, Lee YC, Chiu HM, et al. Prevalence and clinical characteristics of Barrett's esophagus in a Chinese general population. J Clin Gastroenterol. 2008;42:1074–9.
30. Okita K, Amano Y, Takahashi Y, et al. Barrett's esophagus in Japanese patients: its prevalence, form, and elongation. J Gastroenterol. 2008;43:928–34.
31. Amano A, Kinoshita Y. Barrett esophagus: perspectives on its diagnosis and management in Asian populations. Gastroenterology & Hepatol. 2008;4:45–53.
32. Bhattacharyya R, Longcroft-Wheaton G, Bhandari P. The role of acetic acid in the management of Barrett's oesophagus. Clin Res Hepatol Gastroenterol. 2015;39:282–91.
33. Bernstein IT, Kruse P, Andersen IB. Barrett's oesophagus. Dig Dis. 1994; 12:98–105.
34. Toyoda H, Rubio C, Befrits R, Hamamoto N, Adachi Y, Jaramillo E. Detection of intestinal metaplasia in distal esophagus and esophagogastric junction by enhanced-magnification endoscopy. Gastrointest Endosc. 2004;59:15–21.
35. Paull A, Trier JS, Dalton MD, Camp RC, Loeb P, Goyal RK. The histologic spectrum of Barrett's esophagus. N Engl J Med. 1976;295:476–80.
36. Glickman JN, Spechler SJ, Souza RF, Lunsford T, Lee E, Odze RD. Multilayered epithelium in mucosal biopsy specimens from the

gastroesophageal junction region is a histologic marker of
gastroesophageal reflux disease. Am J Surg Pathol. 2009;33:818–25.

37. Chen X, Zhu LR, Hou KH. The characteristics of Barrett's esophagus: an
analysis of 4120 cases in China. Dis Esophagus. 2009;22:348–53.

38. Park JJ, Kim JW, Kim HJ, et al. The prevalence of and risk factors for Barrett's
esophagus in a Korean population: a nationwide multicenter prospective
study. J Clin Gastroenterol. 2009;43:907–14.

39. Lee IS, Choi SC, Shim KN, et al. Prevalence of Barrett's esophagus remains
low in the Korean population: nationwide cross-sectional prospective
multicenter study. Dig Dis Sci. 2010;55:1932–9.

20

Length of Barrett's segment predicts failure of eradication in radiofrequency ablation for Barrett's esophagus

Tyler Luckett[1], Chaitanya Allamneni[1], Kevin Cowley[1], John Eick[2], Allison Gullick[1] and Shajan Peter[1*]

Abstract

Background: We aim to investigate factors that may contribute to failure of eradication of dysplastic Barrett's Esophagus among patients undergoing radiofrequency ablation treatment.

Methods: A retrospective review of patients undergoing radiofrequency ablation for treatment of Barrett's Esophagus was performed. Data analyzed included patient demographics, medical history, length of Barrett's Esophagus, number of radiofrequency ablation sessions, and histopathology. Subsets of patients achieving complete eradication were compared with those not achieving complete eradication.

Results: A total of 107 patients underwent radiofrequency ablation for Barrett's Esophagus, the majority white, overweight, and male. Before treatment, 63 patients had low-grade dysplasia, and 44 patients had high-grade dysplasia or carcinoma. Complete eradication was achieved in a majority of patients (57% for metaplasia, and 76.6% for dysplasia). Failure of eradication occurred in 15.7% of patients. The median number of radiofrequency ablation treatments in patients achieving complete eradication was 3 sessions, compared to 4 sessions for failure of eradication ($p = 0.06$). Barrett's esophagus length of more than 5 cm was predictive of failure of eradication ($p < 0.001$).

Conclusions: Radiofrequency ablation for dysplastic Barrett's Esophagus is a proven and effective treatment modality, associated with a high rate of complete eradication. Our rates of eradication from a center starting an ablation program are comparable to previously published studies. Length of Barrett's segment > 5 cm was found to be predictive of failure of eradication in patients undergoing radiofrequency ablation.

Keywords: Barrett's esophagus, Radiofrequency ablation, Endoscopy, Esophagus

Background

Barrett's Esophagus (BE) is a condition in which the stratified squamous epithelium that lines the distal esophagus is replaced by metaplastic columnar epithelium that predisposes to the development of dysplasia and adenocarcinoma [1]. Esophageal adenocarcinoma (EAC) incidence has been on the rise, most drastically in the Caucasian segment of the American population [2, 3]. Therefore, it is important to adequately address dysplastic precursor lesions to EAC. A relatively recent addition to

gastrointestinal endoscopy is radiofrequency ablation (RFA) using the HALO system (BARRX Medical, Inc., Sunnyvale, CA, USA), which has been shown to be safe and effective for the treatment of BE, including low-grade dysplasia (LGD) and high-grade dysplasia (HGD) [4–6]. Not only is RFA associated with decreased neoplastic progression compared to surveillance endoscopy [7, 8], a recent meta-analysis of the literature showed a pooled complete eradication of intestinal metaplasia (CE-IM) rate of 78% (95% CI 70–86%) and complete eradication of dysplasia (CE-D) rate of 91% (95% CI 87–95%) [9].

Despite high rates of eradication, as many as one-third of patients experience recurrence after complete eradication [10]. Some cited predictors of recurrence are older

* Correspondence: ssugandha@uabmc.edu
[1]Department of Gastroenterology and Hepatology, University of Alabama at Birmingham, 1720 2nd Avenue South, BDB 380, Birmingham, AL 35294, USA

age, non-Caucasian race and longer length of pretreatment BE [11, 12]. Additionally, some patients do not respond to RFA or require multiple sessions to obtain complete eradication. While some have not been able to determine any significant predictors of response to therapy [13], others have found that active reflux disease, longer history of dysplasia, increased hiatal hernia size as well as increased length of BE are all predictors of RFA failure [14–16].

The success of RFA is such that it has become integrated at many large institutions in combination with resection techniques, such as endoscopic mucosal resection (EMR) and endoscopic submucosal dissection (ESD), which are needed to remove macroscopically visible lesions [17]. Given this increased use, it is vital to determine which patients may be at high risk for not responding to RFA and thus neoplastic progression. The current literature is conflicting, as studies that have found predictors of RFA failure differ in their results. For instance, Lyday et al. found CE-IM to be inversely related to BE length [15], while van Vilsteren et al. did not find BE length to be statistically significant [14], leading to the conclusion that further investigation is warranted.

The goals of this study were as follows: (1) to determine factors that may predict failure of CE-IM and CE-D in patients treated with RFA, and (2) to report the rates of CE-IM and CE-D at a large institution that recently began offering RFA and compare them to those previously published in the literature.

Methods
Study design
After the study was reviewed and approved by the University of Alabama at Birmingham Institutional Review Board (IRB), a retrospective review of consecutive patients undergoing RFA between December 2009–February 2015, for treatment of Barrett's Esophagus at the University of Alabama at Birmingham (UAB) was performed. All study participants provided informed written consent prior to study enrollment. Data was entered and stored in a de-identified spreadsheet. Data abstracted for analysis included patient demographic characteristics, medical history, pathological findings, endoscopic findings, endoscopic procedures, adverse events, treatment, and biopsies with histopathology findings on surveillance. A standard four quadrant biopsy protocol based on the Seattle protocol was used for sampling [18]. As part of this protocol, targeted biopsy using narrow band imaging was performed. All biopsies were examined by the same experienced GI pathologist, and were reviewed again by a separate pathologist for documentation of consensus. Histopathology was graded and classified as high grade dysplasia, low grade dysplasia, or intestinal

metaplasia. Both endoscopic inspection and biopsy results were used to determine which patients needed additional rounds of RFA to try to achieve CE. The biopsy protocol at our institution was as follows: We would continue RFA sessions until BE appeared endoscopically cleared, and then biopsies would be obtained at that time. Patients in our study required between two to ten RFA sessions to achieve complete eradication (mean = 3 sessions), and after any number of RFA sessions, if the patient appeared to have endoscopic clearance of BE, then biopsies would be obtained at that time to document complete eradication. Similarly, if a patient had an endoscopically visible lesion that needed targeted biopsy, then biopsies would be obtained at that time. Based on the results of mucosal biopsies after endoscopic treatment, patients were then divided based on histopathology into complete eradication (CE) of dysplasia (CE – D) or intestinal metaplasia (CE – IM). Subsets of patients achieving CE were compared with those not achieving CE. Those patients with mucosal biopsies demonstrating persistent dysplasia or intestinal metaplasia after treatment with RFA were considered failure of CE. Thus, failure was based upon histology, not endoscopy. Patients were considered lost to follow-up if post-treatment biopsies were not obtained.

Procedure description
Patients were placed in the decubitus supine position. All procedures were performed with patients under monitored anesthesia care (MAC). Measurements of BE were done using the Prague Classification [19]. Patients underwent ablation using the circumferential device (HALO^{360} system) or a focal device (HALO^{90} both from Covidien GI Solutions) according to the extent of disease and investigator preference, as previously described. Subsequent ablation sessions were performed every 2 months, until complete endoscopic and histological eradication of Barrett's Esophagus. At each ablation session, if any visible nodular lesions were identified, these were first treated with Endoscopic Mucosal Resection (EMR) using the Band ligation with the Duette Multi-Band Mucosectomy Device (Wilson-Cook, Winston-Salem, NC, USA) as previously described [20]. Then, the gastro-esophageal junction was ablated circumferentially, irrespective of its endoscopic appearance. Our protocol for ablation therapy has been previously described [21]. In more detail, the protocol for circumferential ablation and focal ablation included endoscopy with visual inspection, reading landmarks, sizing balloon, selection of ablation type, first pass ablation, clearing the face, and then second pass ablation. Focal ablation RFA was performed for treating shorter segments or islands of tongues of BE. Energy was delivered at settings of 12 J/cm2. A similar second pulse of energy was given after cleaning the electrode. Each target area received

a total of 4 energy ablations for focal ablation and 2 for cir-cumferential ablation respectively. The average length of each RFA treatment was 15.6 min.

CE-IM and CE-D were defined as complete eradica-tion of IM and dysplasia, respectively, as documented by histopathology from mucosal biopsy obtained by white-light endoscopy (GIF-HQ190 Olympus, Tokyo, Japan). Time to CE-IM or CE-D was measured from the date of first RFA to the first follow-up EGD with normal histopathology reported for biopsy specimens. Recur-rence was defined as the presence of IM or dysplasia in standard surveillance biopsies. The neosquamocolumnar junction was assessed in every case by white-light endos-copy with biopsies. For surveillance, 4-quadrant biopsies were performed at 1 cm intervals of the original extent of the Barrett's Esophagus, starting at 1 cm proximal to the top of the gastric folds. In addition, any suspicious visible lesions were targeted, biopsied, and placed in sep-arate jars. Remission of intestinal metaplasia/ dysplasia was confirmed with endoscopic findings and the four quadrant biopsy protocol.

Statistical analysis

Unadjusted univariate and bivariate comparisons were made, utilizing chi-square or Fisher exact test for cat-egorical variables and two tailed t-tests or Wilcoxon Rank Sums for continuous variables, where appropriate. Negative binomial logistic regression was used to model predictors of failure for CE-IM and CE-D utilizing stepwise selection. Significance was determined by a $p < 0.05$. All statistical analysis was performed using SAS 9.4 (SAS Institute Inc., Cary, NC).

Results

A total of 107 patients underwent RFA for BE. Overall, 96.3% ($n = 103$) of the patients were white, and 86.9% ($n = 93$) were male. The median age was 64 years (range 58–72 years), and the mean length of Barrett's esophagus was 6.7 cm (range 2-8 cm, median 5 cm). Most patients were overweight, with mean BMI 29.1 (range 25.5–32.6). On average, each patient underwent 3 (range 2–10, median 3) RFA procedures. The median time until CE-IM was 238 days (119–474) and the median time until CE-D was 251 days (133–525). There were 20 pa-tients (15.7%) who did not obtain post-treatment biop-sies, and were considered lost to follow up. Of the patients included in the study, 41.1% had HGD, and 58.9% had LGD. After RFA treatment, 57.0% of patients achieved CE-IM, and 76.6% achieved CE-D. 4.7% of pa-tients progressed to esophageal adenocarcinoma. The average time to progression from dysplasia to adenocar-cinoma was 170 days. The initial pathology for all pa-tients that progressed to esophageal adenocarcinoma was HGD. Focal ablation was performed only for shorter

segments of BE, as this tends to be more effective than circumferential ablation for these lesions. Comparing eradication rates between focal and circumferential abla-tion was not the main study objective, so our study did not directly compare differences in circumferential abla-tion versus focal ablation. Also, many longer segment BE lesions initially treated with circumferential ablation were later followed up with focal ablation, making it dif-ficult to directly compare circumferential and focal abla-tion. There were no statistically significant differences in rates of CE-IM or CE-D for patients with HGD versus those with LGD. There were no statistically significant differences in BE segment length in patients with HGD (mean 6.2 ± 4.2 cm) versus LGD (mean 5.3 ± 3.8 cm).

Independent predictors of failure to achieve CE-IM [see Table 1] included age > 64 years, (OR: 2.6, (1.20–5.79); $p < 0.02$), and having a BE segment length greater than 5 cm (OR: 4.03(1.78–9.09); $p < 0.001$). On adjustment, both age (OR: 4.508, (1.72–11.84), $p < 0.0022$) and length of seg-ment (OR: 7.064, (2.62–19.06), p < 0.001) remained signifi-cant predictors of failure to achieve CE-IM.

Independent predictors of failure to achieve CE-D [see Table 2] included having hypertension (OR: 3.33(1.21–9.17); $p = 0.02$), and having a BE segmental length greater than 5 cm (OR: 2.60 (1.04–6.51); $p = 0.04$). On adjustment, both hypertension (OR 3.86; 1.32–11.31, $p < 0.01$) and length of segment (OR 3.08; 1.12–8.46, $p < 0.03$) remained significant predictors of failure to achieve CE-D (see Table 3). The number of patients who developed adenocarcinoma was very small, so no inde-pendent predictors were identified.

There were no major complications from RFA ther-apy in our study population. Specifically, there was no stricturing or bleeding noted on follow-up EGD. Retrospective review from the medical records did not reveal any documented complications related to anesthesia/ sedation.

Discussion

Many studies have analyzed the durability and recur-rence of BE associated with RFA, but few studies to date have examined factors which affect the rate of eradica-tion of CE-IM or CE-D with RFA. We analyzed multiple factors including patient characteristics such as age, co-morbidities such as GERD, hypertension, or diabetes mellitus, risk factors such as tobacco use or duration of reflux, and endoscopic characteristics such as length of Barrett's segment and number of treatments with RFA. The number of patients in our study population who drank alcohol was low, so this risk factor was not ana-lyzed. In our study, the overall rate of CE-IM and CE-D was 57 and 76.6%, respectively. The rates of CE-IM and CE-D in our study are similar to other published studies, which demonstrate rates of CE-IM ranging from 41 to

Table 1 Factors Affecting Complete Eradication of Intestinal Metaplasia

Patient Characteristic	All Patients[a]		Complete Eradication of Intestinal Metaplasia		Incomplete Eradication of Intestinal Metaplasia		p-value[b]
	107	100.0%	61	57.0%	46	43.0%	
Race							
White	103	96.3%	59	96.7%	44	95.7%	0.773
Other	4	3.7%	2	3.3%	2	4.3%	
Sex							
Male	93	86.9%	51	83.6%	40	86.9%	0.242
Female	14	13.1%	10	16.4%	6	13.1%	
Age	[c]64	(58–72)	[c] 63	(57–72)	[c] 67	(59–76)	0.117
BMI	[c] 29.1	(25.5–32.6)	[c] 30.9	(26.5–33.1)	[c] 28.3	(24.5–30)	0.077
Dysplasia							
HGD	44	41.1%	24	39.3%	20	43.5%	0.667
LGD	63	58.9%	37	60.7%	26	56.5%	
Comorbidities							
GERD	75	70.1%	30	49.2%	32	69.6%	0.339
Hyperlipidemia	26	24.3%	17	27.9%	11	23.9%	0.322
Diabetes	25	23.4%	15	24.6%	10	21.7%	0.730
Hypertension	59	55.1%	30	49.2%	31	67.4%	0.154
History of Tobacco Usage							
Yes	60	56.1%	30	49.2%	29	63.0%	0.225
No	33	30.8%	21	34.4%	13	28.3%	
Unknown	14	13.1%	10	16.4%	4	8.7%	
Endoscopic Treatments Received							
EMR	24	22.4%	16	26.2%	8	17.4%	0.326
Length							
Median, IQR	5	(2–7)	3	(2–7)	7	(2–8)	< 0.001
</= 5 cm	64	59.8%	44	72.1%	20	43.4%	< 0.001
> 5 cm	43	40.2%	17	27.9%	26	56.6%	
Number of RFA's							
Median, IQR	3	(2–5)	3	(2–5)	4	(2–5)	0.023
≤ 3	62	57.9%	41	67.2%	21	45.7%	0.008
> 3	45	42.1%	20	32.8%	25	54.3%	

[a]Data presented as N (%) or median (IQR)
[b]p-value ≤0.05 is significant
[c]average; not total number of patients

67% [9]. Some other studies with higher rates of CE-IM and CE-D typically treated shorter lengths of BE than our current study [21, 22] which had 42.1% of patients with BE segment greater than 5 cm. We found that length of Barrett's segment length greater than 5 cm was independently predictive of a higher rate for failure of complete eradication in patients undergoing RFA. Of those patients in our study with failure of CE-IM or CE-D, 56.6 and 60.0% of patients, respectively, had a pretreatment BE length of > 5 cm. Longer segments of BE have been associated with potentially more aggressive behavior and with a resultant higher risk of progression, which may explain the lower rates of CE in our study [11, 12]. These studies demonstrate similar findings with longer segments of BE associated with higher rates of eradication failure and recurrence. In addition, their finding that BE of length 4.8 vs. 3.8 cm had significantly higher recurrence after treatment correlates closely with our data showing that BE length > 5 cm predicts failure with RFA. Although the reasons for the association are unclear, a longer pretreatment segment may be a marker for more severe acid exposure and injury [12]. Recent

Table 2 Factors Affecting Complete Eradication of Dysplasia

	All Patients[a]		Complete Eradication of Dysplasia		Incomplete Eradication of Dysplasia		
	107	100.0%	82	76.6%	25	23.4%	p-value[b]
Patient Characteristics							
Race							
White	103	96.3%	80	97.6%	23	92.0%	0.232
Other	4	3.7%	2	2.4%	2	8.0%	
Sex							
Male	93	86.9%	69	84.1%	24	96.0%	0.180
Female	14	13.1%	13	15.9%	1	4.0%	
Age	[c]64	(58–72)	[c] 64	(57–72)	[c] 66	(59–76)	0.336
BMI	[c] 29.1	(25.5–32.6)	[c] 30.5	(26.5–33.1)	[c] 27.45	(24.5–30)	0.045
Dysplasia							
HGD	44	41.1%	30	36.6%	14	56.0%	0.084
LGD	63	58.9%	52	63.4%	11	44.0%	
Comorbidities				0.0%			
GERD	75	70.1%	60	73.2%	15	60.0%	0.208
Hyperlipidemia	26	24.3%	20	24.4%	6	24.0%	0.968
Diabetes	25	23.4%	18	22.0%	7	28.0%	0.532
Hypertension	59	55.1%	40	48.8%	19	76.0%	0.017
History of Tobacco Usage							
Yes	60	56.1%	43	52.4%	17	68.0%	0.350
No	33	30.8%	28	34.1%	5	20.0%	
Unknown	14	13.1%	11	13.4%	3	12.0%	
Endoscopic Treatments Received							
EMR	24	22.4%	18	22.0%	6	24.0%	0.732
Length							
Median, IQR	5	(2–7)	4	(2–7)	6	(2–8)	0.150
</= 5 cm	64	59.8%	52	63.4%	12	48.0%	0.038
> 5 cm	43	40.2%	30	36.6%	13	52.0%	
Number of RFA's							
Median, IQR	3	(2–5)	3	(2–5)	4	(2–5)	0.066
≤ 3	62	57.9%	52	63.4%	10	40.0%	0.064
> 3	45	42.1%	30	36.6%	15	60.0%	

[a]Data presented as N (%) or median (IQR)
[b]p-value ≤0.05 is significant
[c]average; not total number of patients

studies also show a spatial preference for dysplasia being more common in proximal areas of the Barret's segment [23]. In addition, recent literature studying cryotherapy as a modality for BE refractory to RFA has also revealed that RFA failure groups have longer Barrett's segments. [24, 25]. We believe the length of Barrett's segment ablated was the main reason for the large range of RFA sessions required for eradication of BE, as longer segments tended to require more frequent RFA sessions to achieve eradication. The choice of focal or circumferential ablation was standardized based on the protocol as discussed above, and we feel that the choice of ablation technique was not a contributing cause to the range of RFA sessions required for eradication. A greater BMI seems to be associated with longer segment of BE, however we did not find the BMI to be an independent predictor for failure in our study [26].

Another finding of our study was that having a greater number of RFA treatments was predictive of failure of CE-IM. Those patients who required more than 3 RFA treatments were significantly more likely to have failure of CE-IM. Of the 46 patients who failed to achieve

Table 3 Predictors of Failure

Covariate	Incomplete Eradication of Intestinal Metaplasia						Incomplete Eradication of Dysplasia					
	Univariate Analysis			Multivariate Analysis			Univariate Analysis			Multivariate Analysis		
	OR	95% CI	p-value	OR	95% CI	p-value	OR	95% CI	p-value	OR	95% CI	p-value
Not White	1.34	0.18–9.89	0.77				3.48	0.46–26.07	0.23			
Female	2.06	0.60–7.04	0.25	4.157	0.94–18.40	0.060						
65 years or older	2.63	1.20–5.79	0.02	4.508	1.72–11.84	0.0022	2.16	0.857–5.45	0.10	Ref.	Ref.	0.10
Obese, BMI > 30	2.60	1.11–6.14	0.01				2.29	0.85–6.20	0.08			
HGD	1.19	0.55–2.58	0.67				2.21	0.89–5.47	0.09	2.151	0.80–5.80	0.13
GERD	1.50	0.65–3.45	0.34				Ref.	Ref.	0.21			
Hyperlipidemia	1.59	0.63–3.98	0.32				Ref.	Ref.	0.97			
Diabetes	1.17	0.47–2.92	0.73				1.38	0.50–3.83	0.53			
Hypertension	1.76	0.81–3.85	0.16				3.33	1.21–9.17	0.02	3.86	1.32–11.31	0.01
Tobacco Usage	2.50	0.71–8.85	0.23				1.45	0.36–5.85	0.36			
Length > 5 cm	4.03	1.78–9.09	< 0.01	7.064	2.62–19.06	< 0.01	2.60	1.04–6.51	0.04	3.08	1.12–8.46	0.03
> 3 RFA's	2.16	0.96–4.89	0.06				1.15	0.45–2.93	0.78			
				c statistic:	0.766					c statistic:	0.761	
				r squared	0.285					r squared	0.2215	

CE-IM, 54.3% had greater than 3 RFA treatments. This is similar to findings from other studies such as Agoston et al., which also suggest increased number of treatments predicts failure of eradication [11] [27]. These results may actually be explained by a more aggressive neoplastic phenotype as opposed to a result of treatment, and could explain differences in measured rates of achieving CE-IM. Other notable statistically significant predictors of failure in our study included age greater than 64 years old for CE-IM. While the significance of this finding is unclear, it has been suggested that elderly people may have more prolonged exposure to carcinogens and are therefore more likely to accumulate somatic mutations [12]. Hypertension was also found to be a statistically significant predictor of failure of CE-D. We suspect that this is likely just a statistical finding related to small study size. Further evaluation is necessary to support these factors as predictors of eradication failure.

These findings are important because RFA is used commonly for the treatment of BE. Identifying factors which place patients at higher risk of not responding to RFA may also help identify individuals with a greater risk of progressing to neoplasia. Those patients with longer pretreatment BE are at greater risk of failure of complete eradication with RFA, and may benefit from a more invasive treatment approach such as EMR. Patient's with persistent BE after greater than 3 treatments with RFA are at greater risk of failure of complete eradication, and this could be helpful for directing further therapy as continued RFA sessions may be less beneficial. At this point, other treatment modalities such as APC, cryotherapy, or EMR could be considered. Other contributing factors such as medication noncompliance or lack of appropriate follow-up should also be considered. It should also be noted that studies have shown that RFA is a cost-effective strategy for treatment of dysplastic Barrett's esophagus [28].

Our study had limitations which should be considered when interpreting the data. The study was retrospective in nature, and data was collected entirely from our own single institution: a large, academic, tertiary-care hospital which is relatively new to the technique of radiofrequency ablation for eradication of Barrett's Esophagus. Another limitation is that there was a moderate percentage that were lost to follow up, thus limiting the results. However, in general, our data is similar to that of other large, academic hospitals with high rates of complete eradication of both intestinal metaplasia and dysplasia. The retrospective nature of our study also makes misclassification possible. Also, some patients were lost to follow up for unknown reasons, which could affect the reported rates of eradication.

The lower eradication rate is another limitation of our study. This lower rate is likely related to the number of patients lost to follow-up, as well as the fact that our patient sample is entirely from a tertiary care referral center, likely dealing with the most complex cases.

Conclusion

In conclusion, we have identified pathologic factors as well as endoscopic factors which are associated with a higher risk of failure to achieve CE-IM or CE-D with RFA treatment of BE. Knowledge of these predictors can help identify patients at higher risk for treatment failure and subsequent increased risk for neoplastic progression. This knowledge may be beneficial to prompt a more aggressive initial therapy to prevent unnecessary procedures or neoplastic progression.

Abbreviations
BE: Barrett's Esophagus; BMI: body mass index; CE: Complete eradication; CE-D: Complete eradication of dysplasia; CE-IM: Complete eradication of intestinal metaplasia; EAC: Esophageal adenocarcinoma; EMR: Endoscopic mucosal resection; ESD: Endoscopic submucosal dissection; HGD: High grade dysplasia; LGD: Low grade dysplasia; MAC: Monitored anesthesia care; RFA: Radiofrequency ablation

Funding
This research study received no outside sources of funding. There are no conflicts of interest.

Authors' contributions
TL, JE, KC, and SP made substantial contributions to the conception and project design. TL and KC made substantial contributions to the acquisition and analysis of data. AG and TL made substantial contributions to the statistical analysis of the data. TL, KC, CA, and SP made substantial contributions to the drafting of the manuscript, as well as critical revisions. All parties have given final approval of the version to be published, and agree to be accountable for all aspects of the work.

Competing interests
The authors declare that they have no competing interests.

Author details
[1]Department of Gastroenterology and Hepatology, University of Alabama at Birmingham, 1720 2nd Avenue South, BDB 380, Birmingham, AL 35294, USA. [2]University of North Carolina Internal Medicine Residency, University of North Carolina, Carolina, North, USA.

References
1. Spechler SJ, et al. American Gastroenterological Association medical position statement on the management of Barrett's esophagus. Gastroenterology. 2011;140:1084–91.
2. Brown LM, et al. Incidence of adenocarcinoma of the esophagus among white Americans by sex, stage, and age. J Natl Cancer Inst. 2008;100(16):1184–7.
3. Pohl H, Welch HG. The role of overdiagnosis and reclassification in the marked increase of esophageal adenocarcinoma incidence. J Natl Cancer Inst. 2005;97(2):142–6.
4. Sharma VK, et al. Circumferential and focal ablation of Barrett's esophagus containing dysplasia. Am J Gastroenterol. 2009;104:310–7.
5. Shaheen NJ, et al. Radiofrequency ablation in Barrett's esophagus with dysplasia. N Engl J Med. 2009;360:2277–88.
6. Ganz RA, et al. Circumferential ablation of Barrett's esophagus that contains high-grade dysplasia: a U.S. multicenter registry. Gastrointest Endosc. 2008;68(1):35–40.
7. Small AJ, et al. Radiofrequency ablation is associated with decreased neoplastic progression in patients with Barrett's esophagus and confirmed low-grade dysplasia. Gastroenterology. 2015;
8. Phoa KN, et al. Radiofrequency ablation vs endoscopic surveillance for patients with Barrett esophagus and low-grade dysplasia. JAMA. 2014;311(12):1209–17.
9. Orman ES, et al. Efficacy and durability of radiofrequency ablation for Barrett's esophagus: systematic review and meta-analysis. Clin Gastroenterol Hepatol. 2013;11:1245–55.
10. Gupta M, et al. Recurrence of esophageal intestinal metaplasia after endoscopic mucosal resection and radiofrequency ablation of Barrett's esophagus: results from a US multicenter consortium. Gastroenterology. 2013;145:79–86.
11. Vaccaro BJ, et al. Detection of intestinal metaplasia after successful eradication of Barrett's esophagus with radiofrequency ablation. Dig Dis Sci. 2011;56:1996–2000.
12. Pasricha S, et al. Durability and predictors of successful radiofrequency ablation for Barrett's esophagus. Clin Gastroenterol Hepatol. 2014;12:1840–7.
13. Shaheen NJ, et al. Durability of radiofrequency ablation in Barrett's esophagus with dysplasia. Gastroenterology. 2011;141:460–8.
14. van Vilsteren FG, et al. Predictive factors for initial treatment response after circumferential radiofrequency ablation for Barrett's esophagus with early neoplasia: a prospective multi-center study. Endoscopy. 2013;45:516–25.
15. Lyday WD, et al. Radiofrequency ablation of Barrett's esophagus: outcomes of 429 patients from a multicenter community practice registry. Endoscopy. 2010;42:272–8.
16. Krishnan K, et al. Increased risk for persistent intestinal metaplasia in patients with Barrett's esophagus and uncontrolled reflux exposure before radiofrequency ablation. Gastroenterology. 2012;143:576–81.
17. Blevins CH, Iyer PG. Endoscopic therapy for Barrett's oesophagus. Best Pract Res Clin Gastroenterol. 2015;29:167–77.
18. Spechler SJ, Sharma P, Souza RF, Inadomi JM, Shaheen NJ. American Gastroenterological Association technical review on the Management of Barrett's esophagus. Gastroenterology. 2011;140(3):e18–3. https://doi.org/10.1053/j.gastro.2011.01.031.
19. Sharma, Prateek P (11/2006). "The development and validation of an endoscopic grading system for Barrett's esophagus: the Prague C & M criteria". Gastroenterology (New York, N.Y. 1943) (0016–5085), 131 (5), p. 1392 PMID: 17101315 DOI: https://doi.org/10.1053/j.gastro.2006.08.03.
20. Kothari S, Kaul V. Endoscopic mucosal resection and endoscopic submucosal dissection for endoscopic therapy of Barrett's esophagus-related neoplasia. Gastroenterol Clin N Am 2015;44(2):317–335. doi: https://doi.org/10.1016/j.gtc.2015.02.006. Review. PubMed PMID: 26021197.
21. Peter S, Mönkemüller K. Ablative endoscopic therapies for Barrett's-esophagus-related neoplasia. Gastroenterol Clin N Am 2015;44(2):337–353. doi: https://doi.org/10.1016/j.gtc.2015.02.014. Review. PubMed PMID: 26021198.
22. Haidry RJ, Dunn JM, Thorpe S, et al. Radio frequency ablation is more effective in shorter segments of Barrett's oesophagus for eradication of high grade dysplasia/intramucosal cancer - results from the UK RFA HALO registry. Gastroenterology. 2011;140:S215.
23. Cotton CC, Duits LC, Wolf WA, Peery AF, Dellon ES, Bergman JJ, Shaheen NJ. Spatial predisposition of dysplasia in Barrett's esophagus segments: a pooled analysis of the SURF and AIM dysplasia trials. Am J Gastroenterol. 2015 Oct;110(10):1412–9. https://doi.org/10.1038/ajg.2015.263. Epub 2015 Sep 8. PubMed PMID: 26346864.
24. Weusten BL, Bergman JJ. Cryoablation for managing Barrett's esophagus refractory to radiofrequency ablation?Don't embrace the cold too soon! Gastrointest Endosc. 2015;82:449–51.
25. Trindade AJ, Inamdar S, Kothari S, Berkowitz J, McKinley M, Kaul V. Feasibility of liquid nitrogen cryotherapy after failed radiofrequency ablation for Barrett's esophagus. Dig Endosc. 2017;29:680–5. https://doi.org/10.1111/den.12869.

26. Abdallah J, Maradey-Romero C, Lewis S, Perzynski A, Fass R. The relationship between length of Barrett's oesophagus mucosa and body mass index. Aliment Pharmacol Ther. 2015 Jan;41(1):137–44. https://doi.org/10.1111/apt.12991. Epub 2014 Oct 17. PubMed PMID: 25327893.

27. Agoston AT. Predictors of treatment failure after radiofrequency ablation for Intramucosal adenocarcinoma in Barrett esophagus: a multi-institutional retrospective cohort study. Am J Surg Pathol. 2016;40(4):554–62.

28. Hur C, Choi SE, Rubenstein JH, Kong CY, Nishioka NS, Provenzale DT, Inadomi JM. The cost effectiveness of radiofrequency ablation for Barrett's esophagus. Gastroenterology. 2012;143(3):567–75. https://doi.org/10.1053/j.gastro.2012.05.010. Epub 2012 May 21

21

Treatment of long-segment Barrett's adenocarcinoma by complete circular endoscopic submucosal dissection

Miki Kaneko[1], Akira Mitoro[1*] [iD], Motoyuki Yoshida[1], Masayoshi Sawai[1], Yasushi Okura[1], Masanori Furukawa[1], Tadashi Namisaki[1], Kei Moriya[1], Takemi Akahane[1], Hideto Kawaratani[1], Mitsuteru Kitade[1], Kousuke Kaji[1], Hiroaki Takaya[1], Yasuhiko Sawada[1], Kenichiro Seki[1], Shinya Sato[1], Tomomi Fujii[3], Junichi Yamao[2], Chiho Obayashi[3] and Hitoshi Yoshiji[1]

Abstract

Background: We present the first description of *en bloc* endoscopic submucosal dissection (ESD) for total circumferential Barrett's adenocarcinoma, predominantly of the long-segment Barrett's esophagus (LSBE), with a 2-year follow-up and management strategies for esophageal stricture prevention.

Case presentation: A 59-year-old man was diagnosed with LSBE and Barrett's adenocarcinoma by esophagogastroduodenoscopy (EGD). A 55-mm-long circumferential tumor was completely resected by ESD. Histopathology revealed a well-differentiated adenocarcinoma within the LSBE superficial muscularis mucosa. For post-ESD stricture prevention, the patient underwent an endoscopic triamcinolone injection administration, oral prednisolone administration, and preemptive endoscopic balloon dilatation. Two years later, there is no evidence of esophageal stricture or recurrence.

Conclusions: ESD appears to be a safe, effective option for total circumferential Barrett's adenocarcinoma in LSBE.

Keywords: Barrett esophagus, Adenocarcinoma of esophagus, Endoscopic submucosal dissections, Esophageal stricture

Background

Recently, there has been an increased incidence of Barrett's adenocarcinoma and its resection by endoscopic submucosal dissection (ESD) has been reported [1]. Barrett's esophagus originates from gastroesophageal reflux disease (GERD) and occasionally progresses to esophageal adenocarcinoma. A local resection of cancerous lesions in the Barrett's esophagus mucosal layer (T1a) is recommended as a therapeutic option because it is minimally invasive. ESD is common in Japan because it allows *en bloc* resection of large lesion [2]; however, GERD-induced submucosal fibrosis beneath the cancerous lesion often makes ESD difficult to perform. A lesion occupying the

Barrett's esophagus circumference poses therapeutic difficulties and has a high risk of post-treatment esophageal stenosis. No reliable methods currently exist for esophageal stricture prevention after complete circular ESD for Barrett's adenocarcinoma. We describe a case of long-segment Barrett's esophagus (LSBE), which was mostly replaced by an early esophageal adenocarcinoma, treated by complete circular ESD and followed up for 2 years without esophageal stricture or recurrence.

Case presentation

A 59-year-old man complaining of heart burn for two decades was diagnosed with LSBE with an irregular surface on esophagogastroduodenoscopy (EGD) during a routine check-up. A targeted biopsy of the irregular mucosa revealed an adenocarcinoma. The patient was reported to have a 10-year history of LSBE on his annual

* Correspondence: mitoroak@naramed-u.ac.jp
[1]Third Department of Internal Medicine, Nara Medical University, 840 Shijo-cho, Kashihara, Nara 634-8522, Japan
Full list of author information is available at the end of the article

check-ups, but no irregular mucosa in LSBE had been previously found. No remarkable medical history was elicited. Clinical examination and laboratory studies had unremarkable results. EGD showed a sliding herniation in the esophagus and LSBE was classified as C4M5 according to the Prague C & M criteria (Fig. 1a). LSBE surface mucosa was unevenly reddish and contained an erosive area (Fig. 1b-c). Narrow band imaging (NBI) with magnification revealed a scattered lesion with LSBE mucosal and vasculature irregularities (Fig. 1d-e). The biopsy revealed that most of LSBE was replaced with a well-differentiated adenocarcinoma. Endoscopic ultrasound (20 MHz) revealed thickening of the mucosal layer, although the submucosal layer was intact (Fig. 1f). No metastatic lesions were detected on enhanced CT. Finally, the patient was diagnosed with early esophageal adenocarcinoma corresponding to the LSBE area; the lesion was totally circumferential and longitudinally measured 50 mm. After receiving written informed consent, ESD was performed using an EG-580RD (Fujifilm Medical, Tokyo, Japan) with a distal attachment (D201–11804; Olympus Medical Systems, Tokyo, Japan). A submucosal injection of 0.4% sodium hyaluronate (MucoUp; Johnson and Johnson, Tokyo, Japan) was administered. Marking, incision, and dissection were performed using a hook knife (KD-620QR; Olympus Medical Systems). An electrosurgical generator (VIO300D, ERBE Elektromedizin, Tübingen, Germany) was used with specifications set at dry-cut mode 60 W, effect 3, and spray coagulation mode 60 W, effect 2. Carbon dioxide was used for insufflation. ESD procedure was performed as follows: distal marking at 5 mm caudally from the EG junction (Fig. 2a) and proximal marking 10 mm cranially from the SC junction (Fig. 2b), followed by circumferential incision at the caudal end of the lesion (Fig. 2c). A submucosal tunnel entrance was created by a partial incision at the cranial end of the lesion (Fig. 2d) and submucosal dissection was performed (Fig. 2e), followed by the creation of three submucosal tunnels in the same way (Fig. 2f). Finally, incision between the opening of each tunnel and dissection of the connective submucosal tissue between each tunnel assisted by the thread-traction method was performed. *En bloc* resection was achieved without intraoperative adverse events (Fig. 2g-h). The operation period was 12 h. Histopathological analysis of the resected tissue demonstrated that the adenocarcinoma occupied the entire lumen circumference and was well differentiated. Both the cranial and caudal margins were tumor free (Fig. 3a). The depth of the tumor invasion was the superficial muscularis mucosa without lymphatic vessel and vascular involvement (Fig. 3b-c), and minimal lateral extension under the adjacent squamous epithelium was observed (Fig. 3d). The timeline after ESD is shown in Fig. 4. Postoperative adverse events such as pneumomediastinum, mediastinitis, or bleeding did not occur. The hospitalization period was 4 weeks. An intralesional steroid injection of 40 mg triamcinolone acetonide diluted with saline to a total dose of 20 mL (40 injection points, 0.5 mL per point, 8 points per circle every 10 mm) was completed on the first day post-ESD. Oral prednisolone was administered at an initial dose of 30 mg/day on the third day post-ESD, which was gradually tapered and discontinued 14 weeks later. Prophylactic endoscopic balloon dilation (EBD) with 12–15 mm balloon diameter

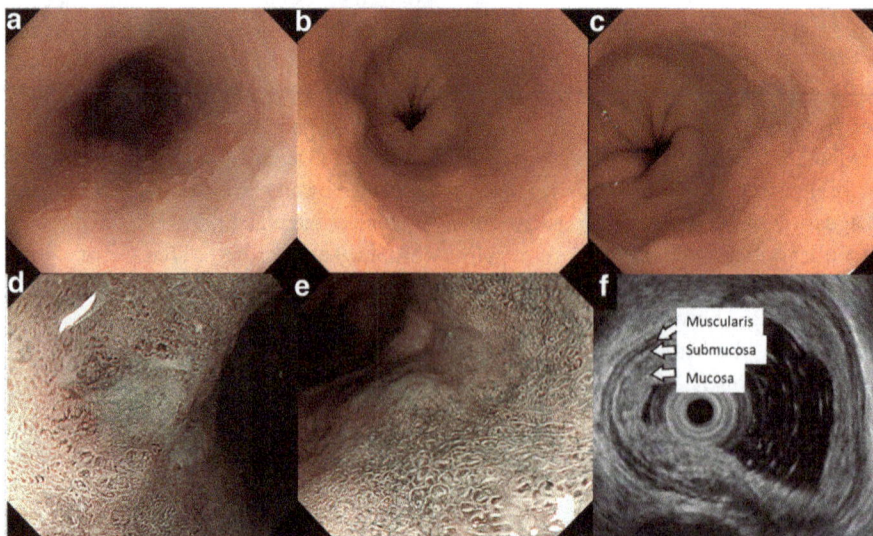

Fig. 1 Endoscopic findings. **a** Long-segment Barrett's esophagus (C4/M5). **b** A reddish and depressed lesion noted at the 7 o'clock position. **c** Rough surface and uneven redness observed. **d**, **e** Irregular structural and vascular patterns detected by magnifying endoscopy with narrow band imaging. **f** Endoscopic ultrasonography (20 MHz) showing the tumor in the mucosal layer with a normal submucosal layer (arrows)

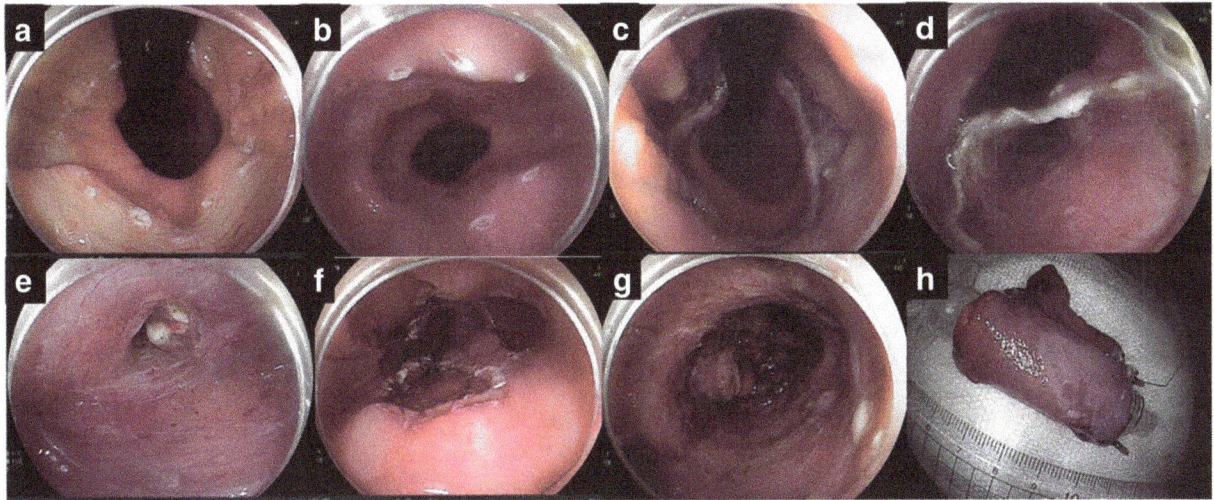

Fig. 2 Endoscopic submucosal dissection (ESD). **a** Anal extent of resection. **b** Adoral extent of resection: 1-cm margin from the SC junction, taking into consideration the progression under the squamous epithelium. **c** Circumferential incision at the caudal end of the lesion. **d** Creation of the entrance of a submucosal tunnel at the cranial end of the lesion. **e** Tunnel creation by submucosal dissection. The upper side of the image is the mucosa and the lower side is the muscle. **f** Creation of three submucosal tunnels. **g** Complete circular ESD was performed. **h** *En bloc* resected cylindrical specimen

(CRE balloon; Boston Scientific, Boston, USA) was commenced on the 10th day post-ESD and was conducted once every 1–8 weeks for 30 weeks (20 sessions). A proton pump inhibitor (PPI), proteinase inhibitor (100 mg camostat mesylate, three times after each meal), and prokinetic agent (5 mg mosapride citrate hydrate, three times after each meal) were orally administered for almost 2 years to prevent the occurrence of GERD and promote the natural healing of the post-ESD ulcer (Fig. 4). At the 2-year follow-up, the post-ESD ulcer had been covered with regenerated squamous epithelium, although small erosions still existed at the center of the post-ESD area (Fig. 5a) and EG junction (Fig. 5b). The patient does not have dysphagia and there is no evidence of esophageal stricture or recurrence 2 years after ESD.

Discussion and conclusions

Endoscopic mucosal resection (EMR) is a therapeutic option for esophageal intramucosal carcinoma (T1a); however, the procedure may be unsuitable for large

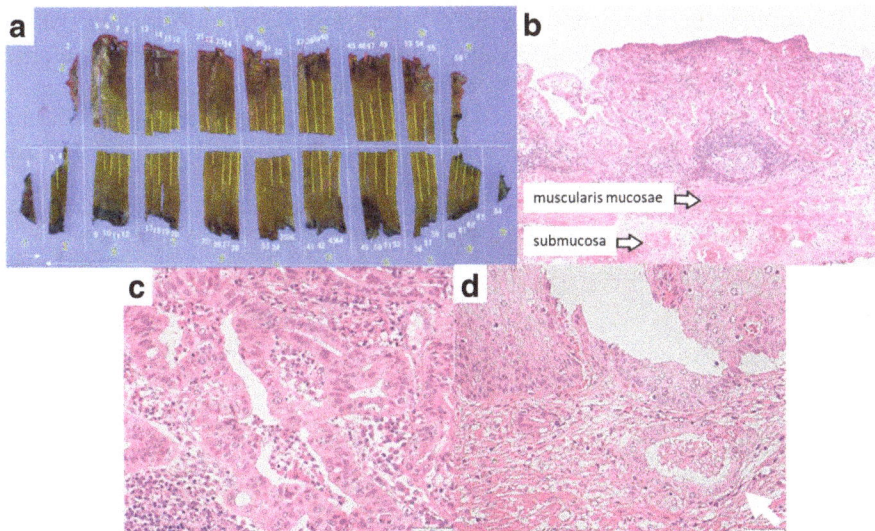

Fig. 3 Macroscopic and histopathological findings. **a** The opened specimen measured 110×55 mm^2 with the tumor occupying the whole luminal circumference. **b** The depth of tumor invasion was superficial muscularis mucosa. **c** Well-differentiated adenocarcinoma. **d** Cancer invasion observed under the adjacent squamous epithelium (arrow)

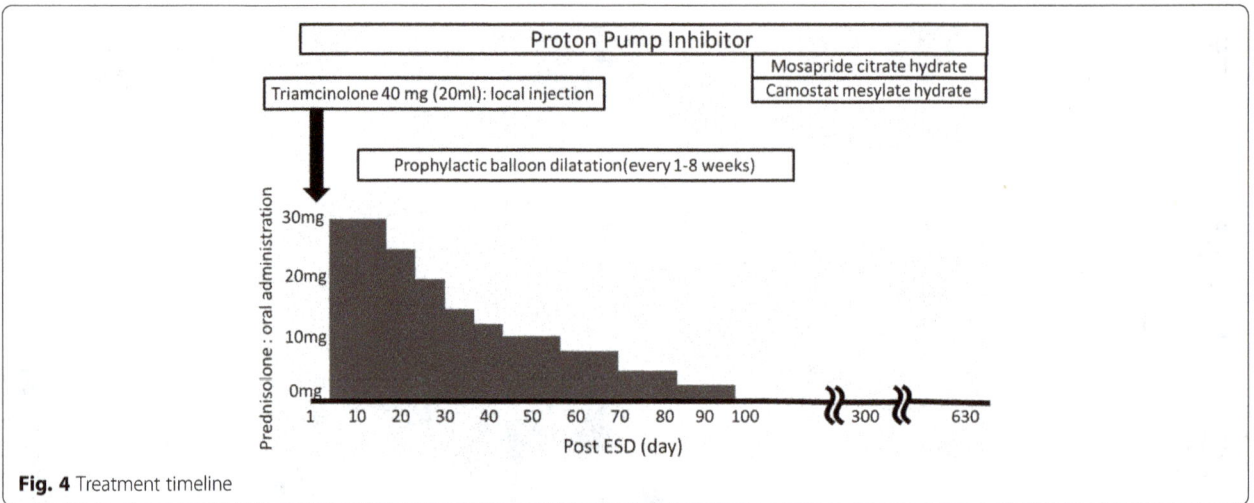

Fig. 4 Treatment timeline

lesions because of the difficulty associated with *en bloc* resection. *En bloc* resection is very important for an exact diagnosis and should be followed by an appropriate planned post-resection management strategy. ESD is the most common treatment method for intramucosal esophageal and gastric cancers (T1a) in Japan and facilitates *en bloc* resection even for large lesions. However, because the lesion in the present case was entirely circumferential and longitudinally measured 50 mm, treatment was presumed to be difficult even with ESD and the risk of post-ESD stricture of esophagus was extremely high. Although the alternative option of reliable treatment was open surgery, it was considered too invasive for such an early-stage Barrett's adenocarcinoma. Therefore, we selected ESD as the treatment strategy for this lesion.

Magnifying endoscopy with NBI facilitates easy detection of early Barrett's adenocarcinoma [3, 4]. However, the diagnosis of the extent of the tumor and attention to subsquamous tumor growth, often observed in patients with Barrett's adenocarcinoma, is required [5]. The resected specimen revealed minimal tumor extension under the adjacent squamous epithelium. The circumferential incision of the cranial end should be undertaken at the oral side of the SC junction.

Submucosal fibrosis might exist in Barrett's esophagus because of the preexisting inflammation of the esophageal wall. Even with ESD, dissecting a long segment of the submucosal layer with fibrosis is challenging. Most of the submucosal layer beneath the lesion showed remarkable fibrosis in the present case. Counter-traction is very important to dissect the fibrous submucosa. We initially created three submucosal tunnels. Endoscopic submucosal tunneling dissection was introduced as a safe, effective treatment for large, circumferential superficial esophageal neoplasia [6, 7]. The creation of tunnels was assisted by counter-traction produced by the surrounding fibrous submucosa. However, it was difficult to distinguish the mucosal side from the muscle side in the submucosal tunnel because both sides were whitish because of fibrosis. Therefore, the orientation of vertical direction might be lost, and this constitutes a risk factor for perforation or incision into the mucosal lesion. To maintain a vertical orientation, we frequently removed

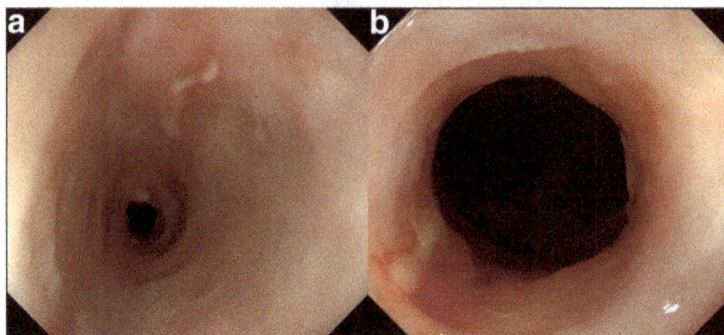

Fig. 5 Endoscopic view of the esophagus 565 days post-ESD. **a** Linear ulcer persists. **b** The EG junction area through which an EGD (9.2-mm diameter endoscope) can be passed

the scope from the submucosal tunnel and reconfirmed the orientation of anatomical direction. We dissected the connective submucosal tissue between each tunnel assisted by the thread-traction method [8], which was very useful for obtaining good counter-traction during the procedure.

It is well known that circumferential resection of more than three quarters of the lumen leads to esophageal stenosis. To avoid this major complication, various strategies have been implemented. However, there is no established prophylactic option for esophageal stenosis after radical resection. We employed intralesional steroid injection and oral steroid therapy [9, 10]. We frequently conducted prophylactic EBD, though it is a controversial option for preventing the esophageal stenosis [11, 12]. Frequent gastric acid and bile juice reflux was presumed in the present case because the patient suffered from esophageal hiatus herniation. Despite treatment with PPI, protease inhibitor, and prokinetic agent, squamous epithelium regeneration was slow and two erosions persisted long-term. We were concerned about the chronic inflammation with subsequent fibrosis at the ESD site. Once a firm strictural fibrosis is established, it might be difficult to relieve using therapeutic EBD. Therefore, we employed prophylactic EBD with intralesional steroid injection and oral steroid therapy. Prophylactic EBD was undertaken more often because of the slow healing of the post-ESD ulcer. To clarify the significance of prophylactic EBD with oral and intralesional steroid therapy, reports from additional cases are desirable.

ESD for LSBE mostly replaced with superficial Barrett's adenocarcinoma (SBA) is challenging. A prophylactic approach for post-ESD esophageal stricture remains unclear. However, compared with other treatment options such as EMR and surgical operation, ESD appears to be a safe and effective option for the treatment of total circumferential long-segment Barrett's adenocarcinoma.

Abbreviations
EBD: Endoscopic balloon dilation; EGD: Esophagogastroduodenoscopy; EMR: Endoscopic mucosal resection; ESD: Endoscopic submucosal dissection; GERD: Gastroesophageal reflux disease; LSBE: Long-segment Barrett's esophagus; PPI: Proton pump inhibitor; SBA: Superficial Barrett's adenocarcinoma

Acknowledgments
Not applicable.

Funding
Only official funding from Nara Medical University was obtained.

Authors' contributions
MK drafted the manuscript. AM critically revised the manuscript. MK, AM, MY, MS, MF, and JY performed the endoscopic treatment for this patient as a team. YO, TN, KM, TA, HK, MK, KK, HT, YS, KS, and SS made substantial contributions in deciding the treatment strategy for this patient. TF and CO made substantial contributions on the histopathological analysis of the resected specimen. HY has given final approval of the version to be published. All authors read and approved the final manuscript.

Competing interests
The authors declare that they have no competing interests.

Author details
[1]Third Department of Internal Medicine, Nara Medical University, 840 Shijo-cho, Kashihara, Nara 634-8522, Japan. [2]Department of Endoscopy, Nara Medical University, 840 Shijo-cho, Kashihara, Nara 634-8522, Japan. [3]Department of Diagnostic Pathology, Nara Medical University, 840 Shijo-cho, Kashihara, Nara 634-8522, Japan.

References
1. Chevaux JB, Piessevaux H, Jouret-Mourin A, Yeung R, Danse E, Deprez PH. Clinical outcome in patients treated with endoscopic submucosal dissection for superficial Barrett's neoplasia. Endoscopy. 2015;47:103–12.
2. Tachimori Y, Ozawa S, Numasaki H, et al. Comprehensive registry of esophageal cancer in Japan, 2009. Esophagus. 2016;13:110–37.
3. Sharma P, Bergman JJ, Goda K, Kato M, Messmann H, Alsop BR, et al. Development and validation of a classification system to identify high-grade dysplasia and esophageal Adenocarcinoma in Barrett's esophagus using narrow-band imaging. Gastroenterology. 2016;150:591–8.
4. Takahashi A, Oyama T. Barrett's esophageal adenocarcinoma diagnosed by narrow-band imaging magnifying endoscopy. Dig Endosc. 2013;25:184–9.
5. Omae M, Fujisaki J, Shimizu T, Igarashi M, Yamamoto N. Magnifying endoscopy with narrow-band imaging findings in the diagnosis of Barrett's esophageal adenocarcinoma spreading below squamous epithelium. Dig Endosc. 2013;25:162–7.
6. Gan T, Yang JL, Zhu LL, Wang YP, Yang L, Wu JC. Endoscopic submucosal multi-tunnel dissection for circumferential superficial esophageal neoplastic lesions (with videos). Gastrointest Endosc. 2016;84:143–6.
7. Arantes V, Albuquerque W, Freitas Dias CA, Demas Alvares Cabral MM, Yamamoto H. Standardized endoscopic submucosal tunnel dissection for management of early esophageal tumors. Gastrointest Endosc. 2013;78:946–52.
8. Koike Y, Hirasawa D, Fujita N, Maeda Y, Ohira T, Harada Y, et al. Usefulness of the thread-traction method in esophageal endoscopic submucosal dissection: randomized controlled trial. Dig Endosc. 2015;27:303–9.
9. Yamaguchi N, Isomoto H, Nakayama T, Hayashi T, Nishiyama H, Ohnita K, et al. Usefulness of oral prednisolone in the treatment of esophageal stricture after endoscopic submucosal dissection for superficial esophageal squamous cell carcinoma. Gastrointest Endosc. 2011;73:1115–21.
10. Hashimoto S, Kobayashi M, Takeuchi M, Sato Y, Narisawa R, Aoyagi Y. The efficacy of endoscopic triamcinolone injection for the prevention of esophageal stricture after endoscopic submucosal dissection. Gastrointest Endosc. 2011;74:1389–93.
11. Isomoto H, Yamaguchi N, Nakayama T, Hayashi T, Nishiyama H, Ohnita K, et al. Management of esophageal stricture after complete circular endoscopic submucosal dissection for superficial esophageal squamous cell carcinoma. BMC Gastroenterol. 2011;11:46.
12. Jain D, Singhal S. Esophageal stricture prevention after endoscopic submucosal dissection. Clin Endosc. 2016;49:241–56.

22

Obesity increases the risk of erosive esophagitis but metabolic unhealthiness alone does not: a large-scale cross-sectional study

Myong Ki Baeg[1], Sun-Hye Ko[2]* ⓘ, Seung Yeon Ko[3], Hee Sun Jung[4] and Myung-Gyu Choi[5]

Abstract

Background: Obesity is a known risk factor for erosive esophagitis (EE) and metabolic unhealthiness has been implicated in EE pathogenesis. However, obesity and metabolic unhealthiness are not synonymous and the associations between obesity, metabolic health, and EE are unclear. Therefore, our aim was to investigate the relationship between EE, obesity, and metabolic health.

Methods: We performed a retrospective cross-sectional study of subjects undergoing health screening at a university hospital. Subjects were classified into 4 groups based on metabolic and obesity criteria: metabolically healthy nonobese (MHNO), metabolically healthy obese (MHO), metabolically unhealthy nonobese (MUNO), and metabolically unhealthy obese (MUO). Multivariable analysis was used to identify EE risk factors with MHNO subjects as reference. To determine if there were synergistic interactions between metabolic health and obesity status, the Rothman's synergy index and attributable proportion of risk were also calculated.

Results: We included 10,338 subjects (5448 MHNO, 1605 MHO, 1600 MUNO, 1685 MUO). The prevalence of EE was 6.5% in MHNO, 12.6% in MHO, 9.3% in MUNO, and 14.3% in MUO. EE risk was increased significantly by obesity (MHO: OR, 1.589, 95% CI, 1.314–1.921, $P < 0.001$; MUO: OR, 1.734, 95% CI, 1.441–2.085, $P < 0.001$), but not in MUNO subjects (OR, 1.224, 95% CI, 0.991–1.511, $P = 0.060$). Male sex, blood leukocyte count, alcohol, and smoking significantly increased EE risk, but *H. pylori* infection was protective. Replacement of obesity with abdominal obesity gave similar results. The Rothman's synergy index was 0.920 (95% CI, 0.143–5.899) and the attributable proportion of risk was − 0.051 (95% CI, − 1.206–1.105), indicating no interaction between metabolic and obesity status on EE risk.

Conclusions: We demonstrated that obesity increased the risk of EE, regardless of metabolic health status. However, EE risk was not significantly increased in MUNO subjects, suggesting that metabolic unhealthiness may not be involved in EE pathogenesis. As observational cross-sectional studies cannot prove causality, prospective longitudinal studies involving obesity and metabolic treatment should be performed to further investigate the association between obesity, metabolic health, and EE risk.

Keywords: Erosive esophagitis, Gastroesophageal reflux disease, Metabolic health status, Obesity, Wildman criteria

* Correspondence: sunhyeko@gmail.com
[2]Department of Internal Medicine, Inje University Haeundae Paik Hospital, Inje University College of Medicine, 875 Haeundaero, Haeundae-Gu, Busan 612-896, South Korea
Full list of author information is available at the end of the article

Background

Gastroesophageal reflux disease (GERD) is a multifactorial disease that has genetic, physiologic and environmental risk factors [1]. One risk factor that has attracted great interest is obesity [2], of which the epidemic increase has paralleled the global increase in GERD [3]. The potential mechanisms linking obesity with GERD are pathophysiologic changes brought on by increased intra-abdominal pressure and metabolic unhealthiness associated with pro-inflammatory cytokine production and the insulin/insulin growth factor pathway [1, 4]. Although obesity has often been regarded as being synonymous with metabolic unhealthiness, not all obese people are metabolically unhealthy and one-third of metabolically unhealthy people are of normal weight [5, 6]. However, the association between obesity, metabolic health, and GERD has not been investigated adequately.

Endoscopically visible breaks in the gastroesophageal junction are a reliable sign of GERD. This is clinically important because healing of such endoscopically confirmed erosive esophagitis (EE) can be regarded as a surrogate for successful therapy and correlates well with symptomatic relief [7]. EE is associated with potentially serious complications such as Barrett's esophagus (BE) and esophageal adenocarcinoma (EAC) [8, 9], which have also been linked with obesity and metabolic unhealthiness [10–12]. Therefore, the aim of our study was to investigate the relationship between EE, obesity, and metabolic health status.

Methods

Study population

We performed a retrospective cross-sectional study of subjects who underwent routine health screening from March 2009 to July 2014 at the Center for Health Promotion of Seoul St. Mary's Hospital (Seochogu, Seoul, South Korea). Subjects underwent health screening voluntarily or as part of annual/bi-annual employee check-ups. Such check-ups cover about 40–50% of the Korean population. Those who underwent screening esophagogastroduodenoscopy and for whom fasting serum insulin results were available were included in this study. Those who underwent multiple visits had only the first set of endoscopy included. We excluded subjects who 1) had a history of current or previous malignancies, 2) had a history of upper gastrointestinal surgery, and 3) were missing medical or social records or anthropometric/laboratory findings. This study was approved by the Institutional Review Board of Seoul St. Mary's Hospital, which permitted the study without informed consent requirements because it was a retrospective study using blinded subject identities (KC14RISI0574).

Data collection

Physical characteristics including weight, height, waist circumference, and blood pressure were measured by trained medical personnel. Blood pressure was measured using an appropriately sized cuff with the subject in a sitting position after at least 10 min of rest. Waist circumference was measured at the midline between the lowest rib and the iliac crest.

Blood samples were taken after an overnight fast of at least 12 h. White blood cell (WBC) counts were analyzed using a Sysmex-XE2100 automated blood cell analyzer (Sysmex, Kobe, Japan). Fasting plasma glucose (FPG), total cholesterol, triglyceride, high-density lipoprotein (HDL) cholesterol, and low-density lipoprotein cholesterol levels were measured using a Hitachi 7600 automated analyzer (Hitachi Co., Tokyo, Japan). Glycated hemoglobin (HbA1c) was measured using a Tosoh HLC-723 HbG7 analyzer (Tosoh Bioscience Ltd., Redditch, UK). *Helicobacter pylori*-specific immunoglobulin G concentration was measured using the Immulite 2000 XPi platform (Siemens Healthcare Diagnostics, Erlangen, Germany).

Esophagogastroduodenoscopy

Esophagogastroduodenoscopy (Olympus GIF-H260; Olympus Ltd., Tokyo, Japan) was performed in subjects who had fasted overnight by endoscopists who were board-accredited gastroenterologists and certified as experts by the Korean Society of Gastrointestinal Endoscopy. EE was defined according to the Los Angeles Classification [13]. All endoscopy results were reassessed visually by two authors who were blinded to the initial endoscopy records.

Definitions

Body mass index was calculated as weight divided by height squared (kg/m^2). Obesity was defined according to the World Health Organization Criteria for East Asians (> 25 kg/m^2) [14]. Abdominal obesity was defined as waist circumference ≥ 90 cm in men and ≥ 80 cm in women, which are the modified criteria for the Asian population [15]. Insulin resistance was computed by the homeostasis model assessment of insulin resistance (HOMA-IR) as follows: fasting insulin (pmol/L) × fasting glucose (mmol/L)/22.5 [16]. Metabolic health status was determined by the modified Wildman criteria, which were as follows: (1) systolic blood pressure ≥ 130 mmHg or diastolic blood pressure ≥ 85 mmHg or use of antihypertensive medication, (2) triglyceride levels ≥ 1.7 mmol/L or use of lipid-lowering drugs, (3) FPG ≥ 5.5 mmol/L or use of antidiabetes therapy, (4) HDL cholesterol levels < 1.0 mmol/L in men and < 1.3 mmol/L in women, and (5) HOMA-IR > 90th percentile in our population (≥ 3.17) [6, 17, 18]. Subjects were defined as metabolically healthy if they met ≤ 1 of the modified

Wildman criteria and metabolically unhealthy if they met ≥ 2 of the criteria. Based on the modified Wildman and obesity criteria, the subjects were classified as (1) metabolically healthy nonobese (MHNO), (2) metabolically healthy obese (MHO), (3) metabolically unhealthy nonobese (MUNO), and (4) metabolically unhealthy obese (MUO).

Statistical analysis

Clinical characteristics and parameters were expressed as mean ± standard deviation or numbers (percentage). Categorical variables were analyzed by Pearson's chi-square test, and continuous variables by analysis of variance. P values < 0.05 were considered significant. Multivariable regression analysis was performed to identify risk factors for EE. Odds ratios (ORs) and 95% confidence intervals (CIs) for EE were calculated for the MHO, MUNO, and MUO groups using the MHNO group as the reference category. A separate analysis was performed, replacing obesity with abdominal obesity to investigate its effects. In addition, we analyzed the interaction between metabolic health and obesity status by calculating the Rothman's synergy index and the attributable proportion of risk [19, 20]. If metabolic health and obesity had an interaction to increase the risk of EE, the synergy index would be greater than 1.0, whereas if there were no additive effects, the value would be below 1. The attributable proportion of risk gives an estimate of the proportion of EE cases that are attributable to any interaction between metabolic health and obesity status beyond each factor alone. If there were any positive interaction, the attributable proportion of risk would be greater than 0 [19].

Results

During routine health screening in the study period, 14,368 Koreans underwent screening esophagogastroduodenoscopy

and fasting insulin measurement. Of these, 4030 were excluded for the following reasons: (1) 150 because of repeat testing, (2) 89 with malignancies, (3) three with prior upper gastrointestinal surgery, and (4) 3788 with missing social or medical records or anthropometric/laboratory data. Of the 10,338 subjects included in the study, there were 5448 in the MHNO group, 1605 in the MHO group, 1600 in the MUNO group, and 1685 in the MUO group (Fig. 1).

The prevalence of EE was 6.5% in the MHNO group, 12.6% in the MHO group, 9.3% in the MUNO group, and 14.3% in the MUO group. There was a significantly higher proportion of males in the obese groups. Indices related to glucose metabolism such as FPG, HbA1c, insulin, and HOMA-IR were lowest in the MHNO group and successively increased in the MHO, MUNO, and MUO groups. The percentage of subjects who drank coffee or alcohol was significantly higher in the obese groups. Other characteristics of the four groups are listed in Table 1.

Characteristics of the subjects based on EE status are shown in Table 2. Subjects with EE were significantly more likely to be male and obese, and included significantly more subjects who drank coffee or alcohol and had a smoking history. Those with EE were significantly less likely to be seropositive for *H. pylori*.

Univariable analysis of EE risk factors found that male sex, higher WBC count, higher glucose metabolism indices, drinking coffee or alcohol, or smoking significantly increasedEE risk. Protective factors for EE were higher HDL cholesterol levels and *H. pylori* seropositivity (Table 3).

Multivariable analysis found that compared with the reference MHNO group, EE risk was significantly higher in the obese groups (MHO: OR, 1.589, 95% CI, 1.314–1.921, $P < 0.001$; MUO: OR, 1.734, 95% CI, 1.441–2.085, $P <$ 0.001), but not in the MUNO group (OR, 1.224, 95% CI,

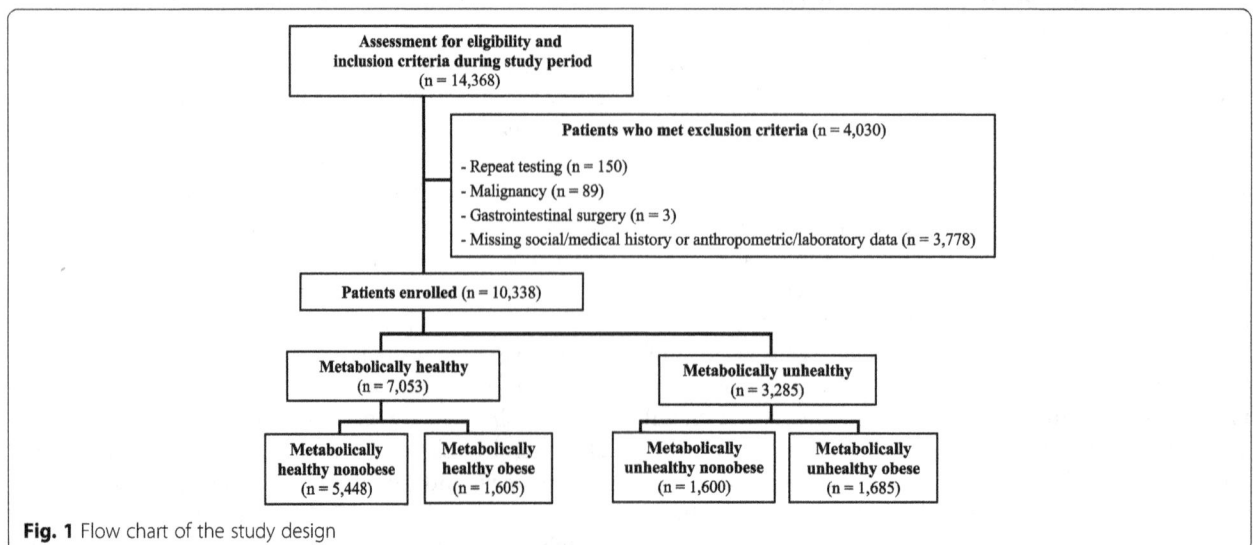

Fig. 1 Flow chart of the study design

Table 1 Characteristics of subjects by metabolic obesity status

	MHNO (n = 5448)	MHO (n = 1605)	MUNO (n = 1600)	MUO (n = 1685)	P
Age (years)	49.5 ± 11.4	51.6 ± 11.1	56.5 ± 10.3	53.9 ± 11.2	< 0.001
Male (n, %)	2339 (42.9%)	1074 (66.9%)	921 (57.6%)	1204 (71.5%)	< 0.001
Diabetes (n, %)	153 (2.8%)	50 (3.1%)	418 (26.1%)	467 (27.7%)	< 0.001
Hypertension (n, %)	582 (10.7%)	328 (20.4%)	616 (38.5%)	682 (40.5%)	< 0.001
BMI (kg/m^2)	21.7 ± 2.0	26.8 ± 1.7	22.9 ± 1.6	27.6 ± 2.3	< 0.001
Abdominal obesity (n, %)	1454 (26.7%)	1127 (70.2%)	574 (35.9%)	1320 (78.3%)	< 0.001
Coffee (n, %)	3664 (67.3%)	1156 (72.0%)	1025 (64.1%)	1240 (73.6%)	< 0.001
Alcohol (n, %)	2337 (42.9%)	932 (58.1%)	735 (45.9%)	949 (56.3%)	< 0.001
Smoking (n, %)	1883 (34.6%)	705 (43.9%)	715 (44.7%)	886 (52.6%)	< 0.001
H.pylori seropositive (n, %)	2757 (50.6%)	839 (52.3%)	863 (53.9%)	922 (54.7%)	0.008
WBC count (× 10^9/L)	5.4 ± 1.7	5.7 ± 1.6	6.0 ± 1.8	6.3 ± 1.7	< 0.001
FPG (mmol/L)	4.9 ± 0.8	5.1 ± 0.7	6.1 ± 1.8	6.2 ± 1.6	< 0.001
HbA1c (%)	5.4 ± 0.5	5.5 ± 0.5	6.0 ± 1.1	6.1 ± 1.0	< 0.001
Insulin (pmol/L)	34.7 ± 21.5	50.0 ± 27.1	54.9 ± 38.9	80.6 ± 61.8	< 0.001
HOMA-IR	1.1 ± 0.7	1.6 ± 0.9	2.2 ± 2.0	3.2 ± 2.5	< 0.001
Total cholesterol (mmol/L)	5.1 ± 0.9	5.2 ± 0.9	5.2 ± 1.0	5.2 ± 1.1	< 0.001
Triglyceride (mmol/L)	0.9 ± 0.5	1.1 ± 0.6	1.8 ± 1.1	2.0 ± 1.3	< 0.001
HDL-cholesterol (mmol/L)	1.5 ± 0.3	1.3 ± 0.3	1.2 ± 0.3	1.1 ± 0.3	< 0.001
LDL-cholesterol (mmol/L)	3.1 ± 0.8	3.3 ± 0.8	3.1 ± 0.9	3.2 ± 0.9	< 0.001
EE (n, %)	356 (6.5%)	202 (12.6%)	149 (9.3%)	241 (14.3%)	< 0.001
EE grade (n, %)					< 0.001
A	310 (5.7%)	172 (10.7%)	127 (7.9%)	186 (11.0%)	
B	37 (0.1%)	27 (1.7%)	19 (1.2%)	45 (2.7%)	
C or D	9 (0.2%)	3 (0.2%)	3 (0.2%)	10 (0.6%)	

Data are presented as either mean ± standard deviation or as number (%)

BMI body mass index, *EE* erosive esophagitis, *FPG* fasting plasma glucose, *HbA1c* glycated hemoglobin, *HDL* high density lipoprotein, *HOMA-IR* homeostasis model assessment of insulin resistance, *MHNO* metabolic healthy nonobese, *MHO* metabolic healthy obese, *MUNO* metabolic unhealthy nonobese, *MUO* metabolic unhealthy obese, *LDL* low density lipoprotein, *TC* total cholesterol, *WBC* white blood cell

0.991–1.511, P = 0.060). Other predictive factors for EE were male sex, higher WBC counts, alcohol, and smoking history while *H. pylori* seropositivity remained protective (Table 4). When obesity was replaced in the analysis with abdominal obesity, the risk factors for EE remained similar. EE risk was significantly higher in the groups with abdominal obesity but not in the metabolically healthy abdominally nonobese group (Table 4). Analyzing obesity and metabolic health separately by multivariable analysis gave similar results, with obesity being a significant risk factor for EE (OR, 1.521, 95% CI, 1.314–1.761, P < 0.001), but metabolic health was not significant (OR, 1.154, 95% CI, 0.992–1.342, P = 0.064).

We calculated the Rothman's synergy index and attributable proportion of risk to identify any interaction between metabolic health and obesity on EE. The Rothman's synergy index and the attributable proportion of risk was 0.920 (< 1, 95% CI, 0.143–5.899) and – 0.051 (< 0, 95% CI, – 1.206–1.105), respectively, which suggest

that there were no synergistic effects or increased risks from the interaction between them.

Discussion

This study demonstrated that obesity increases the risk of EE, regardless of metabolic health status. Nonobese metabolically unhealthy subjects did not have a significant increase in EE risk while there was a significant increase in those who were obese. These findings were consistent when abdominal obesity replaced obesity in the analysis. Our study shows that obesity or abdominal obesity plays a significant role in EE risk, whereas metabolic health may not.

Our study reinforced the classic view that obesity or abdominal obesity increases EE risk [1, 21]. This is most likely because of the increased intraabdominal pressure, increased transient lower esophageal sphincter relaxation and anatomic disruption of the esophagogastric junction brought on by obesity or abdominal obesity [1, 21].

Table 2 Characteristics of subjects with or without erosive esophagitis

	EE (−) (n = 9390)	EE (+) (n = 948)	P
Age (years)	51.7 ± 11.4	51.2 ± 11.6	0.193
Male (n, %)	4780 (50.9%)	758 (80.0%)	< 0.001
Diabetes (n, %)	963 (10.3%)	125 (13.2%)	0.005
Hypertension (n, %)	1960 (20.9%)	248 (26.2%)	< 0.001
Obesity (n, %)	2847 (30.3%)	443 (46.7%)	< 0.001
Abdominal obesity (n, %)	4040 (43.0%)	432 (45.6%)	0.119
Metabolic unhealthiness (n, %)	2895 (30.8%)	390 (41.1%)	< 0.001
Metabolic obesity status (n, %)			< 0.001
Metabolic healthy nonobese	5092 (54.2%)	356 (37.6%)	
Metabolic healthy obese	1403 (14.9%)	202 (21.3%)	
Metabolic unhealthy nonobese	1451 (15.5%)	149 (15.7%)	
Metabolic unhealthy obese	1444 (15.4%)	241 (25.4%)	
Metabolic abdominal obesity status (n, %)			< 0.001
Metabolic healthy abdominal nonobese	4122 (43.9%)	351 (37.0%)	
Metabolic healthy abdominal obese	2373 (25.3%)	207 (21.8%)	
Metabolic unhealthy abdominal nonobese	1228 (13.1%)	165 (17.4%)	
Metabolic unhealthy abdominal obese	1667 (17.8%)	225 (23.7%)	
Smoking (n, %)	3634 (38.7%)	555 (58.5%)	< 0.001
Alcohol (n, %)	4321 (46.0%)	632 (66.7%)	< 0.001
Coffee (n, %)	6386 (68.0%)	699 (73.7%)	< 0.001
Laboratory findings			
Helicobacter pylori seropositive (n, %)	5080 (54.1%)	301 (31.8%)	< 0.001
White blood cell count ($\times 10^9$/L)	5.7 ± 1.7	6.1 ± 1.8	< 0.001
Fasting plasma glucose (mmol/L)	5.3 ± 1.3	5.5 ± 1.6	< 0.001
Glycated hemoglobin (%)	5.6 ± 0.7	5.8 ± 0.9	< 0.001
Insulin (pmol/L)	6.7 ± 5.5	7.8 ± 5.7	< 0.001
HOMA-IR	1.65 ± 1.57	2.01 ± 2.05	< 0.001
Total cholesterol (mmol/L)	5.2 ± 1.0	5.2 ± 0.9	0.719
Triglyceride (mmol/L)	1.2 ± 0.9	1.5 ± 1.1	< 0.001
High density lipoprotein cholesterol (mmol/L)	1.4 ± 0.3	1.3 ± 0.3	< 0.001
Low density lipoprotein cholesterol (mmol/L)	3.2 ± 0.8	3.2 ± 0.8	0.628

Data are presented as either mean ± standard deviation or as number (%)
EE erosive esophagitis, *HOMA-IR* homeostasis model assessment of insulin resistance

Recently, a new perspective has suggested that GERD is also mediated by a metabolic pathway [4]. This is supported by several studies that have reported a positive association between insulin resistance and GERD [22–24]. However, these studies were limited by their small number of subjects, that they included only obese subjects without a nonobese control group or had potential multicollinearity issues [22–24]. Most importantly, obesity and metabolic unhealthiness were not analyzed independently, which may have confounded the outcome. In our study, EE risk was dependent on obesity but not on metabolic status. This suggests that metabolic unhealthiness by itself may not be a sufficient risk factor for EE, but is subordinate to obesity.

Interestingly, our study also found that increased WBC counts may increase EE risk. The WBC count is a biomarker of systemic inflammation and has been associated with increased overall, cancer-related, and vascular disease-related mortality [25]. Though metabolic unhealthiness was not associated with the risk of EE, the significant increase in WBC count in subjects with EE subjects suggests that inflammatory processes may contribute to EE. This is supported by a recent study that reported that subjects with erosive esophagitis had significantly higher standardized ^{18}F-fluorodeoxyglucose uptake values at the esophagogastric junction [26]. It is also supported by studies that have reported that levels of proinflammatory

Table 3 Univariable risk factors of erosive esophagitis

	Odds ratio	95% Confidence interval	P
Age	0.996	0.990–1.002	0.193
Male	3.848	3.265–4.534	< 0.001
Diabetes	1.329	1.089–1.623	0.005
Hypertension	1.343	1.152–1.566	< 0.001
Obesity	2.024	1.768–2.316	< 0.001
Coffee	1.321	1.135–1.536	< 0.001
Alcohol	2.346	2.038–2.701	< 0.001
Smoking	2.237	1.953–2.562	< 0.001
Helicobacter pylori seropositivity	0.395	0.342–0.455	< 0.001
White blood cell count	1.145	1.105–1.185	< 0.001
Fasting plasma glucose	1.006	1.004–1.008	< 0.001
Glycated hemoglobin	1.206	1.121–1.298	< 0.001
Insulin	1.027	1.017–1.037	< 0.001
HOMA-IR	1.1	1.065–1.137	< 0.001
Total cholesterol	1	0.999–1.002	0.719
Triglyceride	1.003	1.003–1.004	< 0.001
High density lipoprotein cholesterol	0.979	0.974–0.985	< 0.001
Low density lipoprotein cholesterol	1.001	0.998–1.003	0.628
Metabolic Obesity status			
Metabolic healthy nonobese	1		
Metabolic healthy obese	2.059	1.716–2.472	< 0.001
Metabolic unhealthy nonobese	1.469	1.203–1.794	< 0.001
Metabolic unhealthy obese	2.387	2.007–2.840	< 0.001
Metabolic abdominal obesity status			
Metabolic healthy abdominal nonobese	1		
Metabolic healthy abdominal obese	1.024	0.856–1.225	0.792
Metabolic unhealthy abdominal nonobese	1.578	1.298–1.919	< 0.001
Metabolic unhealthy abdominal obese	1.585	1.328–1.892	0.001

HOMA-IR homeostasis model assessment of insulin resistance

cytokines such as interleukins 1, 6, and 8 were increased in subjects with GERD [27]. However, as both EE and non-EE subjects had WBC counts within the normal range and MUNO subjects had higher WBC counts than MHO subjects, the association between higher WBC counts and increased EE risk cannot be asserted confidently. Studies involving EE and the inflammatory pathway should be performed to further investigate this association.

Our study is limited by its retrospective cross-sectional design, which allows only inferences to be made regarding obesity/metabolic health status and risk of EE. Another limitation is the lack of data regarding inflammatory factors such as interleukin 1, 6, 8, and tumor necrosis factor alpha, which may have shed more light on the association between inflammation and EE. A third limitation is that we only included subjects for whom both insulin and endoscopy results were available, which may have resulted in a

selection bias. However, because our study included over 10,000 subjects, we believe that the risk of selection bias is low. Finally, we could not investigate the association between BE or EAC and obesity/metabolic health because the prevalence of BE and EAC is very low in Koreans [28, 29].

The main strength of our study is that this is the first study investigating the risk of EE according to a standardized obesity/metabolic health profile to divide the subjects into four distinct obesity/metabolic groups. This enabled us to distinguish the effects of obesity and metabolic health, which contrasts with previous studies whose findings may have been related to underlying obesity rather than to metabolic unhealthiness [22, 24]. Another strength is the large number of subjects included in our study, with at least 1600 subjects in each subgroup. Though this study was of a retrospective cross-sectional design, we believe that the inclusion of a

Table 4 Multivariable risk factors of erosive esophagitis according to metabolic obesity status or metabolic abdominal obesity status

	Odds ratio	95% CI	P	Odds ratio	95% CI	P
Age	1.002	0.996–1.008	0.540	1	0.994–1.006	0.982
Male	2.691	2.196–3.297	< 0.001	3.358	2.727–4.136	< 0.001
Coffee	1.075	0.918–1.258	0.369	1.087	0.929–1.273	0.298
Alcohol	1.338	1.138–1.574	< 0.001	1.346	1.145–1.583	< 0.001
Smoking	1.181	1.007–1.385	0.041	1.171	0.999–1.373	0.052
Helicobacter pylori seropositivity	0.362	0.313–0.419	< 0.001	0.364	0.315–0.422	< 0.001
White blood cell count	1.071	1.029–1.114	0.001	1.068	1.027–1.111	0.001
Metabolic Obesity Status						
Metabolic healthy nonobese	1					
Metabolic healthy obese	1.589	1.314–1.921	< 0.001			
Metabolic unhealthy nonobese	1.224	0.991–1.511	0.06			
Metabolic unhealthy obese	1.734	1.441–2.085	< 0.001			
Metabolic Abdominal Obesity Status						
Metabolic healthy abdominal nonobese				1		
Metabolic healthy abdominal obese				1.585	1.308–1.920	< 0.001
Metabolic unhealthy abdominal nonobese				1.186	0.966–1.455	0.103
Metabolic unhealthy abdominal obese				1.807	1.496–2.182	< 0.001

CI confidence interval

sufficiently large number of subjects lends credibility to our study results. Lastly, we calculated the Rothman's synergy index and attributable proportion of risk to determine if there was any interaction between metabolic health and obesity status. This analysis verified our findings in that there were no significant interactions between metabolic health and obesity status, which also suggests that the risk of EE conferred by obesity was independent of metabolic health status.

Conclusion

Our study found that obesity/abdominal obesity was a risk factor for EE, regardless of metabolic health status. Though EE risk was significantly increased in the MUO group compared with the reference MHNO group, it was not in the MUNO group, which suggests that metabolic health plays a marginal role in EE pathogenesis. Prospective longitudinal studies including body composition and metabolic health analysis as in addition to those involving obesity and metabolic treatment should be performed to further investigate the association between obesity, metabolic health, and EE risk.

Abbreviations

BE: Barrett's esophagus; CI: Confidence interval; EAC: Esophageal adenocarcinoma; EE: Erosive esophagitis; FPG: Fasting plasma glucose; GERD: Gastroesophageal reflux disease; HbA1c: Glycated hemoglobin; HOMA-IR: Homeostasis model assessment of insulin resistance; MHNO: Metabolically healthy nonobese; MHO: Metabolically healthy obese; MUNO: Metabolically unhealthy nonobese; MUO: Metabolically unhealthy obese; OR: Odds ratio; WBC: White blood cell

Funding

This work was supported by the research fund of International St. Mary's Hospital, Catholic Kwandong University.

Authors' contributions

S-HK, MKB, and SYK designed the study. MKB, SYK and HSJ collected the data. HSJ and M-GC analyzed the data. S-HK and MKB wrote the manuscript. S-HK and M-GC edited the manuscript. We also state that all authors have read and approved the manuscript.

Competing interests

The authors declare that they have no competing interests.

Author details

[1]Department of Internal Medicine, International St. Mary's Hospital, College of Medicine, Catholic Kwandong University, Incheon 22711, South Korea. [2]Department of Internal Medicine, Inje University Haeundae Paik Hospital, Inje University College of Medicine, 875 Haeundaero, Haeundae-Gu, Busan 612-896, South Korea. [3]Department of Surgery, Sacred Heart Hospital, Hallym University, Gyeonggi-do, Anyang-si 14068, South Korea. [4]Department of Health Promotion, Seoul St. Mary's Hospital, College of Medicine, The Catholic University of Korea, Seoul 06591, South Korea. [5]Department of Internal Medicine, Seoul St. Mary's Hospital, College of Medicine, The Catholic University of Korea, Seoul 06591, South Korea.

References

1. Boeckxstaens G, El-Serag HB, Smout AJ, Kahrilas PJ. Symptomatic reflux disease: the present, the past and the future. Gut. 2014;63(7):1185–93.
2. Hampel H, Abraham NS, El-Serag HB. Meta-analysis: obesity and the risk for gastroesophageal reflux disease and its complications. Ann Intern Med. 2005;143(3):199 211.
3. Ng M, Fleming T, Robinson M, Thomson B, Graetz N, Margono C, Mullany EC, Biryukov S, Abbafati C, Abera SF, et al. Global, regional, and national

prevalence of overweight and obesity in children and adults during 1980-2013: a systematic analysis for the global burden of disease study 2013. Lancet. 2014;384(9945):766–81.

4. Tilg H, Moschen AR. Visceral adipose tissue attacks beyond the liver: esophagogastric junction as a new target. Gastroenterology. 2010;139(6):1823–6.

5. Stefan N, Kantartzis K, Machann J, Schick F, Thamer C, Rittig K, Balletshofer B, Machicao F, Fritsche A, Haring HU. Identification and characterization of metabolically benign obesity in humans. Arch Intern Med. 2008;168(15):1609–16.

6. Wildman RP, Muntner P, Reynolds K, McGinn AP, Rajpathak S, Wylie-Rosett J, Sowers MR. The obese without cardiometabolic risk factor clustering and the normal weight with cardiometabolic risk factor clustering: prevalence and correlates of 2 phenotypes among the US population (NHANES 1999-2004). Arch Intern Med. 2008;168(15):1617–24.

7. Vakil N, van Zanten SV, Kahrilas P, Dent J, Jones R. The Montreal definition and classification of gastroesophageal reflux disease: a global evidence-based consensus. Am J Gastroenterol. 2006;101(8):1900–20. quiz 1943

8. Shaheen N, Ransohoff DF. Gastroesophageal reflux, Barrett esophagus, and esophageal cancer: scientific review. JAMA. 2002;287(15):1972–81.

9. Lagergren J, Bergstrom R, Lindgren A, Nyren O. Symptomatic gastroesophageal reflux as a risk factor for esophageal adenocarcinoma. N Engl J Med. 1999;340(11):825–31.

10. Duggan C, Onstad L, Hardikar S, Blount PL, Reid BJ, Vaughan TL. Association between markers of obesity and progression from Barrett's esophagus to esophageal adenocarcinoma. Clin Gastroenterol Hepatol. 2013;11(8):934–43.

11. Thrift AP, Hilal J, El-Serag HB. Metabolic syndrome and the risk of Barrett's oesophagus in white males. Aliment Pharmacol Ther. 2015;41(11):1182–9.

12. Di Caro S, Cheung WH, Fini L, Keane MG, Theis B, Haidry R, Di Renzo L, De Lorenzo A, Lovat L, Batterham RL, et al. Role of body composition and metabolic profile in Barrett's oesophagus and progression to cancer. Eur J Gastroenterol Hepatol. 2016;28(3):251–60.

13. Lundell LR, Dent J, Bennett JR, Blum AL, Armstrong D, Galmiche JP, Johnson F, Hongo M, Richter JE, Spechler SJ, et al. Endoscopic assessment of oesophagitis: clinical and functional correlates and further validation of the Los Angeles classification. Gut. 1999;45(2):172–80.

14. WHO Expert Consultation. Appropriate body-mass index for Asian populations and its implications for policy and intervention strategies. Lancet. 2004;363(9403):157–63.

15. Alberti KG, Eckel RH, Grundy SM, Zimmet PZ, Cleeman JI, Donato KA, Fruchart JC, James WP, Loria CM, Smith SC Jr. Harmonizing the metabolic syndrome: a joint interim statement of the international diabetes federation task force on epidemiology and prevention; National Heart, Lung, and Blood Institute; American Heart Association; world heart federation; international atherosclerosis society; and International Association for the Study of obesity. Circulation. 2009;120(16):1640–5.

16. Turner RC, Holman RR, Matthews D, Hockaday TD, Peto J. Insulin deficiency and insulin resistance interaction in diabetes: estimation of their relative contribution by feedback analysis from basal plasma insulin and glucose concentrations. Metabolism. 1979;28(11):1086–96.

17. Kim JW, Kim DH, Roh YK, Ju SY, Nam HY, Nam GE, Kim DW, Lee SH, Lee CW, Han K, et al. Serum ferritin levels are positively associated with metabolically obese normal weight: a Nationwide population-based study. Medicine (Baltimore). 2015;94(52):e2335.

18. Ko SH, Baeg MK, Ko SY, Jung HS, Kim P, Choi MG. Obesity and metabolic unhealthiness have different effects on colorectal neoplasms. J Clin Endocrinol Metab. 2017;102(8):2762–9.

19. Andersson T, Alfredsson L, Kallberg H, Zdravkovic S, Ahlbom A. Calculating measures of biological interaction. Eur J Epidemiol. 2005;20(7):575–9.

20. Knol MJ, VanderWeele TJ, Groenwold RH, Klungel OH, Rovers MM, Grobbee DE. Estimating measures of interaction on an additive scale for preventive exposures. Eur J Epidemiol. 2011;26(6):433–8.

21. El-Serag H. Role of obesity in GORD-related disorders. Gut. 2008;57(3):281–4.

22. Pointer SD, Rickstrew J, Slaughter JC, Vaezi MF, Silver HJ. Dietary carbohydrate intake, insulin resistance and gastro-oesophageal reflux disease: a pilot study in European- and African-American obese women. Aliment Pharmacol Ther. 2016;44(9):976–88.

23. Hsu CS, Wang PC, Chen JH, Su WC, Tseng TC, Chen HD, Hsiao TH, Wang CC, Lin HH, Shyu RY, et al. Increasing insulin resistance is associated with increased severity and prevalence of gastro-oesophageal reflux disease. Aliment Pharmacol Ther. 2011;34(8):994–1004.

24. Tai CM, Lee YC, Tu HP, Huang CK, Wu MT, Chang CY, Lee CT, Wu MS, Lin JT, Wang WM. The relationship between visceral adiposity and the risk of erosive esophagitis in severely obese Chinese patients. Obesity (Silver Spring). 2010;18(11):2165–9.

25. Ruggiero C, Metter EJ, Cherubini A, Maggio M, Sen R, Najjar SS, Windham GB, Ble A, Senin U, Ferrucci L. White blood cell count and mortality in the Baltimore longitudinal study of aging. J Am Coll Cardiol. 2007;49(18):1841–50.

26. Wu YW, Tseng PH, Lee YC, Wang SY, Chiu HM, Tu CH, Wang HP, Lin JT, Wu MS, Yang WS. Association of esophageal inflammation, obesity and gastroesophageal reflux disease: from FDG PET/CT perspective. PLoS One. 2014;9(3):e92001.

27. Rieder F, Biancani P, Harnett K, Yerian L, Falk GW. Inflammatory mediators in gastroesophageal reflux disease: impact on esophageal motility, fibrosis, and carcinogenesis. Am J Physiol Gastrointest Liver Physiol. 2010;298(5):G571–81.

28. Park JJ, Kim JW, Kim HJ, Chung MG, Park SM, Baik GH, Nah BK, Nam SY, Seo KS, Ko BS, et al. The prevalence of and risk factors for Barrett's esophagus in a Korean population: a nationwide multicenter prospective study. J Clin Gastroenterol. 2009;43(10):907–14.

29. Lee IS, Choi SC, Shim KN, Jee SR, Huh KC, Lee JH, Lee KJ, Park HS, Lee YC, Jung HY, et al. Prevalence of Barrett's esophagus remains low in the Korean population: nationwide cross-sectional prospective multicenter study. Dig Dis Sci. 2010;55(7):1932–9.

23

Recurrent esophageal stricture from previous caustic ingestion treated with 40-year self-dilation

C. Gambardella[1*], A. Allaria[1], G. Siciliano[1], C. Mauriello[1], R. Patrone[1], N. Avenia[2], A. Polistena[2], A. Sanguinetti[2], S. Napolitano[3] and G. Conzo[1]

Abstract

Background: Corrosive esophageal strictures are common. The severity of the strictures depends on type, quantity, duration of contact and concentration of the caustic substance ingested. Endoscopic balloon dilation and endoscopic bougienage are a cornerstone in the management of the benign esophageal strictures and are the most widely used treatments, but are expensive and invasive procedures.

Case Presentation: We report the case of an 82-year-old patient with a corrosive esophageal stricture treated for over 40 years by means of home self-bougienage. The procedure has been carried out for the longest lapse of time described in literature, with an excellent control of symptoms. In the case reported, after being carried out for more than 40 years, self-dilation allowed good quality of life and symptoms management, ensuring an excellent nutritional status.

Conclusions: Following an adequate patient training, self-dilatation can be a safe and effective option of treatment, avoiding frequent expensive hospital admissions for endoscopic esophageal dilatation.

Keywords: Self-dilation, Esophageal stricture, Caustic ingestion, Endoscopic dilatation, Self-bougienage, Case report

Background

Esophageal caustic ingestions are among the most challenging emergencies for surgeons, otolaryngologists and gastroenterologists [1]. In Italy 15,000 new cases occur annually. They are mainly observed during childhood, and are unintentional in almost all the cases although. Otherwise, in the 90% of observed in adult population, caustic ingestion has a suicidal purpose. Alkaline and acid caustics are the most common chemical substances utilized, causing esophageal burns and producing tissue destruction through coagulation reactions or liquefaction. Acids ingestion causes a coagulative necrosis leading to eschar formation, preventing their action at a greater depth. On the other hand, alkalis ingestion produces liquefactive necrosis generating proteinates and soaps, leading to full thickness lesions [2]. The severity of the lesions depends on type, quantity, duration of contact and concentration of the caustic substance ingested. Acute complications include mucosal injuries, perforations, fistulae, mediastinitis and peritonitis, while long-term complications include esophageal stricture, pyloric stenosis and esophageal squamous cell carcinoma [3–6]. In the management of caustic injuries, one of the crucial aspect is the prevention of esophageal strictures. Endoscopy should be performed within 24 h to evaluate the severity of the lesions and the prognosis. Insertion of a nasogastric tube, antibiotics, early esophageal dilatation and steroids, the latter not routinely used, are among the most important therapeutic weapons to reduce the risk of a severe esophageal stenosis [1]. Surgical management, including esophagectomy, myocutaneous flaps and esophageal replacement procedures, is complex, and carries significant morbidity and mortality [7]. Herein, we describe a rare case of esophageal self-dilatation after caustic

* Correspondence: claudiog86@hotmail.it
[1]Department of Cardiothoracic Sciences - University of Campania "Luigi Vanvitelli", Via Sergio Pansini 5, 80131 Naples, Italy

soda ingestion by the use of Maloney bougie for the time lapse of about 40 years. We performed a Literature review by a PubMed database search using as keywords "esophageal self-dilation", "self-bougienage", "caustic ingestion", "benign esophageal stenosis".

Case presentation

In November 2015, we observed a woman 82-year-old, with an episode of caustic soda ingestion at the age of twenty-three for suicidal purpose. At that time, she presented to the emergency department with chest pain, vomit and hematemesis. The patient was hemodynamically stabilized and underwent a gastric lavage. Esophagogastroduodenoscopy showed several esophageal burns, ulcerations and liquefactive necrosis. In the following days, the patient experienced dysphagia, odynophagia, heartburn, hematemesis and weight loss. After three months, the symptoms gradually decreased but a cicatricial fibrotic stenosis of the lower third of the esophagus aroused. The patient started self-dilatation with semi-rigid dilators without reaching any relevant symptomatology relief. At one year from the ingestion, she autonomously bought a Maloney dilator of 5 mm of calibre, and started periodically self-dilatations, after an adequate training, consisting of undergoing physician-performed endoscopic dilation and participating in three self-dilation practice sessions supervised by a physician, according to the technique described by Dzeletovic [8]. The periodical self-dilations and semi-liquid nutrition led to a great improvement of her nutritional status (Figs. 1, 2 and 3). The patient had been in good wellness for about 40 years, when she presented to the Emergency department of Surgical Endoscopy for an esophageal obstruction. A food remnant was endoscopically removed, and for the first time the patient underwent an esophageal dilatation with a Savary bougie. For the following 20 years, the woman has practised occasional Savary bougie endoscopic dilatation (maximum calibre 7 mm) alternated with self-bougienage, achieving a good control of symptoms. Moreover, only over the counter, drugs as dimethicone and sodium alginate have been seldom administered. Only during the last year, the patient has experienced dysphagia, heartburn and nocturnal reflux, so an upper gastrointestinal barium examination has been carried out. A stenosis of the middle and lower third of the oesophagus with a delayed emptying was identified (Fig. 4). An endoscopic 7 mm Savary bougie dilatation was performed with a significantly relief of symptoms. Currently, the patient undergoes monthly standard Savary bougie dilatation with an excellent control of the symptoms.

Discussion and conclusions

Caustic ingestion for suicidal purpose is not an uncommon event in Western Countries. The overall prevalence of esophageal stenosis is 129 and 122 per 100.000, for men and woman respectively [7]. Endoscopy within the

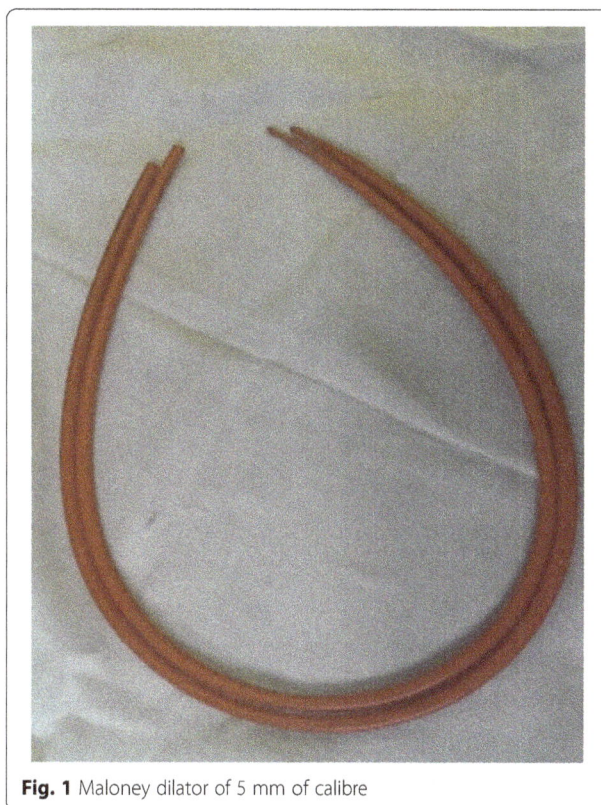

Fig. 1 Maloney dilator of 5 mm of calibre

first 24 h has a paramount importance to see the extent of injury and making treatment decisions like conservative vs surgery [2]. The treatment of esophageal stenosis, the most frequent long-term complication of caustic ingestion, is committed to limit dysphagia, avoiding the complications of esophageal obstruction, and preventing recurrence.

Esophageal strictures may be either simple or complex. Complex strictures are often resistant to dilation and are difficult to treat. Generally, they are caused by caustic ingestion, radiation therapy and esophageal anastomosis. Resistant benign esophageal strictures have a negative impact on the quality of life of the patients, and may lead to weight loss, malnutrition and aspiration. Balloon dilatation or endoscopic bougienage are the most widely used treatment, but are expensive and invasive procedures. In fact, endoscopic dilatation requires frequent hospital admissions and multiple sedation procedures, with inherent associated risks and cost, affecting patient productivity and his daily activity [9]. Moreover, despite repeated endoscopic treatment and medical therapy, 30–40% of patients will develop symptoms recurrence within the first year [8]. Patients with recurrent strictures will need repeated monthly or weekly physicians performed dilations, leading to a total dependence of the patient on the medical team. In order to prolong the dysphagia-free period, and to decrease the frequency of

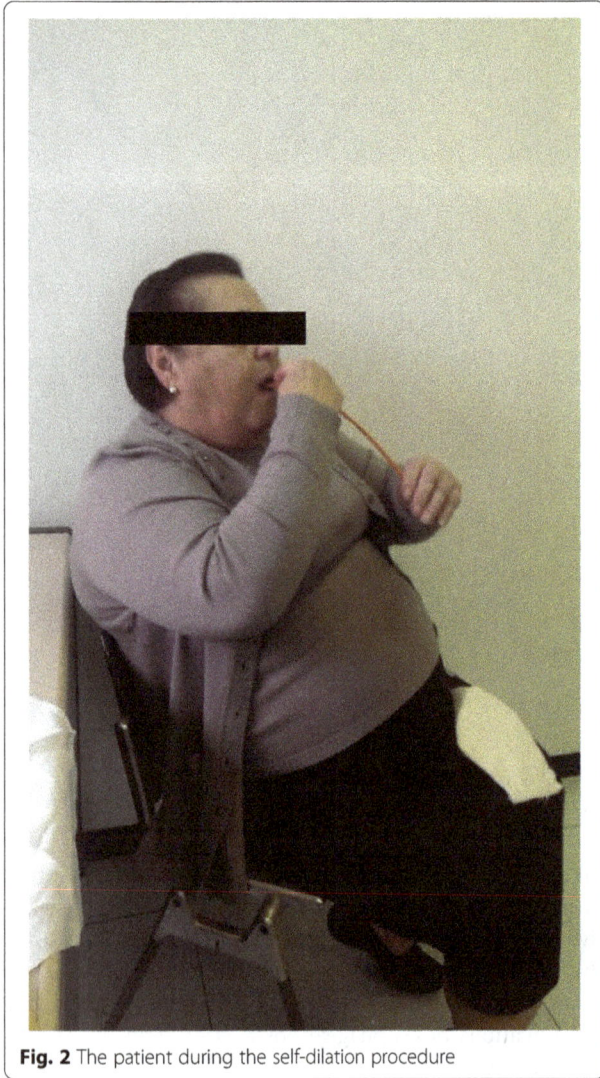

Fig. 2 The patient during the self-dilation procedure

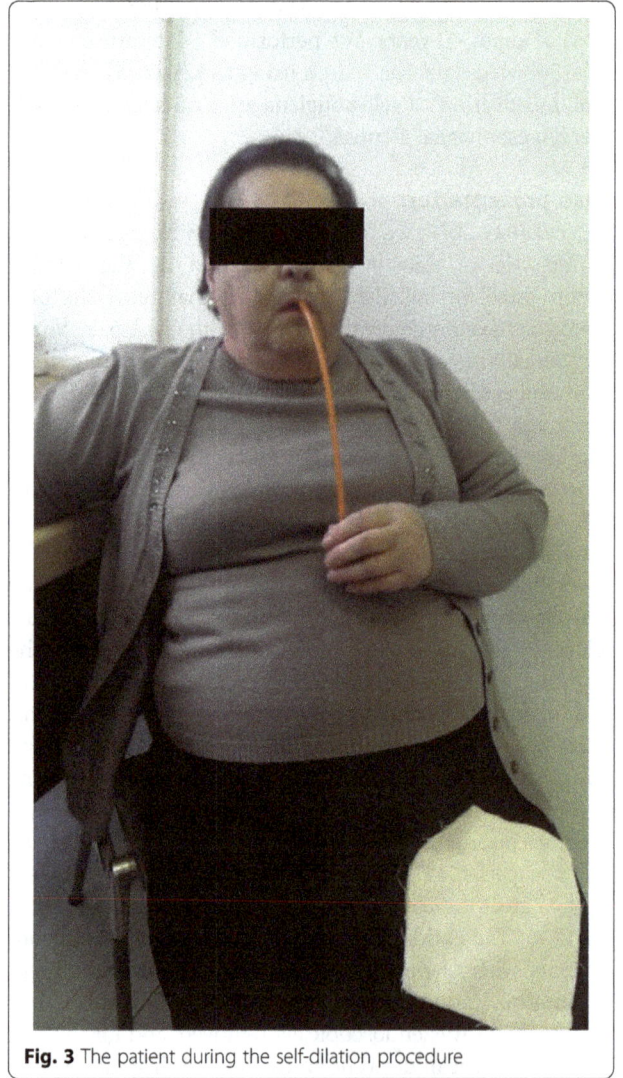

Fig. 3 The patient during the self-dilation procedure

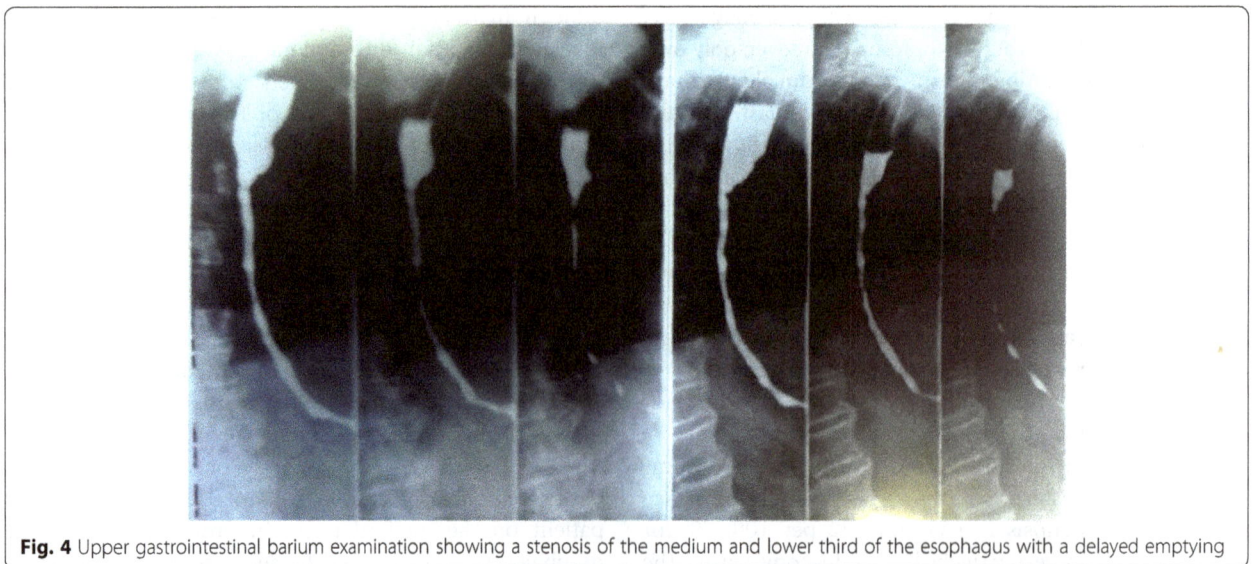

Fig. 4 Upper gastrointestinal barium examination showing a stenosis of the medium and lower third of the esophagus with a delayed emptying

repeated dilations compared with conventional endo-scopic dilations, intramuscular injections of mitomycin C and steroids were suggested. Mitomycin C is a chemotherapeutic agent derived from some Streptomyces species which reduces scars formation when topically applied to a mucosal lesion, and theoretically should prevents esophageal stenosis in selected cases [10, 11]. Nevertheless, there is evidence that triamcinolone and other steroids injection in combination with endoscopic dilation is able to reduce the risk of recurrent dysphagia in refractory benign esophageal strictures of peptic origin, with results coming from small-sized studies with poorly defined population and not concerning caustic ingestion [12].

A safe, cost saving and useful option in patients who require multiple and frequent dilations to maintain esophageal patency is self-dilation [8, 13]. Home bougienage is generally performed with Maloney dilator of 45 ÷ 60 French, causing only a little discomfort to patients. The best patients for this procedure are those who are self-motivated, compliant, with a normal pharyngeal function and who may be poorly surgically treated. Self-dilatation is cost-effective and safe after a short period of training by experienced surgeons and nurses, consisting of viewing the self-dilation teaching-video, meeting with other patients who perform self-dilation, undergoing physician-performed endoscopic dilation and participating to at least three self-dilation practice sessions supervised by a physician [8–11]. Esophageal perforation, bleeding, bacteremia and aspiration pneumonia, with an overall incidence of 0.3%, are the extremely rare self-dilatation complications [13]. The incidence of perforation, the most dangerous adverse effect, is uncommon and has been reported to be 0.14% [7, 14]. In addition, the inadvertent passage of the dilator into the airways is a rare event that could hesitate in pneumonia or pneumothorax [14].

Few cases of self-bougienage have been previously described in literature, and to our knowledge, the case reported describe the procedure carried out for the longest lapse of time. In fact, for about 40 years the patient has been practicing only the self-dilation, with an excellent symptomatology control, while, following an acute episode of obstruction, occasional Savary bougie endoscopic dilatation alternated with home self-dilation have been performed for other 20 years. Bapat et al., reported a long term symptomatic relief in 51 patients treated with self bougienage for corrosive esophageal strictures as final step of management, with only one case of retraining for procedure failing, after which the patient remained asymptomatic [15]. The same results are reported by Gilmore, Kim and Lee in patients requiring frequent dilatations. [9, 16–18]. Gundogdu et al. reported a higher success rate in patients < 8-year-old, in strictures caused by caustic, in stenosis of the upper third of the esophagus and with

stricture length < 5 cm [19]. Dzeletovic et al. reported a more enjoyable life and less interference with daily and social activities for the patients treated with self-dilation, with an improved long-term (32 months) overall health-related quality of life in 90% of cases [7, 13]. Finally, studies from India and China showed favourable results using a Foley catheter and gum elastic bougies [20, 21].

In the case reported, self-dilation, carried out for more than 40 years, allowed a good quality of life and symptoms control ensuring an excellent nutritional status. Even if self-dilation has not received much mention by surgeons and gastroenterologists and remains under-recognized, it can be a safe and effective option of treatment. In selected cases, following an adequate patient instruction and performing periodic instrumental and clinical controls, frequent hospital admissions for endoscopic esophageal dilatation should be avoided, reducing the costs related and favouring a better patient quality of life.

Authors' contributions

GaC and AA contributed equally to this work, participating substantially in conception, drafting and editing of the manuscript.; SG, MC, PR designed the report; GaC, AA, AN, PA, CoG analyzed and collected the data; GaC and NS wrote the paper. All authors have read and approved the manuscript.

Authors' information

Gambardella C is PhD student in Medical, Clinical and Sperimental Sciences at University of Campania "Luigi Vanvitelli" – Naples, Italy.

Competing interests

The authors declare that they have no competing interests.

Author details

[1]Department of Cardiothoracic Sciences - University of Campania "Luigi Vanvitelli", Via Sergio Pansini 5, 80131 Naples, Italy. [2]Endocrine Surgery Unit, University of Perugia, Perugia, Italy. [3]Italian Air Force Medical Corps, Ministry of Defence, Rome, Italy.

References

1.   Shahi AS, Behdad B, Esmaeili A, Moztarzadeh M, Peyvandi H. Esophageal stenting in caustic injuries: a modified technique to avoid laparotomy. Gen Thorac Cardiovasc Surg. 2015;63(7):406–12.
2.   Sugawa C, Lucas CE. Caustic injury of the upper gastrointestinal tract in adults: a clinical and endoscopic study. Surgery. 1989;106(4):802–6.
3.   Assal A, Saloojee N, Dhaliwal H. Esophageal stricture due to magnesium citrate powder ingestion: a unique case. Can J Gastroenterol Hepatol. 2014; 28(11):585–6.
4.   Abaskharoun RD, Depew WT, Hookey LC. Nonsurgical management of severe esophageal and gastric injury following alkali ingestion. Can J Gastroenterol. 2007;21(11):757–60.
5.   Ramasamy K, Gumaste VV. Corrosive ingestion in adults. J Clin Gastroenterol. 2003;37(2):119–24.
6.   Zargar SA, Kochhar R, Mehta S, Mehta SK. The role of fiberoptic endoscopy in the management of corrosive ingestion and modified endoscopic classification of burns. Gastrointest Endosc. 1991;37(2):165–9.
7.   Dzeletovic I, Fleischer DE. Self-dilation for resistant, benign esophageal strictures. Am J Gastroenterol. 2010;105(10):2142–3.

8. Dzeletovic I, Fleischer DE, Crowell MD, Kim HJ, Harris LA, Burdick GE, McLaughlin RR, Spratley RV Jr, Sharma VK. Self dilation as a treatment for resistant benign esophageal strictures: outcome, technique, and quality of life assessment. Dig Dis Sci. 2011;56:435–40.

9. Lee HJ, Lee JH, Seo JM, Lee SK, Choe YH. A single center experience of self-bougienage on stricture recurrence after surgery for corrosive esophageal strictures in children. Yonsei Med J. 2010;51(2):202–5.

10. Zhang Y, Wang X, Liu L, Chen JP, Fan ZN. Intramuscular injection of mitomycin C combined with endoscopic dilation for benign esophageal strictures. J Dig Dis. 2015;16(7):370–6.

11. Machida H, Tominaga K, Minamino H, Sugimori S, Okazaki H, Yamagami H, Tanigawa T, Watanabe K, Watanabe T, Fujiwara Y, Arakawa T. Locoregional mitomycin C injection for esophageal stricture after endoscopic submucosal dissection. Endoscopy. 2012;44(6):622–5.

12. Van Boeckel PGA, Siersema PD. Recfractory esophageal strictures: what to do when dilation fails. Curr Treat Options Gastroenterol. 2015;13(1):47–58.

13. Dzeletovic I, Fleischer DE, Crowell MD, Pannala R, Harris LA, Ramirez FC, Burdick GE, Rentz LA, Spratley RV Jr, Helling SD, Alexander JA. Self-dilation as a treatment for resistant, benign esophageal strictures. Dig Dis Sci. 2013; 58:3218–23.

14. Kashima ML, Eisele DW. Complication of esophageal self-dilation for radiation-induced hypopharyngeal stenosis. Dysphagia. 2003;18:92–5.

15. Bapat RD, Bakhshi GD, Kantharia CV, Shirodkar SS, Iyer AP, Ranka S. Self-bougienage: long-term relief of corrosive esophageal strictures. Indian J Gastroenterol. 2001;20(5):180–2.

16. Sherkin-Langer F, Langer JC, Zupancic J, Winthrop AL, Issenman RM. Home esophageal self-dilatation in children. Gastroenterol Nurs. 1993;16(1):5–8.

17. Kim CH, Groskreutz JL, Gehrking SJ. Recurrent benign esophageal strictures treated with self-bougienage: report of seven cases. Mayo Clin Proc. 1990; 65(6):799–803.

18. Gilmore IT, Sheers R. Oesophageal self-bougienage. Lancet. 1982;1(8272):620–1.

19. Gündoğdu HZ, Tanyel FC, Büyükpamukçu N, Hiçsönmez A. Conservative treatment of caustic esophageal strictures in children. J Pediatr Surg. 1992; 27(6):767–70.

20. Shad SK, Gupta S, Chattopadhyay TK. Self-dilatation of cervical oesophagogastric anastomotic stricture: a simple and effective technique. Br J Surg. 1991;78:1254–5.

21. Manjunath S, Ramachandra C, Veerendra Kumar KV, Prabhakaran PS. Simple dilatation of anastomotic strictures following oesophagectomy in unsedated patients. Eur J Surg Oncol. 2006;32:1015–7.

24

Metabolomic and BH3 profiling of esophageal cancers: novel assessment methods for precision therapy

R. Taylor Ripley[1]* , Deborah R. Surman[1], Laurence P. Diggs[1], Jane B. Trepel[4], Min-Jung Lee[4], Jeremy Ryan[2], Jeremy L. Davis[1], Seth M. Steinberg[3], Jonathan M. Hernandez[1], Choung Hoang[1], Cara M. Kenney[1], Colleen D. Bond[1], Tricia F. Kunst[1], Anthony Letai[2] and David S. Schrump[1]

Abstract

Background: Esophageal cancers accounted for nearly 16,000 deaths in 2016. The number of patients with esophageal cancers increases every year. Neoadjuvant chemoradiotherapy (nCRT) prior to esophagectomy is a standard treatment for esophageal cancers. The patients who have no residual tumor (pathological complete response (pCR)) at surgery are the most likely to experience long term survival. Accurately determining which patients will have a pCR will improve prognostic information for patients and families, confirm lack of response to nCRT, or avoid surgery if no residual tumor is present. Imaging, endoscopy, and liquid biomarkers have all failed to detect pCR without performing an esophagectomy.

Methods: In this study, we are enrolling patients with esophageal adenocarcinoma and squamous cell carcinoma. Patients will undergo standard evaluation including CT scans, laboratory tests, endoscopy with biopsies, and evaluation by a thoracic surgeon. Tissue biopsy is required for enrollment that will be sent for BH3 profiling and metabolomics. Patients will be treated with standard nCRT followed by surgery. Patients with metastatic disease are not eligible. Surgery at the National Cancer Institute will be minimally-invasive robotic surgery. Patients will remain on study indefinitely with regular clinic visits and imaging tests.

Discussion: The mitochondria are critically involved in the intrinsic pathway apoptosis. Bcl-2 homology domain 3 (BH3) profiling is a technique to measure a cell's susceptibility to apoptosis. BH3 profiling measures the relative interactions of proteins that induce or block apoptosis. The collective balance of these proteins determines whether a cell is near the threshold to undergo apoptosis. If the cell is near this threshold, then the tumor may be more likely to die when treated with nCRT. The mitochondria secrete metabolites that may be detectable as biomarkers. Metabolomics is a global assessment of all metabolite changes that has been performed for detection, monitoring, prognosis, and treatment response in cancers. Stratification of patients based on whether pCR occurs or not may elucidate metabolomic signatures that may be associated with response. We are asking whether BH3 profiling or a metabolomic signature will correlate with tumor death after nCRT for esophageal cancer.

Keywords: Esophageal adenocarcinoma, Esophageal squamous cell carcinoma, Pathologic complete response, BH3 profiling, Metabolomics

* Correspondence: Taylor.Ripley@nih.gov
[1]Thoracic and GI Oncology Branch, Center for Cancer Research, National Cancer Institute, Building 10; 4-3952, 10 Center Drive, MSC 1201, Bethesda, MD 20892-1201, USA

Background

Esophageal adenocarcinomas (EAC) and esophageal squamous cell cancers (ESCC) accounted for nearly 17,000 new diagnoses and 16,000 deaths in 2016 [1]. EAC is the dominant histology in the United States and its incidence continues to rise [2]. Neoadjuvant chemoradiotherapy (nCRT) followed by surgical removal of the esophagus (esophagectomy) demonstrated a 47% five-year survival compared to a 34% five-year survival for patients who underwent surgery alone in the CROSS trial [3]. Patients having received nCRT who had no residual tumor at the time of the esophagectomy, referred to as a pathological complete response (pCR), were most likely to achieve long-term survival [4–8]. pCR occurs in about 20% of patients with EAC and 50% of patients with ESCC [9–13]. Accurately predicting response to neoadjuvant therapy may improve prognostic information for patients and families, confirm lack of response to ineffective regimens, and avoid esophagectomy when pCR occurs [14]. Currently, the only means to identify pCR are 18F-FDG-PET scan and endoscopy with biopsies. These tests have been studied extensively and neither reliably predict pCR with a combined positive predictive value of 36% [15, 16]. To date, no reliable biomarker has been developed. Therefore, the only accurate assessment of pathological response is obtained via examination of the excised esophagus [10, 17]. We hypothesize that a metabolomic signature or bcl-2 homology domain 3 (BH3) profiling will correlate with pCR.

Metabolomics is a method of global detection of small molecule metabolites. It allows for analysis of metabolite changes under many conditions including stress, changes in diet, treatment response, or other biological conditions. Increasingly, metabolomics has been used in patients with cancer for tumor detection as well as assessment of prognosis, progression, and treatment response [18]. Clinical examples of utility of metabolomics include monitoring the progression of prostate cancer [19, 20], determining prognosis of glioblastoma and anaplastic astrocytoma [21], and predicting response to imatinib in chronic myelogenous leukemia [22]. We hypothesize that metabolic differences exist between patients who achieve a pCR versus those who do not, therefore, a metabolomic signature should be associated with differences in pathological responses.

Bcl-2 homology domain 3 (BH3) profiling is a technique to measure a cell's readiness to die by the intrinsic pathway of apoptosis. Apoptosis is a mechanism of cell death that prevents damaged cells from becoming cancerous. The inability of damaged cells to undergo apoptosis is a well-established hallmark of cancer [23]. The intrinsic pathway of apoptosis induces mitochondrial outer membrane permeabilization (MOMP) which results in a series of events culminating in cell death.

MOMP is regulated by the Bcl-2 family of proteins that are broadly divided into pro-apoptotic and anti-apoptotic proteins. The interactions of certain Bcl-2 proteins occur at the BH3 domains [24, 25]. BH3 profiling measures the relative interactions of pro- and anti-apoptotic proteins to determine whether a tumor cell is near the threshold to activate apoptosis. Cells are considered 'primed' or 'unprimed' based on whether they are near or far from this threshold, respectively [24–27]. BH3 profiling has been used to successfully predict response to chemotherapy and resistance to targeted therapy in both clinical samples and laboratory cell culture models [28]. BH3 profiling significantly correlated with progression-free survival after treatment with carboplatin and paclitaxel in patients with ovarian adenocarcinoma [28]. We hypothesize that BH3 profiling will correlate with pCR after nCRT for patients with esophageal cancers.

Approximately 50–70% of esophageal cancers harbor mutations in the TP53 gene (p53 protein) which is the most commonly mutated gene in cancer [29]. These mutations result in both loss of tumor suppressor activity and acceleration of tumor growth [30, 31]. EAC patients with p53 mutations respond poorly to chemotherapy and have worse outcomes after either surgery alone or nCRT [32, 33]. Evaluation of p53 mutations will help determine whether patients need different treatment strategies based on p53 status.

The primary aim of this trial is to determine whether a metabolomic signature and BH3 profiling correlates with pCR. The secondary aim of this trial is to determine whether p53-mutational status of the tumors alters the metabolomic signatures or BH3 profiling. Additional secondary aims are to correlate these findings with overall and disease-free survivals. In summary, we anticipate that BH3 profiles or metabolomic signatures will be associated with treatment response to nCRT in esophageal cancer to serve as a basis for precision-based, personalized strategies for future treatment.

Methods
Study Type
Prospective, observational, two-armed (EAC and ESCC) trial.

Aim
Primary objective

- To determine whether a metabolomic signature or BH3 profiles correlates with pathological complete response (pCR) after neoadjuvant chemoradiotherapy (nCRT) for patients with esophageal adenocarcinoma (EAC) or squamous cell carcinoma (ESCC).

Secondary objectives

- To examine if metabolomic signatures or BH3 profiles correlate with disease-free survival (DFS) or overall survival (OS).
- To explore whether specific p53 mutations correlate with metabolomic signatures or BH3 profiles.

Design
Inclusion criteria

- Histologically confirmed EAC or ESCC.
- Stage appropriate for treatment by both nCRT and surgery.
- Disease deemed resectable by surgeon assessment and imaging.

Exclusion criteria

- Patients for whom nCRT followed by surgery is not the appropriate management:
  - Early stage disease requiring local therapy without nCRT.
  - Metastatic disease.
- Performance status that precludes nCRT and/or surgery.
- Biopsy prior to starting nCRT not obtainable.

Statistics
The primary objective is to determine whether a metabolomic signature in tumor, blood, or urine or whether BH3 profiling of pre-neoadjuvant tumor biopsy correlates with the outcome of pCR after nCRT for patients with EAC or ESCC. The measurement of the primary endpoint is whether or not viable tumor is present after surgical resection – pCR. Similarly, a secondary objective is to identify whether metabolomic signatures in tumor, blood, or urine or BH3 profiling in tumor of EAC and ESCC patients correlate with major responses (Mandard score of 1 and 2) versus minimal response (Mandard score 3–5). This analysis is also based on pathological findings of the surgical resection. The patients with major responses include < 10% viable tumor and pCR versus patients with any grade over 10% viable tumor. Another secondary objective is descriptive to evaluate metabolomic profiles of these patients as an exploratory analysis to determine whether certain pathways are significantly upregulated in esophageal cancer.

Sample size calculations
Since this trial is an exploratory biomarker trial, the true number of patients to power this study is unknown. Sreekumar and colleagues compared 16 prostate normal tissue samples to 12 samples of localized prostate cancer to 14 metastatic prostate samples and successfully identified metabolites associated with progression in prostate cancer [20].

We will plan to accrue 10 patients with pCR for both EAC and ESCC in order to have a minimal number of patients with pCRs to compare against the other subjects. For patients with EAC or ESCC, the percentage of patients with a pCR after nCRT is well-documented and significantly different. Therefore, patients with EAC and ESCC will be evaluated independently in two cohorts. Patients with EAC are reported to have 17–27% of patients pCR. Assuming 20% of patients have a pCR with EAC, 66 patients will be accrued in order to have an 86% probability of obtaining 10 patients with pCR. Thus, the accrual goal for Arm 1 for EAC will be set at 66 evaluable patients, and will have an accrual ceiling of 80 patients to allow for up to 14 inevaluable cases. Patients with ESCC are reported to have 40–64% of pCR after neoadjuvant CRT. Assuming 40% of patients have a pCR with ESCC, 32 evaluable patients will be accrued in order to have an 88% probability of obtaining 10 patients with pCR. Thus, the accrual goal for arm 2 will be set at 32 evaluable patients, and will have an accrual ceiling of 40 patients to allow for unevaluable cases. The overall accrual ceiling of the entire study will be 120 patients to allow for to 22 unevaluable patients.

To allow for a small number of unevaluable patients, the accrual ceiling will be set to 120 patients for the entire study. The accrual ceiling will be 80 patients for EAC. If one patient every month enrolls onto this study, accrual is expected to be completed in 6–7 years. The accrual ceiling will be 40 patients for ESCC. If one patient every 2 months enrolls onto this study, the accrual is expected to be completed in 6 years.

The secondary outcomes will be the association of overall survival (OS), disease-free survival (DFS), pathological stage (ypStage), and p53 mutational status with a metabolic signature. Additionally, the patients will be divided by pathological major response (Mandard 1–2) compared to minor or no response (Mandard 3–5). This analysis is similar to comparison of pCR to non-pCR, however, patients with < 10% viable tumor will be included in the favorable group; therefore, this group will be slightly larger than 10 patients with pCR. The OS and DFS will be calculated by Dr. Seth Steinberg using Kaplan-Meier and log-rank tests. The final, pathological stage will be reviewed by the PI prior to any analysis. Given that multiple stages are possible, the additional subgroup analysis of ypStage will be reported as descriptive statistics only without metabolic analysis.

Analysis of data
Analyses involving the actual metabolomics profiles, as well as the analyses involving metabolic signatures, will

be done in conjunction with the company, Metabolon, who will receive, process, and analyze deidentified patient samples (www.metabolon.com). Metabolon uses an authenticated biochemical reference library as standards for known metabolites with LC/MS methodology. This library enables comparisons to identify differences in metabolites in our patient cohorts. The bioinformatic analysis of metabolomic profiles between those with a pCR and the other patients will be done by propriety software that compares the mass spectral ion features of their library to our cohorts. This data is further processed by mapping to known cellular pathways.

Intervention

Assessment prior to initiation of neoadjuvant chemoradiotherapy:

- Complete history and physical examination.
- Nutritional assessment and routine laboratory evaluations.
- CT and/or PET-CT scan of chest, abdomen and pelvis.
- Esophagogastroduodenoscopy (EGD) with confirmation of histology and specimens for metabolomic and BH3 profiling.
  After neoadjuvant therapy, patients will undergo standard preoperative assessment including:
- Complete history and physical examination with clinical assessment for fitness for surgery.
- Pulmonary function tests (PFTs) if indicated.
- Cardiac evaluation and/or EKG if indicated.
- CT, PET or PET-CT scan of chest, abdomen and pelvis.
- Routine preoperative laboratory evaluations.

Surgery and post-operative care:

- Robotically-assisted, minimally-invasive esophagectomy (RAMIE) will be performed if feasible.
- For those for whom a minimally-invasive procedure is contraindicated, a traditional open approach will be performed.
- Jejunostomy tubes are placed in all patients for post-operative nutritional support.
- Patients will receive routine post-esophagectomy care including initial monitoring in ICU.

Follow-up of Study

- Routine clinic appointments and CT scans will be performed at 3, 6, 9, 12, 18, and 24 months then yearly for at least 5 years.
- Patients will be followed for the secondary endpoints of disease-free survival and overall survival.
- Patients will continue surveillance and may remain on study indefinitely.

Discussion

Esophageal cancer is an increasing health burden both in the United States and worldwide. The phase III CROSS trial noted a survival benefit of neoadjuvant chemoradiotherapy (nCRT) followed by surgery, but the patients who experienced the best outcomes in this trial had almost no residual tumor after nCRT [3]. Evaluation after nCRT by PET scans and endoscopy have been studied by multiple groups which have consistently reported that these tests correlate poorly with final pathology [13, 15, 16, 34]. Similarly, biomarker discovery has not yielded a predictive marker for treatment response. Currently, the only method to assess treatment response after nCRT is removal of the esophagus [10, 17]. nCRT and surgery are standard recommendations for treatment of locally-advanced esophageal cancers, however, this treatment strategy is associated with significant morbidity, especially in older patients who often have additional comorbidities. The ability to predict whether nCRT is efficacious has several advantages that could significantly improve patient outcomes by personalizing treatment strategies. First, predicting which patients will respond will help counsel patients and families about expected outcomes. Second, determining if nCRT is not effective will allow discontinuation of toxic regimens in order to proceed to surgery more quickly. Third, if patients achieve pathological complete response (pCR), then surgery is not indicated and these patients can avoid removal of the esophagus.

The most common mechanism of cell death secondary to chemotherapy and radiation therapy is activation of the intrinsic pathway of apoptosis. Apoptosis is a programmed cell death that kills the cell in an orderly manner without induction of inflammation. The intrinsic pathway activates pre-formed proteins that alter the mitochondria leading to cell death. In an individual patient or an individual tumor, the mitochondria may be susceptible or resistant to apoptosis. This concept is analogous to a cell or mitochondria being 'primed' or 'unprimed' for cell death [23–27]. The mitochondria generate energy for cellular function and building blocks for tumor growth. These processes are associated with several metabolic pathways that secrete metabolites with each step. Differences in these pathways may impart the resistance to apoptosis and these differences should secrete different levels of metabolites that could be detected by metabolomics. The metabolic signature of a tumor sensitive to nCRT should be quite different than a resistant tumor [18, 22]. Unlike the global detection of metabolite secretion by metabolomic analysis, BH3 profiling directly measures the functional interactions of the proteins that both induce and block apoptosis. For example, if a tumor contains a high amount of functional Bcl-xL, an anti-apoptotic protein, this tumor may be resistant to nCRT and BH3 profiling should correlate with lack of efficacy of nCRT [27]. Additionally, BH3 profiling provides a test that can be performed within 24 h of biopsy which makes this assessment ideal for patient treatment decisions. Despite the differences between metabolomic signatures and BH3 profiling, they are expected to provide independent evaluations of mitochondrial susceptibility to cell death.

Predicting apoptosis by metabolomic signatures or BH3 profiling focuses on downstream cellular processes independent of tumor mutational status. However, esophageal cancers, similar to other cancers induced by environmental exposures, have a high burden of somatic mutations [35]. Mutations in the TP53 gene are detected in greater than 50% of esophageal cancers whereas the next most common mutations occur in less than 12% of esophageal cancers [32]. Wild-type p53 has multiple functions including the induction of apoptosis whereas p53 mutations may block apoptosis and therefore 'unprime' a tumor cell. p53 mutations may affect both metabolomic signatures as well as BH3 profiling [30, 31]. Therefore, all tumors will be sequenced for TP53 gene mutations and data analysis will account for the mutation type.

Our goal is to determine whether metabolomic signatures or BH3 profiling correlate with treatment response to nCRT. If these techniques can achieve this goal, we may improve patient care by personalizing treatment regimens. Furthermore, if these techniques are successful, future trials will be based on altering the mitochondrial threshold for apoptosis to increase the susceptibility for standard therapeutics. Mitochondrial priming is dynamic, therefore, its threshold for apoptosis can be decreased by selecting tumor specific therapies. For example, blocking Bcl-xL in a tumor that is reliant on this anti-apoptotic protein may 'prime' that cell for death. Alternatively, if p53 mutational status blocks apoptosis, inhibition of p53 may be required to increase the efficacy of standard nCRT. This current observational trial will help design future interventional trials aimed at increasing the pathological response rates which will improve the overall survival of patients with esophageal cancers.

Funding

Funding provided through the Intramural Research Program of the National Cancer Institute/CCR, NIH.

Availability of data and materials

Description of the scope of genetic/genomic analysis:

- The p53 mutational status will be determined using tissue samples. Future whole genome/whole exome studies:

- Patient samples may undergo whole genome sequencing for future studies to potentially predict response and/or toxicities to other investigational agents.

- No additional sample will be drawn for this purpose. Privacy and confidentiality of medical information/biological specimens:

- Confidentiality will be maintained at all times during the study. Samples transferred to independent companies will be stripped of all patient identifiers (e.g., medical record number, patient name or initials) and will be labeled with a unique ID that can be linked only by the principal investigator or associate investigators of the study.

- No personally identifiable information will be released to third parties and samples and data will only be shared with other researchers with the permission of the IRB and under the proper Material Transfer Agreements.

- To provide confidentiality of patient information, we have obtained a Certificate of Confidentiality which helps to protect personally identifiable research information. This certificate allows investigators on this trial to refuse to disclose identifying information related to the research participants, should such disclosure have adverse consequences for patients or damage their financial standing, employability, insurability, or reputation. Management of Results:

- The analyses performed in various NCI laboratories under this protocol are for research purposes only. These tests are not as sensitive as the tests performed by a laboratory certified to perform genetic testing for clinical purposes. We do not plan to inform participants of the results of testing on the tissue and blood that is performed in our research lab. However, in the unlikely event that clinically relevant incidental findings are discovered, subjects will be contacted if a clinically actionable gene variant is discovered.

- Clinically actionable findings for this study are defined as disorders appearing in the American College of Medical Genetics and Genomics recommendations for the return of incidental findings that is current at the time of primary analysis.

- A list of current guidelines is maintained on the CCR intranet: https://ccrod.cancer.gov/confluence/display/CCRCRO/Incidental+Findings+Lists

- Patients that remain in the study will be contacted at that time with a request to provide a blood sample to be sent to a CLIA certified laboratory. If the research findings are verified, patients will be referred to an NCI CCR Genetics Branch certified genetic health care provider for the disclosure of the results. Human Data Sharing Plan:

- Human data generated will be completely de-identified and shared in an NIH-funded or approved public repository shortly after publication of our results. Genomic Data Sharing Plan:

- Unlinked genomic data will be deposited in public genomic databases such as dbGaP in compliance with the NIH Genomic Data Sharing Policy.

Authors' contributions

RTR is the principal investigator of this study and drafted the manuscript. RTR and DSS are responsible for concept and design of the trial and final approval for the version of the manuscript to be published. RTR, DSS, JLD, JMH, CMK, TFK, CB made significant contributions to the development of the clinical protocol. RTR, DRS, LPD, JR, JBT, MJL, JPD, CH, and AL made significant contributions to the design, technical expertise, and data interpretation of tissue handling and laboratory processes. SMS developed the statistical considerations for the trial. All authors contributed to the protocol validity, scientific accuracy, and the final revisions of the manuscript.

Authors' information

Principal Investigator:
R. Taylor Ripley, M.D., National Cancer Institute/CCR, NIH.
10 Center Drive, CRC Room 4–3952.
Bethesda, MD 20892.
Taylor.Ripley@nih.gov
https://ccr.cancer.gov/Thoracic-and-Gastrointestinal-Oncology-Branch/r-taylor-ripley
Research Nurse/Coordinator:
Cara M. Kenney, RN, OCD, CCR, NCI.
10 Center Drive, CRC Room 4–3752.
Bethesda, MD 20892.
kenneycara@mail.nih.gov

Competing interests

The authors declare that they have no competing interests.

Author details

[1]Thoracic and GI Oncology Branch, Center for Cancer Research, National Cancer Institute, Building 10; 4-3952, 10 Center Drive, MSC 1201, Bethesda, MD 20892-1201, USA. [2]Dana-Farber Cancer Institute, Harvard Medical School, Boston, MA, USA. [3]Biostatistics and Data Management Section, Center for Cancer Research, National Cancer Institute, Bethesda, MD, USA. [4]Developmental Therapeutics Branch, Center for Cancer Research, National Cancer Institute, Bethesda, MD, USA.

References

1. Siegel RL, Miller KD, Jemal A. Cancer statistics, 2016. CA Cancer J Clin. 2016;66(1):7–30.
2. Siegel RL, Miller KD, Jemal A. Cancer statistics, 2015. CA Cancer J Clin. 2015;65(1):5–29.
3. van Hagen P, et al. Preoperative chemoradiotherapy for esophageal or junctional cancer. N Engl J Med. 2012;366(22):2074–84.
4. Davies AR, et al. Tumor stage after neoadjuvant chemotherapy determines survival after surgery for adenocarcinoma of the esophagus and esophagogastric junction. J Clin Oncol. 2014;32(27):2983–90.
5. Holscher AH, et al. Prognostic classification of histopathologic response to neoadjuvant therapy in esophageal adenocarcinoma. Ann Surg. 2014;260(5):779–84. discussion 784–5
6. Berger AC, et al. Complete response to neoadjuvant chemoradiotherapy in esophageal carcinoma is associated with significantly improved survival. J Clin Oncol. 2005;23(19):4330–7.
7. Chirieac LR, et al. Posttherapy pathologic stage predicts survival in patients with esophageal carcinoma receiving preoperative chemoradiation. Cancer. 2005;103(7):1347–55.
8. Donohoe CL, Ryan AM, Reynolds JV. Cancer cachexia: mechanisms and clinical implications. Gastroenterol Res Pract. 2011;2011:601434.
9. Shaikh T, et al. Increased time from neoadjuvant chemoradiation to surgery is associated with higher pathologic complete response rates in esophageal cancer. Ann Thorac Surg. 2015;99(1):270–6.
10. van Rossum PS, et al. The incremental value of subjective and quantitative assessment of 18F-FDG PET for the prediction of pathologic complete response to preoperative Chemoradiotherapy in esophageal Cancer. J Nucl Med. 2016;57(5):691–700.
11. Piessen G, et al. Is there a role for surgery for patients with a complete clinical response after chemoradiation for esophageal cancer? An intention-to-treat case-control study. Ann Surg. 2013;258(5):793–9. discussion 799–800
12. Lee JL, et al. A single institutional phase III trial of preoperative chemotherapy with hyperfractionation radiotherapy plus surgery versus surgery alone for resectable esophageal squamous cell carcinoma. Ann Oncol. 2004;15(6):947–54.
13. Yuan H, et al. PET/CT in the evaluation of treatment response to neoadjuvant chemoradiotherapy and prognostication in patients with locally advanced esophageal squamous cell carcinoma. Nucl Med Commun. 2016;37(9):947–55.
14. Hellmann MD, et al. Pathological response after neoadjuvant chemotherapy in resectable non-small-cell lung cancers: proposal for the use of major pathological response as a surrogate endpoint. Lancet Oncol. 2014;15(1):e42–50.
15. Bruzzi JF, et al. Detection of interval distant metastases: clinical utility of integrated CT-PET imaging in patients with esophageal carcinoma after neoadjuvant therapy. Cancer. 2007;109(1):125–34.
16. Elliott JA, et al. Value of CT-PET after neoadjuvant chemoradiation in the prediction of histological tumour regression, nodal status and survival in oesophageal adenocarcinoma. Br J Surg. 2014;101(13):1702–11.
17. Cheedella NK, et al. Association between clinical complete response and pathological complete response after preoperative chemoradiation in patients with gastroesophageal cancer: analysis in a large cohort. Ann Oncol. 2013;24(5):1262–6.
18. Nagrath D, et al. Metabolomics for mitochondrial and cancer studies. Biochim Biophys Acta. 2011;1807(6):650–63.
19. Cao DL, et al. Efforts to resolve the contradictions in early diagnosis of prostate cancer: a comparison of different algorithms of sarcosine in urine. Prostate Cancer Prostatic Dis. 2011;14(2):166–72.
20. Sreekumar A, et al. Metabolomic profiles delineate potential role for sarcosine in prostate cancer progression. Nature. 2009;457(7231):910–4.
21. Yan H, et al. IDH1 and IDH2 mutations in gliomas. N Engl J Med. 2009; 360(8):765–73.
22. Spratlin JL, Serkova NJ, Eckhardt SG. Clinical applications of metabolomics in oncology: a review. Clin Cancer Res. 2009;15(2):431–40.
23. Hanahan D, Weinberg RA. Hallmarks of cancer: the next generation. Cell. 2011;144(5):646–74.
24. Certo M, et al. Mitochondria primed by death signals determine cellular addiction to antiapoptotic BCL-2 family members. Cancer Cell. 2006;9(5):351–65.
25. Potter DS, Letai A. To prime, or not to prime: that is the question. Cold Spring Harb Symp Quant Biol. 2016;81:131–40.
26. Ryan JA, Brunelle JK, Letai A. Heightened mitochondrial priming is the basis for apoptotic hypersensitivity of CD4+ CD8+ thymocytes. Proc Natl Acad Sci U S A. 2010;107(29):12895–900.
27. Ni Chonghaile T, et al. Pretreatment mitochondrial priming correlates with clinical response to cytotoxic chemotherapy. Science. 2011;334(6059):1129–33.
28. Montero J, et al. Drug-induced death signaling strategy rapidly predicts cancer response to chemotherapy. Cell. 2015;160(5):977–89.
29. Stachler MD, et al. Paired exome analysis of Barrett's esophagus and adenocarcinoma. Nat Genet. 2015;47(9):1047–55.
30. Muller PA, Vousden KH. Mutant p53 in cancer: new functions and therapeutic opportunities. Cancer Cell. 2014;25(3):304–17.
31. Galluzzi L, et al. Targeting p53 to mitochondria for cancer therapy. Cell Cycle. 2008;7(13):1949–55.
32. Madani K, et al. Prognostic value of p53 mutations in oesophageal adenocarcinoma: final results of a 15-year prospective study. Eur J Cardiothorac Surg. 2010;37(6):1427–32.
33. Kandioler D, et al. The biomarker TP53 divides patients with neoadjuvantly treated esophageal cancer into 2 subgroups with markedly different outcomes. A p53 research group study. J Thorac Cardiovasc Surg. 2014; 148(5):2280–6.
34. Bruzzi JF, et al. Detection of Richter's transformation of chronic lymphocytic leukemia by PET/CT. J Nucl Med. 2006;47(8):1267–73.
35. Lawrence MS, et al. Mutational heterogeneity in cancer and the search for new cancer-associated genes. Nature. 2013;499(7457):214–8.

25

A rare case of skin blistering and esophageal stenosis in the course of epidermolysis bullosa

Agata Michalak[1], Halina Cichoż-Lach[1]* (iD), Beata Prozorow-Król[1], Leszek Buk[2] and Monika Dzida[2]

Abstract

Background: Epidermolysis bullosa (EB) constitutes a heterogenous group of rare multisystem genetically transmitted disorders comprising several blistering muco-cutaneous diseases with a monogenic basis and either autosomal dominant or autosomal recessive mode of inheritance. EB manifestation is not only limited to the skin. Systemic signs might involve the nose, ear, eye, genitourinary tract and upper gastrointestinal tract. The presence of particular symptoms is directly determined by a type of altered skin protein. Gastrointestinal manifestation of EB is most commonly reflected by esophageal stenosis due to recurrent esophageal blistering, followed by consequent scarring.

Case presentation: Here we present a case of a man with dystrophic EB and dysphagia, skin blistering, joints contractures and missing nails. To our knowledge, the presented man is the oldest one diagnosed with EB living in Poland.

Conclusions: Management of an esophageal stricture in such circumstances is based on endoscopic dilatation. However, in most severe cases, placement of a gastrostomy tube is required. Despite great advances in medicine, a targeted therapy in the course of EB has not been established yet.

Keywords: Epidermolysis bullosa, Esophageal stricture, Dysphagia, Endoscopic dilatation

Background

Epidermolysis bullosa (EB) is a broad entity which encompasses several types of genetically transmitted blistering disorders: EB simplex (EBS), junctional EB (JEB), dystrophic EB (DEB) and Kindler syndrome (KS). The division is mainly based on the level of skin cleavage. Extensive skin blistering as a result of minimal mechanical trauma is a key feature in the course of EB. Degeneration of particular types of skin proteins determines the presence of extracutaneous manifestation, whose range varies among EB subtypes [1, 2] (Fig. 1).

* Correspondence: lach.halina@wp.pl
[1]Department of Gastroenterology with Endoscopy Unit, Medical University of Lublin, Jaczewski Str, Lublin 820-954, Poland

Case presentation

A fourty-year-old man with DEB diagnosed at the age of eight was admitted to the department of gastroenterology because of the dysphagia for two previous months. The diagnosis of DEB was established due to the presence of single blisters on the whole body since the sixth month of life. His sister was also diagnosed with DEB and had similar symptoms of the disease. To our knowledge, the presented patient and his sister are the oldest diagnosed with EB living in Poland. At the age of four the patient started experiencing heartburn occasionally. Five years later dysphagia appeared for the first time. It was an episodal and periodical ailment. He reported a deterioration of dysphagia at the age of nineteen; he mostly consumed liquids and soft consistency meals during that time. Nonetheless, the patient admitted that this esophageal discomfort still was not a constant one and there were time intervals

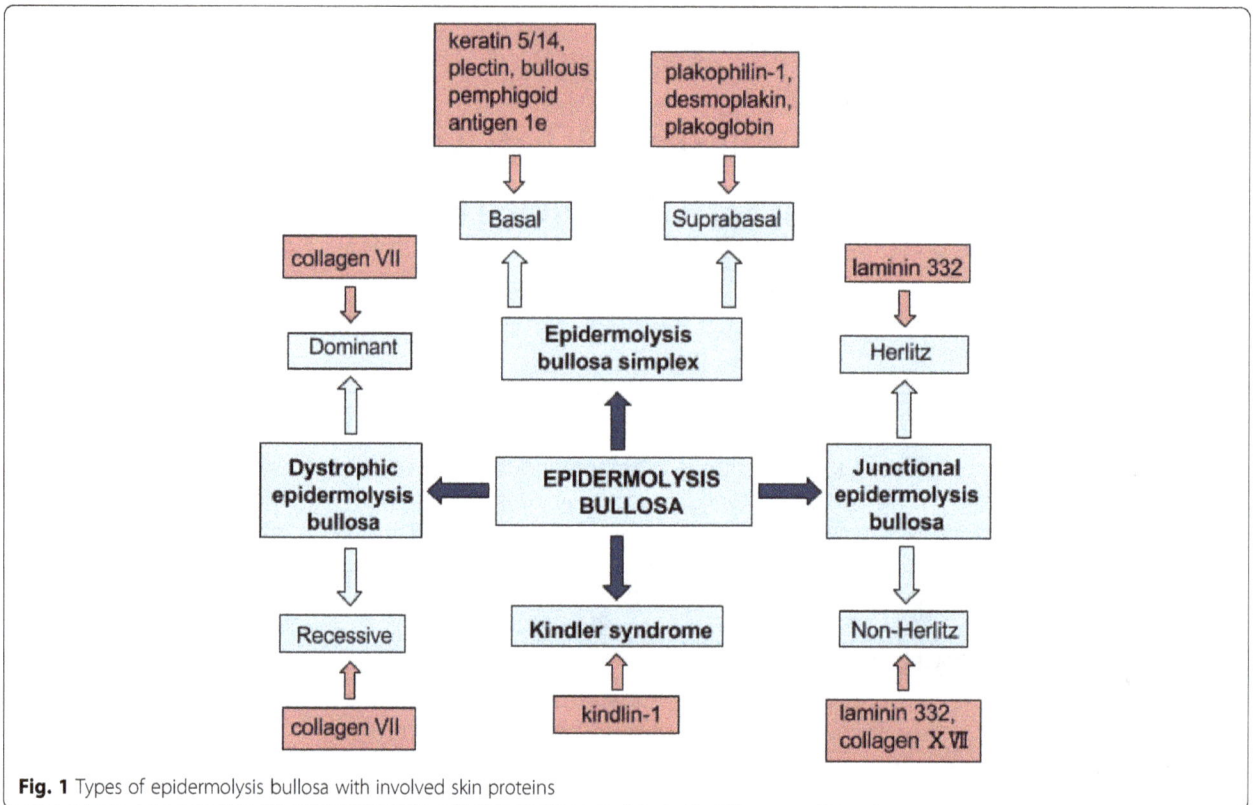

Fig. 1 Types of epidermolysis bullosa with involved skin proteins

without this ailment. In the past there were also episodes of mild esophageal bleeding. The only one endoscopic esophageal dilatation in this patient took place in 1997; a stenosis was located then approximately 18 cm from incisors. The performed procedure ameliorated swallowing difficulty. A barium swallow test obtained one year after the endoscopic dilatation of the esophagus also revealed esophageal constriction on the same level. In 2014 the patient was diagnosed because of hematochezia and pain in hypogastrium. Tissue samples obtained in colonoscopy revealed the presence of nonspecific inflammatory infiltration in the ascending colon and terminal part of the ileum. Interestingly, 3 years ago he complained of hemoptysis and there was a suspicion of bleeding to pulmonary alveoli in the course of DEB. However, a CT scan did not confirm bleeding. On admission to our department the patient was complaining of painful swallowing of solids. Two months earlier he was diagnosed in the cardiology unit because of the chest pain and elevated level of troponin I. An electrocardiogram did not show any abnormalities. The patient refused to undergo coronarography and no more cardiological diagnostic procedures were performed Additional file 1. On admission to our unit he did not complain of the chest pain. On physical examination he appeared comfortable, afebrile with pulse 90 beats per minute, blood pressure 125/90 mmHg, respiratory rate 19 per minute and the body mass index (BMI) was 24.7 kg/

m^2. The patient presented blisters, skin reddening and crust formation on the upper and lower limbs. There were also contractures and disabled movement in his hand joints together with a loss of a finger and toenails (Fig. 2). The apex of the tongue and left palatine arch were covered by superficial ulcerations. During his hospital stay, performed laboratory tests did not reveal any abnormalities. A CT scan of the chest and abdomen showed a thickening of the esophageal wall at maximum to 7 mm on the level from the fourth cervical vertebra to the fourth thoracic vertebra (Fig. 3). A probe of gastroscopy under sedation with benzodiazepine failed due to an esophageal stenosis. An attempt of examination with paediatric endoscope was also unsuccessful. A barium swallow test revealed a narrowing of upper esophageal lumen to 7 mm along the length of 4 cm together with two diverticula on the right side not emptying of contrast. During swallowing other two diverticula appeared which were emptying of contrast (Fig. 4). A barium swallow test also showed a noticeable weakening of the esophageal mucous membrane. After the performed investigation the patient was qualified to endoscopic dilatation of esophageal stenosis and endoscopic management of diverticula. However, he did not agree to undergo this procedure during current hospital stay. In our unit the patient was treated with proton pump inhibitor (PPI) and prokinetic drugs

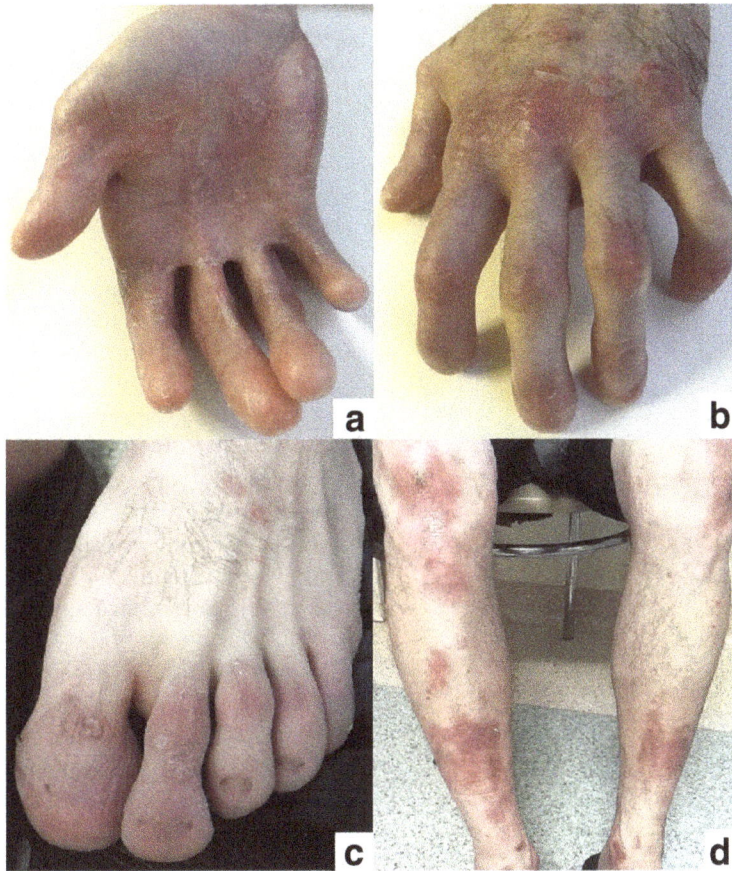

Fig. 2 Contractures in hand joints and crust formation (**a**), blisters (**b**), loss of a finger and toenails (**b** and **c**), skin reddening (**d**)

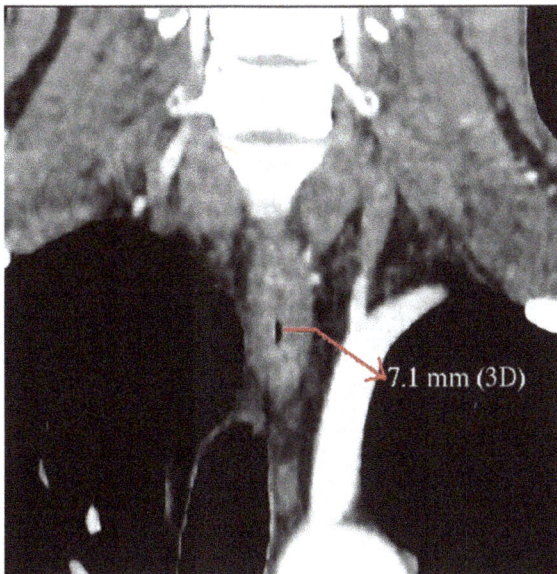

Fig. 3 A thickening of the esophageal wall in a CT scan

administered intravenously, which caused an amelioration of esophageal discomfort. He was discharged in a good general condition with a recommendation of a diet based on soft consistency meals, oral PPI and prokinetic drugs administration and the next follow-up in a month.

Discussion and conclusions

In the 1886 German dermatologist Heinrich Koebner formed an idea of EB, a heterogenous group of genetically transmitted disorders comprising several blistering muco-cutaneous diseases with a monogenic basis and either autosomal dominant or autosomal recessive mode of inheritance. EBS is the most common form in western countries and in general has less severe skin lesions in comparison to JEB or DEB. The herlitz subtype of JEB is less prevalent than the nonherlitz JEB, but both might involve enamel hypoplasia. Skin scarring is a crucial symptom of the herlitz JEB subtype. What is more, mucosal surfaces of the esophagus, upper airway and cornea might also be affected. On the other hand, extracutaneous manifestation is not typical for the nonherlitz JEB. Dominant form of DEB is associated with the formation of skin

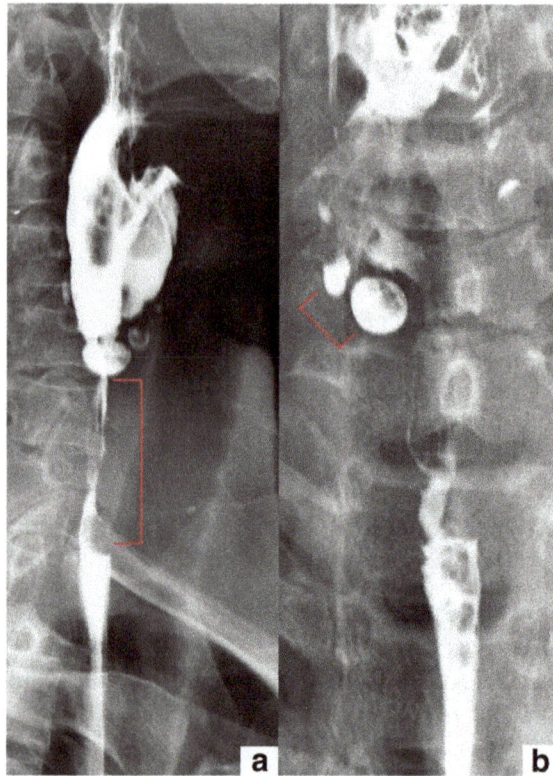

Fig. 4 A narrowing of upper esophageal lumen (red line in picture **a**) and two esophageal diverticula (red line in picture **b**) in a barium swallow test

blisters at birth [3, 4]. Recurrent involvement of the esophagus with subsequent scarring and stenosis can be observed among these patients. Recessive form of DEB is the most severe type of EB and finally leads to disfiguring skin scars, hand and foot deformities, growth retardation and failure to thrive. In addition to skin blistering, photosensitivity and skin pigmentation are characteristic features of KS. EB might involve extra-cutaneous manifestation, leading to severe complications in the eye, nose, oral cavity, ear, larynx and upper respiratory tract. Genitourinary complications (scarring of the glans penis or vaginal vestibule, urethral strictures leading to hydroureter and hydronephrosis) together with musculoskeletal involvement reflected by joints contractures, muscular dystrophy and pseudosyndactyly due to extensive blistering and scarring in DEB are also possible [5–7]. Anemia, usually present in patients with JEB and recessive DEB, heart involvement caused by micronutrient deficiencies and transfusion related iron overload might result in cardiomyopathy. There is also a tendency to develop skin cancers (squamous cell carcinoma, basal cell carcinoma and melanoma) among patients with

EB. Gastrointestinal manifestation might occur in several EB subtypes and the esophagus is the most commonly affected due to repeated blistering and scarring, eventually followed by stenosis. Dysphagia, odynophagia and malnutrition belong to the most typical symptoms. They can be even exacerbated by accompanying gastroesophageal reflux disease. Pyloric atresia, painful perianal blistering and anal canal stenosis together with constipation might also occur [8–14]. In presented patient an extra-cutaneous manifestation of EB was reflected by long-lasting esophageal involvement and its stenosis. It is worth emphasizing that this patient is to our knowledge the oldest one in Poland diagnosed with EB. Nowadays an effective therapy for curing EB does not exist. No drugs are known to correct the underlying molecular defects. Even an anti-collagenase strategy, investigated in various surveys, based on phenytoin or tetracyclines, did not improve the blistering or epithelial disadhesion in EB significantly or consistently. Other recent studies focus on the suppression of transforming growth factor beta-1 (TGF-β1) and reduction of fibrosis in this mechanism. Losartan, an angiotensin II type 1 receptor antagonist was proved to down regulate TGF-β1 activators (e. g. thrombospondin 1) and to improve the course of RDEB. Immunosuppressant drugs like cyclosporine, mycophenolate mofetil and tumor necrosis alpha (TNF-α) inhibitor etanercept were also trialled, however none of them was indicated in chronic therapy of EB. Numerous potential therapies based on cell therapies (allogeneic fibroblasts, mesenchymal stromal cells, bone marrow transplantation), protein replacement and genes modification have been explored. However, further investigations must still be conducted to clarify this issue [15–18]. A modification of diet texture to soft, puree and liquids is the first step in the management of dysphagia in EB patients. If esophageal dilatation is required, endoscopic procedures are usually performed - with the use of a balloon catheter or a bougie. Nevertheless, in the most severe cases of esophageal stenosis, placement of a gastrostomy tube is recommended. Because of a broad range of complications, the treatment of EB patients must be based on a coordinated multidisciplinary approach and extend from psychological support together with dressings and padding blisters to the management of systemic complications [19–22]. Despite great advances in medicine, a targeted therapy in the course of EB has not been established yet.

Abbreviations

BMI: Body mass index; DEB: Dystrophic epidermolysis bullosa; EB: Epidermolysis bullosa; EBS: Epidermolysis bullosa simplex; JEB: Junctional epidermolysis bullosa; KS: Kindler syndrome; PPI: Proton pump inhibitor; TGF-β1: Transforming growth factor beta-1; TNF-α: Tumor necrosis alpha

Acknowledgements
Not applicable.

Funding
No funding was received.

Authors' contributions
AM and BPK analyzed and interpreted the patient data, LB and MD performed radiological investigations, AM and HCL were major contributors in writing the manuscript. All authors read and approved the final manuscript

Competing interests
The authors declare that they have no competing interests.

Author details
[1]Department of Gastroenterology with Endoscopy Unit, Medical University of Lublin, Jaczewski Str, Lublin 820-954, Poland. [2]Department of Radiology and Nuclear Medicine, Medical University of Lublin, Jaczewski Str, Lublin 820-954, Poland.

References
1. Esposito S, Guez S, Orenti A, Tadini G, Scuvera G, Corti L, et al. Autoimmunity and cytokine imbalance in inherited epidermolysis bullosa. Int J Mol Sci. 2016;17:10.
2. El Hachem M, Giancristoforo S, Diociaiuti A. Inherited epidermolysis bullosa. G Ital Dermatol Venereol. 2014;149:651–62.
3. Fine JD, Bruckner-Tuderman L, Eady RA, Bauer EA, Bauer JW, Has C, et al. Inherited epidermolysis bullosa: updated recommendations on diagnosis and classification. J Am Acad Dermatol. 2014;70:1103–26.
4. McGrath JA. Recently identified forms of epidermolysis bullosa. Ann Dermatol. 2015;27:658–66.
5. Has C, Nyström A. Epidermal basement membrane in health and disease. Curr Top Membr. 2015;76:117–70.
6. Watkins J. Diagnosis, treatment and management of epidermolysis bullosa. Br J Nurs. 2016;25:428–31.
7. Bruckner-Tuderman L, Has C. Disorders of the cutaneous basement membrane zone - the paradigm of epidermolysis bullosa. Matrix Biol. 2014;33:29–34.
8. Soro L, Bartus C, Purcell S. Recessive dystrophic epidermolysis bullosa: a review of disease pathogenesis and update on future therapies. J Clin Aesthet Dermatol. 2015;8:41–6.
9. Zidorio AP, Dutra ES, Leão DO, Costa IM. Nutritional aspects of children and adolescents with epidermolysis bullosa: literature review. An Bras Dermatol. 2015;90:217–23.
10. Shinkuma S. Dystrophic epidermolysis bullosa: a review. Clin Cosmet Investig Dermatol. 2015;8:275–84.
11. Gorell ES, Nguyen N, Siprashvili Z, Marinkovich MP, Lane AT. Characterization of patients with dystrophic epidermolysis bullosa for collagen VII therapy. Br J Dermatol. 2015;173:821–3.
12. Bruckner-Tuderman L, McGrath JA, Robinson EC, Uitto J. Progress in epidermolysis bullosa research: summary of DEBRA International research conference 2012. J Invest Dermatol. 2013;133:2121–6.
13. Boeira VL, Souza ES, Rocha Bde O, Oliveira PD, Oliveira Mde F, Rêgo VR, et al. Inherited epidermolysis bullosa: clinical and therapeutic aspects. An Bras Dermatol. 2013;88:185–98.
14. Elluru RG, Contreras JM, Albert DM. Management of manifestations of epidermolysis bullosa. Curr Opin Otolaryngol Head Neck Surg. 2013;21:588–93.
15. Rashidghamat E, McGrath JA. Novel and emerging therapies in the treatment of recessive dystrophic epidermolysis bullosa. Intractable Rare Dis Res. 2017;6:6–20.
16. El-Darouti MA, Fawzy MM, Amin IM, Abdel Hay RM, Hegazy RA, Abdel Halim DM. Mycophenolate mofetil: a novel immunosuppressant in the treatment of dystrophic epidermolysis bullosa, a randomized controlled trial. J Dermatolog Treat. 2013;24:422–6.
17. Gubinelli E, Angelo C, Pacifico V. A case of dystrophic epidermolysis bullosa improved with etanercept for concomitant psoriatic arthritis. Am J Clin Dermatol. 2010;11(Suppl 1):53–4.
18. Nyström A, Thriene K, Mittapalli V, Kern JS, Kiritsi D, Dengjel J. Losartan ameliorates dystrophic epidermolysis bullosa and uncovers new disease mechanisms. EMBO Mol Med. 2015;7:1211–28.
19. De Giuseppe R, Venturelli G, Guez S, Salera S, De Vita C, Consonni D, et al. Homocysteine metabolism in children and adolescents with epidermolysis bullosa. BMC Pediatr. 2016;16:173.
20. Webber BR, Tolar J. From marrow to matrix: novel gene and cell therapies for epidermolysis bullosa. Mol Ther. 2015;23:987–92.
21. Wu W, Lu Z, Li F, Wang W, Qian N, Duan J, et al. Efficient in vivo gene editing using ribonucleoproteins in skin stem cells of recessive dystrophic epidermolysis bullosa mouse model. Proc Natl Acad Sci U S A. 2017;114:1660–5.
22. Bremer J, Bornert O, Nyström A, Gostynski A, Jonkman MF, Aartsma-Rus A, et al. Antisense oligonucleotide-mediated exon skipping as a systemic therapeutic approach for recessive dystrophic epidermolysis bullosa. Mol Ther Nucleic Acids. 2016;5:10.

26

A long-surviving patient with advanced esophageal basaloid squamous cell carcinoma treated only with radiotherapy

Toshiya Maebayashi[1]*[iD], Naoya Ishibashi[1], Takuya Aizawa[1], Masakuni Sakaguchi[1], Homma Taku[2], Moritaka Ohhara[3], Toshirou Takimoto[4] and Yoshiaki Tanaka[5]

Abstract

Background: Esophageal basaloid squamous cell carcinoma (EBSCC) is a rare malignant disease. Advanced EBSCC (AEBSCC) has a poorer prognosis than the more common esophageal squamous cell carcinoma, but no treatment policy has yet been established. This is the first reported case with AEBSCC treated only with radiotherapy. Thus, our long-surviving patient merits consideration. We therefore reviewed cases with the same stage of AEBSCC for further investigation.

Case presentation: An 85-year-old man with a chief complaint of difficulty swallowing foods was diagnosed with AEBSCC, cT3N1M0, stage III, by thorough examination. The basaloid carcinoma extended from the upper thoracic esophagus to the middle thoracic esophagus based on imaging studies, endoscopy and biopsy. Morphologically, the tumor was an elevated ulcerative area. We conducted radiotherapy to relieve symptoms, as the patient and his family refused aggressive treatment. He has remained alive without recurrence for 2 years, to date, after completing radiotherapy.

Conclusions: Basaloid carcinoma might be highly sensitive to radiotherapy. Thus, radiotherapy for local control might be beneficial for elderly patients with complications and those refusing aggressive treatment.

Keywords: Esophageal basaloid squamous cell carcinoma, Radiation therapy

Background

Wain et al. reported basaloid carcinoma for the first time among patients with head and neck cancers [1]. It is a rare histological form of esophageal cancer and reportedly accounts for 0.1% of cases with esophageal cancers [2, 3]. Advanced esophageal basaloid squamous cell carcinoma (AEBSCC) has a poorer prognosis than the more common esophageal squamous cell carcinoma (ESCC), but no treatment policy has yet been established [4].

According to our literature search, this is the first reported case with AEBSCC treated only with radiotherapy. Basaloid carcinoma might be highly sensitive to radiotherapy. Thus, radiotherapy for local control might be beneficial for elderly patients with complications and those refusing aggressive treatment. We evaluated 10 AEBSCC patients at the same disease stage for which detailed descriptions were available (Table 1).

Case presentation

An 85-year-old man with a 1-month history of difficulty swallowing foods presented to our department and was diagnosed with AEBSCC, cT3N1M0, stage III, by thorough examination (Figs. 1, 2, 3, 4 and 5). The basaloid carcinoma extended from the upper thoracic esophagus to the middle thoracic esophagus based on imaging studies (Figs. 1, 3 and 4), endoscopy (Fig. 2), positron emission tomography–computed tomography (Fig. 4) and biopsy (Fig. 5). Morphologically, the tumor was an

* Correspondence: maebayashi.toshiya@nihon-u.ac.jp
[1]Department of Radiology, Nihon University School of Medicine, 30-1 Oyaguchi Kami-cho, Itabashi-ku, Tokyo 173-8610, Japan

Table 1 Clinical characteristics of 10 Japanese cases with stage III esophageal basaloid squamous cell carcinoma: site, morphology, metastasis, survival period, current status and treatment

Site	Morphology	Metastasis	Survival period (months)	Current status	Treatment
Upper and middle	Type 1 (Erosive elevation)	Bone	13	Dead	Surgery alone
Lower	Type 2	Lung, liver, lymph nodes	8	Dead	Chemoradiotherapy after surgery
Upper	Type 2	Lung, brain	22	Dead	Chemotherapy after surgery
Lower	Type 3	Liver	10	Dead	Surgery alone
Lower	Type 1	Liver	36	Alive	1. Chemotherapy after surgery 2. Chemotherapy after liver metastasis resection
Middle	Type 1	Liver, lymph nodes	9	Dead	Surgery after pre-operative chemotherapy
Lower	Type 1	Liver	27	Alive	1. Surgery 2. Surgery after hepatic arterial injection chemotherapy for liver metastasis
Middle	Type 2	Liver, lymph nodes	10	Dead	Chemotherapy after surgery
None	None	Mediastinal lymph modes, solitary lung	61	Alive	1. Surgery 2. Mediastinal lymph node radiation 3. Surgery after chemotherapy for lung metastasis
Upper	Type 3	None	25	Alive	Radiotherapy alone

elevated ulcerative area. Furthermore, the tumor was found to have spread into the submucosa (Figs. 1 and 3). Immunohistochemical staining showed the tumor to be negative for p16. The patient had been diagnosed with prostate cancer 10 years earlier and had received hormone therapy for 5 years. There had been no recurrence of the prostate cancer. His medical history also included pulmonary tuberculosis and spinal stenosis. He smoked 20 cigarettes per day for the prior 12 years and drank 2 *go* (approximately 361 mL) of alcohol daily. We initially recommended surgery as aggressive treatment because his general condition was good and the prognosis of AEBSCC is poor. However, he refused aggressive treatments including chemotherapy. We thus administered

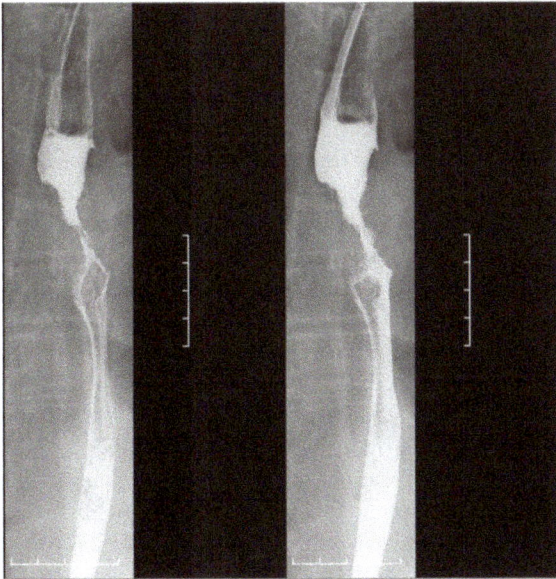

Fig. 1 Esophagography: Extensive narrowing is seen on the oral side from the carina, and mild extension is present in the esophagus on the oral side. Passage of the contrast medium is possible and there are no fistulas in the carina

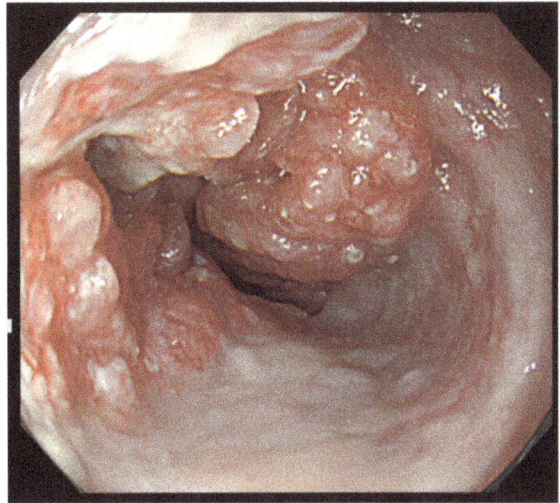

Fig. 2 Upper gastrointestinal endoscopy: Macroscopic type 3 advanced esophageal cancer, which appears to be nearly circumferential, can be seen 22 cm from the gums. The tumor was speculated to have developed and then extended into the submucosal layer

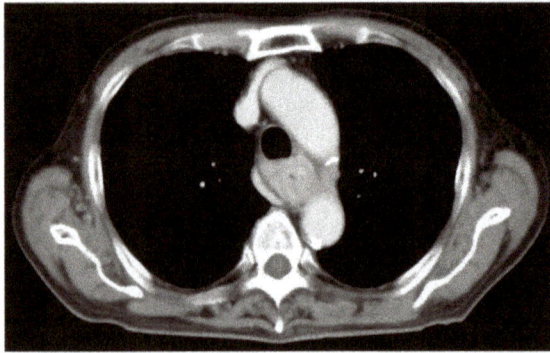

Fig. 3 Computed tomography of the chest: An esophageal tumor, which appears to compress the membranous portion of the trachea, is considered to be indicative of advanced esophageal cancer as an *en bloc* mass with lymph node metastasis

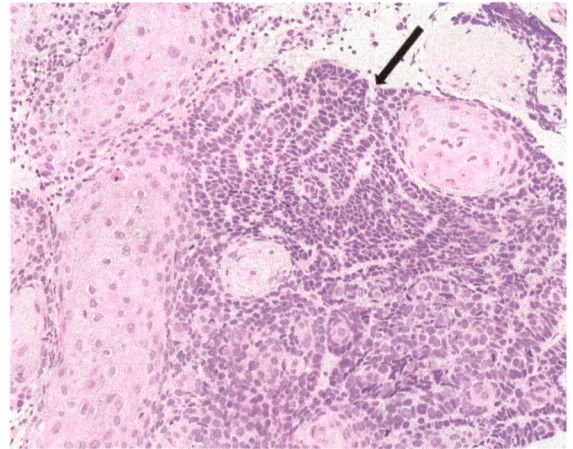

Fig. 5 Biopsy histopathological image (Hematoxylin-Eosin staining: 20 X magnification): Small and spindle-shaped tumor cells with scanty cytoplasm are arranged in cords, forming a tumor nest similar to basal cells with no keratin pattern formation (narrow). Proliferation of atypical squamous epithelium is present around the nest and there are also components of squamous cell carcinoma

radiotherapy for symptom relief. The radiation field ranged from the supraclavicular lymph node region to the entire esophagus, and radiation was delivered at a dose of 60 Gy in 2-Gy fractions (Fig. 6), allocated as 40 Gy to the regional field and 20 Gy to the boost field. To date, approximately 2 years have passed since radiotherapy completion. For follow-up of this patient with AEBSCC after radiation therapy, we obtained a detailed history and performed a full physical examination, computed tomography and upper gastrointestinal endoscopy every 3–6 months. The disease course has been good with neither recurrence nor metastasis and there were no adverse effects related to radiation therapy (Fig. 7). There were no late adverse events related to radiation therapy.

Discussion and conclusions

Esophageal squamous cell carcinoma (ESCC) is the predominant form of esophageal cancer in Japan. Squamous-cell tumors comprise 98% of malignancies in the upper and middle third of the esophagus [5, 6].

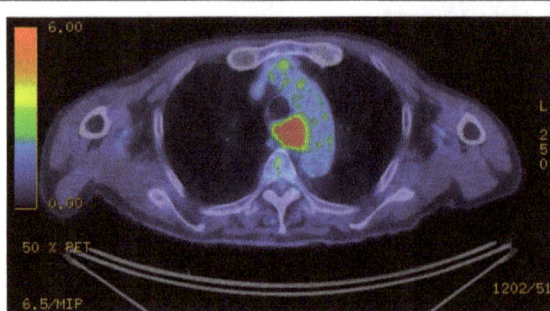

Fig. 4 Positron emission tomography–computed tomography: There is radionuclide accumulation in the portion where the *en bloc* mass forms an esophageal tumor compressing the membranous portion of the trachea and lymph node metastasis is present, but there is no evidence of distant metastasis

Esophageal basaloid squamous cell carcinoma (EBSCC) is a rare histological form of esophageal cancer and reportedly accounts for 0.1% of cases with such cancers [2, 3]. Basaloid squamous cell carcinoma (BSCC) is a high-grade variant of squamous cell carcinoma of the head and neck [7]. Esophageal basaloid carcinoma is derived from esophageal epithelial basal cells or undifferentiated cells with similar multipotential features [8]. Therefore, it is considered to be difficult to identify this type of cancer by biopsy [9] and some reports have indicated that it constitutes 11.3% of esophageal tumors [10].

EBSCC generally shows high-grade malignancy, but no treatment policy has yet been established [11]. Surgery should thus be recommended even if the cancer is superficial [11]. Most reports have indicated that EBSCC is mainly treated with surgery [4, 12]. In terms of chemotherapy, sporadic reports have shown that chemoradiotherapy or chemotherapy can be expected to show efficacy [13–15]. The survival rate of patients with stage I or II EBSCC is considered to be similar to that of those with ESCC [4, 12]. However, the 5-year survival rate in stage III or IV AEBSCC patients is reportedly 10.5%, which indicates that AEBSCC carries a significantly poorer prognosis than the more common ESCC [4]. In Japan, the combination of preoperative chemotherapy and surgery is accepted as standard treatment for stage II or III ESCC based on findings from a Japan Clinical Oncology Group trial (JCOG9907) [16]. The 3-year survival rate of patients who did not undergo surgery for stage II or III ESCC is reportedly 45% [17]. Therefore, multimodal treatment is considered to be important for AEBSCC and some reports have stated that aggressive

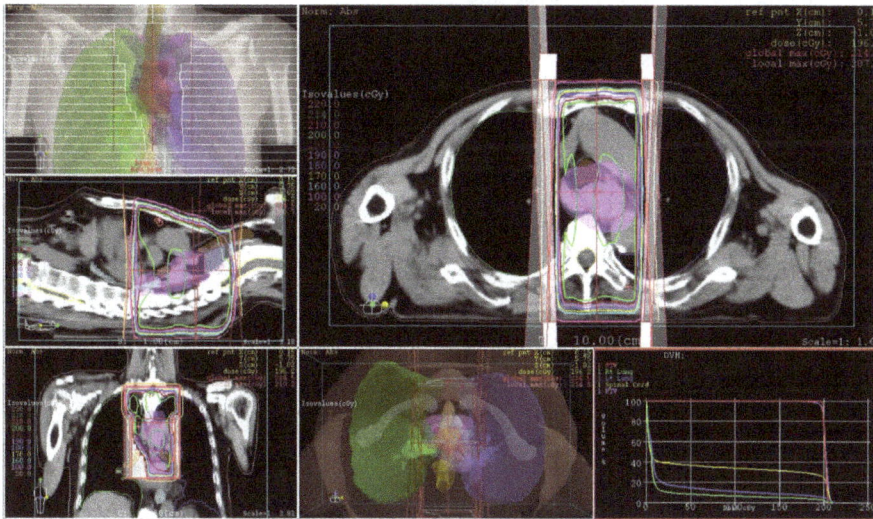

Fig. 6 The irradiated fields and dose distributions for advanced esophageal basaloid squamous cell carcinoma irradiation using 10MV X-rays. He was prescribed a dose of 60 Gy in 2-Gy fractions, allocated as 40 Gy to the regional field and 20 Gy to the boost field. (holding the spinal cord dose below 40Gy)

treatment of metastatic sites led to long-term survival [18, 19]. However, there are no reports referring to radiotherapy, according to our literature search. Our present patient has maintained recurrence-free survival for approximately 2 years since completion of radiotherapy, suggesting that radiotherapy might be effective as local treatment. There are three reports suggesting radiotherapy to be effective, although the patients were not treated with radiotherapy only. One report described a patient with 5-year survival administered radiotherapy when mediastinal lymph node metastasis appeared after surgery for stage III AEBSCC [20] (Table 1). Another report documented 4-year survival in a patient in whom the therapeutic effects on stage IVA AEBSCC were favorable, but radiotherapy was performed only at the site of local recurrence [21]. A patient with long-term survival who underwent stereotactic radiotherapy for a solitary lung metastasis was also reported [13]. However, a stage III AEBSCC patient for whom chemotherapy was performed after surgery reportedly died, 8 months later,

of lung and liver metastases [22] (Table 1); the lesion site was the lower esophagus in that patient reported by Nishida et al. Other patients with upper and middle esophageal lesions had better outcomes [4]. This would explain why the aforementioned patient survived.

We evaluated nine case reports [18, 19, 22–28] describing patients with AEBSCC in the same stage (III) as that in our patient, 10 cases in total, and found the median survival time to be 13 months. Surgery was performed in all cases, but radiotherapy was performed only in three cases. Two of these three, including ours, experienced long-term survival. However, little can be inferred from so few case reports. With multimodal treatment, efficacy of pre-operative chemoradiotherapy and even chemoradiotherapy without surgery can be anticipated (Table 1).

The question of whether EBSCC is rare and accounts for approximately 10% of all esophageal cancers [10] was not discussed in previous reports. EBSCC is histologically characterized by a submucosal tumor-like growth,

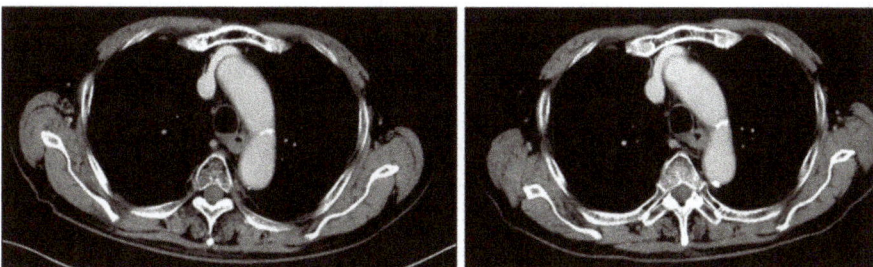

Fig. 7 Computed tomographic images obtained 16 (right figure) and 25 months (left figure) after completion of radiotherapy for esophageal basaloid squamous cell. There has been no evidence of recurrence or metastasis since the initiation of this treatment

due to tumor nests invading the submucosal layer and deeper structures, and the formation of an elevated lesion. Therefore, patients with type I esophageal carcinoma may be diagnosed with squamous cell carcinoma based on biopsy findings only from the superficial layer of the tumor, raising the possibility of including those with basaloid carcinoma. If EBSCC is included in the category of type I advanced esophageal carcinomas, the proportion of this tumor among all esophageal cancers may well increase. In the future, if a tumor is mainly a type I advanced esophageal cancer, we should advocate biopsy in the deep portions of the tumor, considering the possibility of EBSCC.

Our clinical experience suggests that type I esophageal carcinoma is highly sensitive to radiotherapy. Accordingly, there is only one report [29] suggesting radiotherapy to exert beneficial effects on type I advanced esophageal carcinoma. EBSCC is considered to have a high metastatic potential because the tumor spreads to the submucosa. However, Thariat et al. [7] reported that patients with BSCC of the head and neck receiving irradiation did not have poorer outcomes than those with squamous cell carcinoma of the head and neck with positive lymph node status. Therefore, radiotherapy might be beneficial as a local treatment for basaloid carcinoma.

In conclusion, this is the first reported case with AEBSCC treated only with radiotherapy. This is a rare disease, but we intend to make efforts to increase the diagnostic yield. The radiosensitivity of AEBSCC needs to be further examined in future studies.

Abbreviations
AEBSCC: Advanced esophageal basaloid squamous cell carcinoma; BSCC: Basaloid squamous cell carcinoma; EBSCC: esophageal basaloid squamous cell carcinoma; ESCC: esophageal squamous cell carcinoma

Acknowledgements
The authors thank Bierta Barfod for her contribution to the language editing of this manuscript.

Authors' contributions
MT drafted the manuscript; TT and HT diagnosed the advanced esophageal basaloid squamous cell carcinoma; OM examined the patient and initially suggested radiation therapy; MT, IN, SM, AT, and TY examined the patient, then planned and carried out the radiation therapy. All authors read and approved the final manuscript.

Authors' information
TM, NI, TA, MS and YT are radiation oncologists. TH and TT are pathologists. MO is a surgeon. All of the authors currently work in Japan. YT is a former professor at the Department of Radiology at the Nihon University School of Medicine.

Competing interests
We declare that we have no significant competing financial, professional or personal interests that might have influenced the performance or presentation of the work described in this manuscript. The authors have no competing interest to declare.

Author details
[1]Department of Radiology, Nihon University School of Medicine, 30-1 Oyaguchi Kami-cho, Itabashi-ku, Tokyo 173-8610, Japan. [2]Department of Human Pathology, Division of Pathology and Microbiology, Nihion University School of Medicine, Itabashi-ku, Tokyo 173-8610, Japan. [3]Department of Digestive Surgery, Kasukabe Medical Center, Kasukabe, Saitama 344-8588, Japan. [4]Department of Pathology, Kasukabe Medical Center, Kasukabe, Saitama 344-8588, Japan. [5]Department of Radiation Oncology, Kawasaki Saiwai Hospital, Kawasaki, Kanagawa 212-0014, Japan.

References
1. Wain SL, Kier R, Vollmer RT, Bossen EH. Basaloid-squamous carcinoma of the tongue, hypopharynx, and larynx: report of 10 cases. Hum Pathol. 1986;17:1158–66. 3770734
2. Suzuki H, Nagayo T. Primary tumors of the esophagus other than squamous cell carcinoma–histologic classification and statistics in the surgical and autopsied materials in Japan. Int Adv Surg Oncol. 1980;3:73–109. 3770734
3. Tsukayama S, Hirano M, Murakami N, Uno Y Nozawa H. A case report of basaloid-squamous carcinoma of the esophagus. Jpn J Gastroenterol Surg. 2000;33:462–6. [Article in Japanese] PMID: 11383213.
4. Zhang BH, Cheng GY, Xue Q, Gao SG, Sun KL, Wang YG, Mu JW, He J. Clinical outcomes of basaloid squamous cell carcinoma of the esophagus:a retrospective analysis of 142 cases. Asian Pac J Cancer Prev 2013;14:1889–1894. PMID: 23679289.
5. Sawada G, Niida A, Uchi R, Hirata H, Shimamura T, Suzuki Y, Shiraishi Y, Chiba K, Imoto S, Takahashi Y, Iwaya T, Sudo T, Hayashi T, Takai H, Kawasaki Y, Matsukawa T, Eguchi H, Sugimachi K, Tanaka F, Suzuki H, Yamamoto K, Ishii H, Shimizu M, Yamazaki H, Yamazaki M, Tachimori Y, Kajiyama Y, Natsugoe S, Fujita H, Mafune K, Tanaka Y, Kelsell DP, Scott CA, Tsuji S, Yachida S, Shibata T, Sugano S, Doki Y, Akiyama T, Aburatani H, Ogawa S, Miyano S, Mori M, Mimori K. Genomic landscape of esophageal squamous cell carcinoma in a Japanese population. Gastroenterology 2016;150:1171–1182. PMID: 26873401. doi: 10.1053/j.gastro.2016.01.035.
6. Satoh T, Sakata Y. On the path to standardizing esophageal cancer treatment in Japan. Gastrointest Cancer Res. 2009;3:77–9. 19461911
7. Thariat J, Ahamad A, El-Naggar AK, Williams MD, Holsinger FC, Glisson BS, Allen PK, Morrison WH, Weber RS, Ang KK, Garden AS. Outcomes after radiotherapy for basaloid squamous cell carcinoma of the head and neck: a case-control study. Cancer. 2008;15;112(12):2698–709. PMID: 18429002. doi: doi: 10.1002/cncr.23486.
8. Takubo K, Mafune K, Tanaka Y, Miyama T, Fujita K. Basaloid squamous carcinoma of the esophagus with marked deposition of basement membrane substance. Acta Pathol Jpn. 1991;41:59–64. 2031457
9. Nakamura R, Omori T, Takeuchi H, Kawakubo H, Takahashi T, Wada N, Saikawa Y, Kameyama K, Kitagawa Y. Characteristics and diagnosis of esophageal basaloid squamous cell carcinoma. Esophagus. 2016;13:48–54. doi: 10.1007/s10388-015-0490-8.
10. Sarbia M, Verreet P, Bittinger F, Dutkowski P, Heep H, Willers R, Gabbert HE. Basaloid squamous cell carcinoma of the esophagus: diagnosis and prognosis. Cancer 1997;79:1871–1878. PMID: 9149011.
11. Takii M, Takemura M, Kaibe N, Ohshima T, Kikuchi S, Sasako M. Two Resected Cases with Superficial Basaloid Squamous Carcinoma of the Esophagus. Gan To Kagaku Ryoho 2016;43(11):1381–1384. [Article in Japanese] PMID: 27899779.
12. Yoshioka S, Tsujinaka T, Fujitani K, Kawahara K. Prognostic analysis of four cases of basaloid cell carcinoma of the esophagus and 60 reported cases in Japan. Jpn J Gastroenterol Surg. 2004;37(3):290 295. [Article in Japanese].
13. Saito S, Hosoya Y, Zuiki T, Hyodo M, Lefor A, Sata N, et al. A clinicopathological study of basaloid squamous carcinoma of the esophagus. Esophagus. 2009;6:177–81. doi: 10.1007/s10388-009-0202-3.
14. Tokura M, Yoshimura T, Murata T, Matsuyama T, Hoshino M, Goto H, Kakimoto M, Koshiishi H. A Case of Long-Term Survival of Advanced Esophageal Basaloid Squamous Carcinoma Invading the Trachea. Gan To Kagaku Ryoho. 2015;42(12):1893–5. [Article in Japanese] PMID: 26805208.

A long-surviving patient with advanced esophageal basaloid squamous cell carcinoma treated...

185

15. Yamauchi M, Shinozaki K, Sumioka M, Nishisaka T. Long-term survival of a patient with stage IV basaloid squamous carcinoma of the esophagus with lung metastases following combined modality therapy. Nihon Shokakibyo Gakkai Zasshi. 2015;112:1503–9. [Article in Japanese] PMID: 26250130. doi:10.11405/nisshoshi.112.1503.

16. Ando N, Kato H, Igaki H, Shinoda M, Ozawa S, Shimizu H, Nakamura T, Yabusaki H, Aoyama N, Kurita A, Ikeda K, Kanda T, Tsujinaka T, Nakamura K, Fukuda H. A randomized trial comparing postoperative adjuvant chemotherapy with cisplatin and 5-fluorouracil versus preoperative chemotherapy for localized advanced squamous cell carcinoma of the thoracic esophagus (JCOG9907). Ann Surg Oncol 2012;19(1):68–74. PMID: 21879261. doi: 10.1245/s10434-011-2049-9.

17. Kato K, Muro K, Minashi K, Ohtsu A, Ishikura S, Boku N, Takiuchi H, Komatsu Y, Miyata Y, Fukuda H; Gastrointestinal oncology study Group of the Japan Clinical Oncology Group (JCOG). Phase II study of chemoradiotherapy with 5-fluorouracil and cisplatin for stage II-III esophageal squamous cell carcinoma: JCOG trial (JCOG 9906). Int J Radiat Oncol Biol Phys 2011;81(3):684–690. PMID: 20932658. doi: 10.1016/j.ijrobp.2010.06.033.

18. Sanda Y, Kaneda K, Miura Y, Nakayama S, Kawaguchi K. Case of Resected Metachronous Liver Metastasis of Basaloid Cell Carcinoma of the Esophagus. Nihon Rinsho Geka Gakkai Zasshi (Journal of Japan Surgical Association). 2013;4:1488–94. doi: 10.3919/jjsa.74.1488. (in Japanese with English abstract).

19. Sasaki K, Izumi Y, Hanashi T, Yoshida M, Takahashi T. Liver metastasis of basaloid-squamous cell carcinoma of the esophagus successfully resected after intra-hepatoarterial chemotherapy. Report of a case. Nihon Rinsho Geka Gakkai Zasshi (Journal of Japan Surgical Association). 2002;63:608–12. [Article in Japanese] doi: 10.3919/jjsa.63.608.

20. Kosaka T, Mogi A, Yamaki E, Miyazaki T, Kuwano H. Surgical resection of a solitary pulmonary metastasis from basaloid squamous cell carcinoma of the esophagus: a case report. Ann Thorac Cardiovasc Surg 2014;20:646–649. PMID: 2408891 doi: 10.5761/atcs.cr.13-00100.

21. Tokura M, Yoshimura T, Murata T, Matsuyama T, Hoshino M, Goto H, Kakimoto M, Koshiishi H. A Case of Long-Term Survival of Advanced Esophageal Basaloid Squamous Carcinoma Invading the Trachea. Gan To Kagaku Ryoho. 2015;42:1893–5. [Article in Japanese] PMID: 26805208.

22. Nishida Y, Kushibuchi T, Nishimura S, Shibata J, Akira Kawaguchi A, Kodama M. A Case Report of Basaloid-(Squamous) Carcinoma of the Esophagus. Jpn J Gastroenterol Surg. 1995;28:1829–33. [Article in Japanese].

23. Mizukami Y, Nimura Y, Hayakawa N, Torimoto Y, Hirai T, Yasui A, Tokoro A, Kohno H, Akita Y, Nagano M, Shionoya S. A case of basaloid cell carcinoma of the esophagus. Jpn J Gastroenterol Surg. 1989;22:2681–2684. [Article in Japanese].

24. Murakami S, Hashimoto T, Takeno S, Hazamada S, Uchida Y, Yokoyama S. A case of basaloid-squamous carcinoma of the esophagus. Nihon Rinsho Geka Gakkai Zasshi (Journal of Japan Surgical Association). 1998;59:1829–32.

25. Moriya H, Katada N, Mieno H, Hoshoda K, Yamashita K, Kikuti S, Ohbu M, Watanabe M. Clinicopathological characteristics of patients with basaloid squamous cell carcinoma of the esophagus. The Kitasato Medical Journal. 2014;44:19–24. [Article in Japanese].

26. Tsukayama S, Hirano M, Murakami N, Uno Y, Nozawa H, Yoshino H, Orta N, Kikkawa H, Masuda S. A Case Report of Basaloid-Squamous carcinoma of the Esophagus. The Japanese Journal of Gastroenterological Surgery. 2000;33:462–466. [Article in Japanese] doi:10.5833/jjgs.33.462.

27. Kosaka T, Mogi A, Yamaki E, Miyazaki T, Kuwano H. Surgical resection of a solitary pulmonary metastasis from basaloid squamous cell carcinoma of the esophagus:a case report. Ann Thorac Cardiovasc Surg 2014;20:646–649. PMID: 24088918. doi: 10.5761/atcs.cr.13-00100.

28. Ozaki K, Maeda Y, Suzuki K, Namiki S, Kimura S, Takeuchi TA. Case of basaloid cell carcinoma of the esophagus of which preoperative diagnosis was poorly differentiated squamous cell carcinoma. Surgery. 2009;71:1120–

29. Yoshii T, Inokuchi Y, Sue S, Ohkawa S. Analysis of endoscopic evaluation of primary responses to CRT in advanced esophageal cancer. Progress of Digestive Endoscopy. 2011;79:41–5. 10.11641/pde.79.2_41.

Permissions

The contributors of this book come from diverse backgrounds, making this book a truly international effort. This book will bring forth new frontiers with its revolutionizing research information and detailed analysis of the nascent developments around the world.

We would like to thank all the contributing authors for lending their expertise to make the book truly unique. They have played a crucial role in the development of this book. Without their invaluable contributions this book wouldn't have been possible. They have made vital efforts to compile up to date information on the varied aspects of this subject to make this book a valuable addition to the collection of many professionals and students.

This book was conceptualized with the vision of imparting up-to-date information and advanced data in this field. To ensure the same, a matchless editorial board was set up. Every individual on the board went through rigorous rounds of assessment to prove their worth. After which they invested a large part of their time researching and compiling the most relevant data for our readers.

The editorial board has been involved in producing this book since its inception. They have spent rigorous hours researching and exploring the diverse topics which have resulted in the successful publishing of this book. They have passed on their knowledge of decades through this book. To expedite this challenging task, the publisher supported the team at every step. A small team of assistant editors was also appointed to further simplify the editing procedure and attain best results for the readers.

Apart from the editorial board, the designing team has also invested a significant amount of their time in understanding the subject and creating the most relevant covers. They scrutinized every image to scout for the most suitable representation of the subject and create an appropriate cover for the book.

The publishing team has been an ardent support to the editorial, designing and production team. Their endless efforts to recruit the best for this project, has resulted in the accomplishment of this book. They are a veteran in the field of academics and their pool of knowledge is as vast as their experience in printing. Their expertise and guidance has proved useful at every step. Their uncompromising quality standards have made this book an exceptional effort. Their encouragement from time to time has been an inspiration for everyone.

The publisher and the editorial board hope that this book will prove to be a valuable piece of knowledge for researchers, students, practitioners and scholars across the globe.

List of Contributors

Valter Nilton Felix
Digestive Surgery Division, São Paulo University ,Head of the Nucleus of General and Specialized Surgery, São Paulo, Brazil. School of Medicine, São Paulo University, R. Frei Caneca, 1407 – cj 221, São Paulo, SP, Brazil

Ioshiaki Yogi, Daniel Senday, Fernando Tadeu Vannucci Coimbra, David Pares Vinicius Garcia and Carlos Eduardo Garcia
Nucleus of General and Specialized Surgery, São Paulo, Brazil

Ning Wu, Yongjun Zhu, Liewen Pang, Gang Chen and Zhiming Chen
Department of Cardio-thoracic Surgery, HuaShan Hospital of Fudan University, Shanghai 200040, People's Republic of China

Dhruba Kadel
Department of General Surgery, HuaShan Hospital of Fudan University, Shanghai 200040, China

Hiroaki Takahashi, Satoshi Okahara and Junichi Kodaira
Department of Gastroenterology, Keiyukai Daini Hospital, Hondori-13, Shiroishi-ku, Sapporo 003- 0027, Japan

Yoshiaki Arimura and Yasuhisa Shinomura
Department of Gastroenterology, Rheumatology, and Clinical Immunology, Sapporo Medical University, S-1, W-16, Chuo-ku, Sapporo 060-8543, Japan

Kaku Hokari and Hiroyuki Tsukagoshi
Department of Gastroenterology, Keiyukai Sapporo Hospital, Hondori-14, Shiroishi-ku, Sapporo 003-0027, Japan

Masao Hosokawa
Department of Surgery, Keiyukai Sapporo Hospital, Hondori-14, Shiroishi-ku, Sapporo 003-0027, Japan

Lidia Ciobanu, Oliviu Pascu and Marcel Tantau
Regional Institute of Gastroenterology and Hepatology, University of Medicine and Pharmacy, Croitorilor Street 19-21, Cluj-Napoca 400162, Romania

Oana Pinzariu
Emergency Clinic Country Hospital, Cluj-Napoca 400006, Romania

Bogdan Furnea
Regional Institute of Gastroenterology and Hepatology, Cluj-Napoca 400162, Romania

Emil Botan
Department of Pathology, Emergency Clinic Country Hospital, Cluj-Napoca 400006, Romania

Marian Taulescu
Department of Pathology, Faculty of Veterinary Medicine, University of Agricultural Science and Veterinary Medicine, Cluj-Napoca 400372, Romania

Bin Deng, Xue-Feng Gao, Yun-Yun Sun, Yuan-Zhi Wang, Da-Cheng Wu, Wei-Ming Xiao, Jian Wu and Yan-Bing Ding
Department of Gastroenterology, the Second Clinical College of Yangzhou University, Yangzhou, Jiangsu 225001, China

Yan-Bing Ding
Department of Gastroenterology, Yangzhou No. 1 People's Hospital, 368# of HanJiang middle road, Yangzhou, Jiangsu 225001, China

Siddharth Singh, Swapna Devanna and Jithinraj Edakkanambeth Varayil
Division of Gastroenterology and Hepatology, Department of Internal Medicine, Mayo Clinic, 200 First Street SW, Rochester 55905MN, USA

Mohammad Hassan Murad
Department of Preventive Medicine, Mayo Clinic, Rochester, USA

Prasad G Iyer
Knowledge and Evaluation Research Unit, Mayo Clinic, Rochester, MN, USA

Ryu Ishihara, Noriko Matsuura, Noboru Hanaoka, Sachiko Yamamoto, Tomofumi Akasaka, Yoji Takeuchi, Koji Higashino, Noriya Uedo and Hiroyasu Iishi
Department of Gastrointestinal Oncology, Osaka Medical Center for Cancer and Cardiovascular Diseases, 1-3-3 Nakamichi Higashinari-ku, Osaka 537-8511, Japan

Wei-Cheng Huang
Divisions of Gastroenterology, Wan Fang Hospital, Taipei Medical University, No. 111, Section 3, Hsing Long Road, Taipei 116, Taiwan

Chih-Hsin Lee
Divisions of Pulmonology, Department of Internal Medicine, Wan Fang Hospital, Taipei Medical University, Taipei, Taiwan

Fat-Moon Suk
Department of Internal Medicine, School of Medicine, College of Medicine, Taipei Medical University, Taipei, Taiwan

Sohaib Abu-Farsakh and Zhongren Zhou
Department of Pathology and Laboratory Medicine, University of Rochester, Box 626601 Elmwood Ave, Rochester, NY 14642, USA

Tongtong Wu and Amy Lalonde
Department of Biostatistics and Computational Biology, University of Rochester Medical Center, 265 Crittenden Boulevard CU 420630, Rochester, NY 14642-0630, USA

Jun Sun
Department of Medicine, Division of Gastroenterology and Hepatology, University of Illinois College of Medicine, 840 South Wood Street MC 716, Chicago, IL 60612, USA

Qazi Masood and Iffat Hassan
Postgraduate Department of Dermatology, STDs & Leprosy, Government Medical College, Srinagar, Jammu and Kashmir, India

Jaswinder Singh
Department of Gastroenterology, SKIMS, Soura, Srinagar, Kashmir, India

Tasleem Arif
Postgraduate Department of Dermatology, STDs and Leprosy, Jawaharlal Nehru Medical College (JNMC), Aligarh Muslim University (AMU), Aligarh, India

Zhongren Zhou and Jiqing Ye
Departments of Pathology and Laboratory Medicine, University of Rochester, Rochester, 601 Elmwood Ave, Rochester, NY 14642, USA

Santhoshi Bandla and Jeffrey H Peters
Departments of Surgery, University of Rochester, Rochester, NY, USA

Yinglin Xia
Biostatistics and Computational Biology, University of Rochester, Rochester, NY, USA

Jianwen Que
Biomedical Genetics, University of Rochester, Rochester, NY, USA

James D Luketich and Arjun Pennathur
Department of Cardiothoracic Surgery, University of Pittsburgh Medical Center, Pittsburgh, PA, USA

Dongfeng Tan
Department of Pathology, The University of Texas MD Anderson Cancer Center, Houston, TX, USA

Tony E Godfrey
Department of Surgery, Boston University School of Medicine, Boston, MA, USA

Jovana Arand and Peter Malfertheiner
Clinic of Gastroenterology, Hepatology, and Infectious Diseases, Otto-von-Guericke University, Leipziger Str. 44, D 30120 Magdeburg, Germany

Ulrich Peitz
Clinic of Gastroenterology, Raphaelsklinik, Münster, Germany

Michael Vieth
Institute of Pathology, Klinikum Bayreuth, Bayreuth, Germany

Matthias Evert
Institute of Pathology, University Regensburg, Regensburg, Germany

Albert Roessner
Institute of Pathology, Otto-von-Guericke University, Magdeburg, Germany

Chuanzhen Zhang, Shanshan Wang, Changqing Xu, Wenjun Du, Changhong Liu, Meijuan Zhang, Ruiping Hou and Ziping Chen
Digestive Department, Shandong Provincial Qianfoshan Hospital, Shandong University, Jingshi Road 16766#, Jinan 250014, China

Daojie Yan
Infectious Diseases Hospital, Laiwu Hospital, Taishan Medical College, Laiwu, China

Tao Ning
Key Laboratory of Carcinogenesis and Translational Research (Ministry of Education), Laboratory of Genetics, Peking University School of Oncology, Beijing Cancer Hospital & Institute, Beijing, China

Kengo Nagai, Ryu Ishihara,Takeshi Yamashina, Kenji Aoi, Noriko Matsuura, Takashi Ito, Mototsugu Fujii, Sachiko Yamamoto, Noboru Hanaoka, Yoji Takeuchi, Koji Higashino, Noriya Uedo, Hiroyasu Iishi and Masaharu Tatsuta
Departments of Gastrointestinal Oncology, Osaka Medical Center for Cancer and Cardiovascular Diseases, 3-3, Nakamichi 1-chome, Higashinari-ku, Osaka 537-8511, Japan

Shingo Ishiguro
PCL Osaka Inc., Osaka, Japan

Takashi Ohta
Department of Gastroenterology, NTT West Osaka Hospital, Osaka, Japan

Hiromitsu Kanzaki
Department of Gastroenterology and Hepatology, Okayama University Graduate School of Medicine, Okayama, Japan

Yasuhiko Tomita
Departments of Pathology, Osaka Medical Center for Cancer and Cardiovascular Diseases, Osaka, Japan

Takashi Matsunaga
Departments of Medical Informatics, Osaka Medical Center for Cancer and Cardiovascular Diseases, Osaka, Japan

M. Venerito, C. Helmke, T. Wex, R. Rosania, K. J. Weigt and P. Malfertheiner
Department of Gastroenterology, Hepatology and Infectious Diseases, Otto-von-Guericke University Hospital, Leipziger Str. 44, 39120 Magdeburg, Germany

D. Jechorek
Institute of Pathology, Otto-von-Guericke University Hospital, Leipziger Str. 44, 39120 Magdeburg, Germany

Antweiler
Department of Biometrics and Medical Informatics, Otto-von-Guericke University Hospital, Leipziger Str. 44, 39120 Magdeburg, Germany

Mi Jin Gu and Joon Hyuk Choi
Department of Pathology, Yeungnam University College of Medicine, Daegu, Republic of Korea

Masanori Suzuki
Department of Gastroenterology, Kanma Memorial Hospital, 2-5, Nasushiobara city, Tochigi 325-0046, Japan

Kuangi Fu, Peng Jin, Yuqi He and Jianqiu Sheng
Department of Gastroenterology, PLA Army General Hospital, Beijing 100700, China

Byeong Geun Song, Yang Won Min, Ra Ri Cha, Hyuk Lee, Byung-Hoon Min, Jun Haeng Lee, Poong-Lyul Rhee and Jae J. Kim
Department of Medicine, Samsung Medical Center, Sungkyunkwan University School of Medicine, 81 Irwon-ro, Gangnam-gu, Seoul 06351, South Korea

Yating Sun, Shiyang Ma, Jinhai Wang and Lei Dong
Department of Gastroenterology, the Second Affiliated Hospital of Xi'an Jiaotong University, No. 157 Xiwu Road, Xi'an, Shaanxi 710004, China

Li Fang
Endoscopy Center, Ankang People's Hospital, Ankang 401147, China

Tyler Luckett, Chaitanya Allamneni, Kevin Cowley, Allison Gullick and Shajan Peter
Department of Gastroenterology and Hepatology, University of Alabama at Birmingham, 1720 2nd Avenue South, BDB 380, Birmingham, AL 35294, USA

John Eick
University of North Carolina Internal Medicine Residency, University of North Carolina, Carolina, North, USA

Miki Kaneko, Akira Mitoro, Motoyuki Yoshida, Masayoshi Sawai, Yasushi Okura, Masanori Furukawa, Tadashi Namisaki, Kei Moriya, Takemi Akahane, Hideto Kawaratani, Mitsuteru Kitade, Kousuke Kaji, Hiroaki Takaya Yasuhiko Sawada Kenichiro Seki Shinya Sato and Hitoshi Yoshiji
Third Department of Internal Medicine, Nara Medical University, 840 Shijo-cho, Kashihara, Nara 634-8522, Japan

Junichi Yamao
Department of Endoscopy, Nara Medical University, 840 Shijo-cho, Kashihara, Nara 634-8522, Japan

Tomomi Fujii and Chiho Obayashi
Department of Diagnostic Pathology, Nara Medical University, 840 Shijo-cho, Kashihara, Nara 634-8522, Japan

Myong Ki Baeg
Department of Internal Medicine, International St. Mary's Hospital, College of Medicine, Catholic Kwandong University, Incheon 22711, South Korea

Sun-Hye Ko
Department of Internal Medicine, Inje University Haeundae Paik Hospital Inje University College of Medicine, 875 Haeundaero, Haeundae-Gu, Busan 612-896, South Korea

Seung Yeon Ko
Department of Surgery, Sacred Heart Hospital, Hallym University, Gyeonggi-do, Anyang-si 14068, South Korea

Hee Sun Jung
Department of Health Promotion, Seoul St. Mary's Hospital, College of Medicine, The Catholic University of Korea, Seoul 06591, South Korea

Myung-Gyu Choi
Department of Internal Medicine, Seoul St. Mary's Hospital, College of Medicine, The Catholic University of Korea, Seoul 06591, South Korea

C. Gambardella, A. Allaria, G. Siciliano, C. Mauriello, R. Patrone and G. Conzo
Department of Cardiothoracic Sciences - University of Campania "Luigi Vanvitelli", Via Sergio Pansini 5, 80131 Naples, Italy

N Avenia, A. Polistena and A. Sanguinetti
Endocrine Surgery Unit, University of Perugia, Perugia, Italy

S. Napolitano
Italian Air Force Medical Corps, Ministry of Defence, Rome, Italy. Received: 31 August 2016 Accepted

R. Taylor Ripley, Deborah R. Surman, Laurence P. Diggs, Jeremy L. Davis, Jonathan M. Hernandez, Choung Hoang, Cara M. Kenney, Colleen D. Bond, Tricia F. Kunst and David S. Schrump
Thoracic and GI Oncology Branch, Center for Cancer Research, National Cancer Institute, Building 10; 4-3952, 10 Center Drive, MSC 1201, Bethesda, MD 20892-1201, USA

Jeremy Ryan and Anthony Letai
Dana-Farber Cancer Institute, Harvard Medical School, Boston, MA, USA

Seth M. Steinberg
Biostatistics and Data Management Section, Center for Cancer Research, National Cancer Institute, Bethesda, MD, USA

Jane B. Trepel and Min- Jung Lee
Developmental Therapeutics Branch, Center for Cancer Research, National Cancer Institute, Bethesda, MD, USA

Agata Michalak, Halina Cichoż-Lach and Beata Prozorow-Król
Department of Gastroenterology with Endoscopy Unit, Medical University of Lublin, Jaczewski Str, Lublin 820-954, Poland

Leszek Buk and Monika Dzida
Department of Radiology and Nuclear Medicine, Medical University of Lublin, Jaczewski Str, Lublin 820-954, Poland

Toshiya Maebayashi, Naoya Ishibashi, Takuya Aizawa and Masakuni Sakaguchi
Department of Radiology, Nihon University School of Medicine, 30-1 Oyaguchi Kami-cho, Itabashi-ku, Tokyo 173-8610, Japan

Homma Taku
Department of Human Pathology, Division of Pathology and Microbiology, Nihion University School of Medicine, Itabashi-ku, Tokyo 173-8610, Japan

Moritaka Ohhara
Department of Digestive Surgery, Kasukabe Medical Center, Kasukabe, Saitama 344-8588, Japan

Toshirou Takimoto
Department of Pathology, Kasukabe Medical Center, Kasukabe, Saitama 344-8588, Japan

Yoshiaki Tanaka
Department of Radiation Oncology, Kawasaki Saiwai Hospital, Kawasaki, Kanagawa 212-0014, Japan.

Index